CHASING MEN ON FIRE

MW00835419

CHASING MEN ON FIRE

The Story of the Search for a Pain Gene

Stephen G. Waxman

The MIT Press
Cambridge, Massachusetts
London, England

© 2018 Massachusetts Institute of Technology

All rights reserved. No part of this book may be reproduced in any form by any electronic or mechanical means (including photocopying, recording, or information storage and retrieval) without permission in writing from the publisher.

This book was set in Helvetica LT Std and Times New Roman by Toppan Best-set Premedia Limited. Printed and bound in the United States of America.

Library of Congress Cataloging-in-Publication Data is available.

Names: Waxman, Stephen G., author.
Title: Chasing men on fire : the story of the search for a pain
    gene / Stephen G. Waxman ; foreword by James E. Rothman.
Description: Cambridge, MA : The MIT Press, [2018] | Includes bibliographical
    references and index.
Identifiers: LCCN 2017026622 | ISBN 9780262037402 (hardcover : alk. paper)
Subjects: | MESH: Pain--genetics | Pain Management | NAV1.7 Voltage-Gated
    Sodium Channel
Classification: LCC RB127 | NLM WL 704 | DDC 616/.0472--dc23 LC record available at https://lccn.loc.gov/2017026622

10   9   8   7   6   5   4   3   2   1

For P, G, and those who shared their DNA.

And for M, W, RT, and JD; for D, J, CJ, and L; and of course for M…

CONTENTS

FOREWORD

If you are interested in how scientific medicine is done, this is cause enough to read this book. Whether you are a layperson or a scientist, if you are interested in the brain and the nervous system, you will also be interested because Waxman explains the ideas and their history so clearly and simply and yet accurately. Indeed the book is so well written that it reads like a detective novel, making it irresistible to turn the next page (or swipe the screen of your Kindle).

The explicit focus is Waxman's lifelong pursuit as a neurologist of how pain arises, how we can better understand it, and how new medicines for pain can be developed to treat it. He has had remarkable success in this pursuit initially through the discovery of a gene that controls pain. Waxman's decades-long path of discovery offers important lessons concerning how important progress in medicine is achieved: taking a risk in tackling a seemingly insurmountable problem, staying the course, following the scientific method with rigor and enthusiasm.

I have had the opportunity of following the bookends of the story close up, first as Steve Waxman's colleague at Stanford Medical School in the late 1970s, near the beginning, and now at Yale School of Medicine. Waxman, trained both as a neurologist and a molecular neuroscientist, begins by noting, "Two soldiers may both have missile wounds injuring the same nerve. One is disabled by neuropathic pain, unable to touch the injured limb because feather-light contact triggers immense discomfort, while the other notices numbness but no pain at all." And he then poses the question, "Might the difference lie in their genes?"

Genes can teach us much about human health and disease. One way to pinpoint critically important genes is to locate and study families in which an experiment of nature—a mutated gene—causes inherited disease. This approach has famously led to the discovery of genes influencing many diseases ranging from cystic fibrosis in children to Alzheimer's disease in the aging. Waxman has followed this path in a worldwide search—a hunt that spanned forty years and thousands of miles—for families with inherited pain. Within these very unusual families there was a secret, a gene that encodes a master switch that can turn pain on or off.

Interestingly, the story is told via two intertwined narratives. The scientific narrative is relayed by a series of research papers intended for professional scientists that illustrate the steps forward in the search for a pain gene. These papers provide an excellent example of "bench to bedside" research that, in this case, reaches from genes, to molecules that enable neurons to signal each other, then to pain-signaling nerve cells that shriek when they should be whispering, and finally to people who feel they are on fire, people suffering from excruciating pain due to alterations in a single gene. These "people on fire" provide a genetic model of neuropathic pain.

Happily for the nonspecialist, the primary research papers are accompanied by commentaries that explain what the research means, why it needed to be done, and how it was done. Here we get a rare glimpse, provided by a working scientist, into how scientific collaborations arise, how discoveries are made, how a finding on one disease can inform research on other disorders, and how research is "translated" from the laboratory bench to the clinic. These personal accounts tell a story of "how science happens."

The identification of a pain gene may be relevant to many of us. Following up on the identification of one specific gene as a central player in the man on fire syndrome, research on that gene has extended to the broader general population, where it is important in common disorders such as trigeminal neuralgia that can affect any of us. Research on this gene also provides a vivid example of the developing strategy of precision medicine, guided by genomics, that has the promise of relieving pain "first time around." It may also point the way toward development of a new class of pain medications that are more effective and that do not have addictive potential. While much remains to be accomplished before the scourge of chronic pain can be effectively treated in most people, we now have a strong scientific foundation that in the fullness of time will enable this, thanks in significant part to the passionate and effective contributions chronicled here.

James E. Rothman
Nobel Laureate in Physiology or Medicine (2013)
Professor, Yale University

This volume had its origin when several people suggested that I write a book on my search for a pain gene, a gene that controls pain sensibility in humans. Each suggested that the topic was timely, but each imagined a book for a different audience. A colleague forwarded the idea of a text for scientists-in-training and physicians-in-training, another suggested a book for a lay readership interested in pain, and still another suggested a volume for scientists and physicians. In the end, after consulting with colleagues, book publishers, and editors, and ultimately with Bob Prior of MIT Press, I decided to take a hybrid approach, combining some of my primary papers with commentaries that place them in a broader context in order to reach all these audiences.

Chronic pain affects more than 250 million sufferers around the world, is a leading cause of disability, and occurs more frequently than cancer, heart disease, and diabetes combined. The available pain medications are often ineffective or only partially effective. The number of patients needed to be treated, in order to achieve a 50% reduction in pain, is more than four for most of the currently available medications. And, many of the currently available pain medications produce side effects that impair quality of life and limit their use. There is a pressing need for new and better pain medications, and that, in turn, requires that we understand pain at a fundamental level.

The cells within our bodies, including pain-signaling nerve cells, are built largely of protein molecules. The blueprints for these essential building blocks are contained within the human genome, within more than 20,000 genes. Thus genes can tell us how pain-signaling nerve cells work, and might show us how to design new medications.

This type of genetic approach propelled the development of the statin medications, which regulate our lipid levels and have had an immense impact on health. In the case of the statins, it was the discovery and study of very rare families with inherited hypercholesterolemia that pointed the way to drugable molecular targets and ultimately to a new class of medicines. Rare genetic disorders can teach us important lessons about more common diseases. By analogy to the statins, the discovery of a "pain gene" would almost certainly teach us important lessons about chronic pain and how it arises. It also might facilitate the development of more effective pain medications, hopefully devoid of "central" side effects such as confusion, loss of balance, sleepiness, and addictive potential.

This book provides a personal account of the search for a pain gene. By a "pain gene" I mean a gene that encodes protein molecules that are central players in pain, and that, when gone mutant in very rare families, causes severe pain or, conversely, inability to sense pain. The search was propelled by these questions: "Why does one soldier with a nerve injury experience incapacitating pain, while another soldier with a similar injury does not? Why does one person with diabetic neuropathy suffer from debilitating burning pain, while another person with diabetic neuropathy notices numbness and tingling without significant discomfort? And, most importantly, can we develop new therapeutic strategies that might help those who suffer from chronic pain?"

The chapters in this book tell two intertwined stories. The scientific story is told by eleven primary papers documenting steps forward in the search for a pain gene and in the quest to cure pain. These papers are accompanied by personal accounts that explain what the research means, why it needed to be done, and how it was done. These commentaries tell the story *behind* the science—a story of "how science happens."

There are four sections to this book. The chapters in the first section, "Dissecting God's Megaphone," set the stage. Within the second section, "Chasing Men on Fire: The Search," the first two chapters trace the path to discovery of the pain gene. The following two chapters describe the beauty and intricacy of the channel encoded by the pain gene; these chapters will be of interest to readers with a passion for detail, although others may choose to skip them. The third section of this book, "Beyond the Search: Expanding Horizons," shows how the search for a pain gene in a rare disease has informed research on more common disorders. And the final section, "Muting God's Megaphone: From the Squid toward the Clinic," shows how discovery of the pain gene is being used to develop new treatments for pain.

Scientific papers are often filled with jargon. I have tried, wherever possible, to avoid jargon in the commentaries that accompany the primary papers in this book. Nevertheless, a few words of explanation are in order: A focus of this book is a rare medical disorder called erythromelalgia, which has also been termed erythermalgia in the medical literature and the "man on fire" syndrome in the lay literature. Since it is quite rare, only a minority of physicians have seen patients with erythromelalgia. But once they have seen a patient, the physician remembers this rare disorder because the clinical picture is striking: People with erythromelalgia—even in the absence of a hot stimulus—suffer from intense burning pain. They describe the pain as a sensation of being scalded, or having their body filled with hot lava. Men and women with the inherited form of erythromelalgia—a subset of about 5% of individuals with erythromelalgia, in whom there is a genetic cause—pointed the way to the pain gene.

Throughout this book, I refer to "DRG neurons." This term refers to dorsal root ganglion neurons. These are the primary sensory neurons, with cell bodies located in clusters outside the spinal cord, that innervate our body surface and organs. DRG neurons play a central role in inherited erythromelalgia and in other pain disorders and are the cells where $Na_V1.7$, a molecule essential for the sensation of pain, is highly expressed.

The identification of a pain gene is especially timely now. In the wake of identification of one specific gene as a major player in the man on fire syndrome, research on that gene has extended from rare genetic disorders to the general population, where it is important in common disorders that can affect all of us. Research on this gene may pave the way for pharmacogenomics, which will transform pain management from trial and error to "first time around." It may also point the way toward development of novel, more effective pain medications.

As important as a pain gene was, it was not easy to find. Neurologists see chronic pain frequently in clinical practice, but most neurologists have never encountered, and never will encounter, families with genetic pain disorders. The search for a pain gene spanned thousands of miles, from New Haven to Alabama to Beijing and then to the Netherlands. It required the coordinated efforts of geneticists, neurophysiologists, pharmacologists, molecular and cell biologists, as well as clinicians, and it was facilitated by collaborations of researchers on three continents. It was also propelled by the patients themselves, by the DNA that they shared with researchers and by the personal accounts they provided of their pain. The story behind the search reaches from genes, to the protein molecules they produce, to pain-signaling neurons that scream when they should be silent, and then to actual people—people who feel they are on fire. And the story points the way to molecules that produce pain not only in the man on fire syndrome, but also more broadly in "the rest of us" within the general population.

This book tells that story.

ACKNOWLEDGMENTS

None of us lives or works in a vacuum, and I certainly have not. I owe an immense debt to my teachers and mentors. These have included J. David Robertson and Howard Hermann of Harvard Medical School and J. Z. Young of University College London. My mentors at the Albert Einstein College of Medicine, neurophysiologist Dominick Purpura and electron microscopist George Pappas, showed by example that neuroscience is not constrained by any single set of methods but can, on the contrary, be truly multidisciplinary; Michael Bennett, also a professor at Einstein, provided an example of rigor in electrophysiology and, both at Einstein and during summers at the Marine Biological Laboratory in Woods Hole, pointed my research compass in the direction of axons. As a medical student, I also had the good fortune to work at University College London with Patrick Wall, one of the fathers of modern pain research. I was the only student in his laboratory at the time, and he introduced me to the mystery of pain. As a resident at the Harvard Neurology Unit at Boston City Hospital and subsequently as a faculty member at Harvard Medical School, I had the privilege of being mentored by Norman Geschwind. And in my early studies at MIT, I was encouraged by Jerry Lettvin, an incisively creative neuroscientist who taught me to leave tradition behind, and by John Moore, a tough-minded and incisive biophysicist who showed by example that one could leave scientific tradition behind without sacrificing scientific rigor.

In the more recent past, my search for a pain gene has been fueled by interactions with gifted colleagues around the world, including especially productive collaborations with Joost Drenth at Radboud University, Catharina Faber and Ingemar Merkies at the University of Maastricht, and John Wood at University College London. I never thought I would have role models as an adult. They have proved me wrong on this. Without them, the hunt for a pain gene would still be at an earlier stage.

I owe an immense debt—more than can be put into words—to a team of talented and energetic coworkers at Yale University. Jeff Kocsis's prowess with the microelectrode enabled early studies on injured axons. Sulayman Dib-Hajj, gifted with a unique talent for unlocking the mysteries of large genes, is a good friend and a colleague who contributed in many ways to the search for a pain gene. Joel Black's skill as a cell biologist and microscopist also contributed to our progress; immunocytochemistry is fraught with potential pitfalls, but Joel always got it right. Highly talented channel biologists, including Ted Cummins, Tony Rush, Chongyang Han, Jianying Huang, Yang Yang, Mark Estacion, Dmytro Vasylyev, Xiaoyang Cheng, and others in my laboratory were essential to the research described in this book. Paul Geha, of Yale's Department of Psychiatry, expanded our research repertoire to include functional brain imaging. And Betsy Schulman, in her role as clinical research coordinator, has become an invaluable link between our research group and our research subjects. The progress described in this book represents the crystals from the sweat of these colleagues, and credit for this work ultimately belongs to them.

Medical research teaches us about the body and its workings and also can take us from theory toward therapy. In this regard I have been privileged to work together with talented colleagues in the biopharmaceutical industry including Douglas Krafte, Ruth McKernan, Aoibhinn McDonnell, Richard Butt,

Simon Tate, Valerie Morrisett, and their coworkers. I am confident that, working together, academia and the biopharmaceutical sector will make more effective, nonaddictive pain therapies a reality.

The search for a pain gene began in the "premolecular era," in 1966. Constructing a history of discoveries that began fifty years ago is not easy. I thank Gayla Kanaster and Pam Costa for filling in some details. Joost Drenth and Al George filled in others. Any errors or omissions in telling of the story are, of course, mine.

Scientific research depends on funding. In this regard I am indebted to many agencies, organizations, and people. The Department of Veterans Affairs has, over the decades, supported research that has benefited not just veterans, but also many millions of Americans in general. Patricia Dorn and Audrey Kusiak of the VA have been strong supporters and have pushed me hard. I thank them for both. I thank the Paralyzed Veterans of America, a remarkable organization, for its unflagging support of research on spinal cord dysfunction and its consequences including pain and spasticity, for building the research facility where I work, and for invaluable continued support. Early on, as our work progressed within this facility, James Pelkey provided funding for a laboratory focusing specifically on sensory neurons, and underscored the importance of finding a cure for chronic pain. The Erythromelalgia Association provided an early grant, and its membership has provided advice since we launched our battle against this disorder. The Nancy Taylor Foundation, Michelson Foundation, and Kenneth Rainin Foundation provided funding that facilitated various stages of the work described here. Dundas and Sandra Flaherty, who endowed the professorship that I hold at Yale, have become good friends and a constant source of encouragement.

In writing this book I benefited greatly from the editorial acumen of Matthew Futterman; he helped me to focus on the important parts of the story and to tell it clearly. Merle Waxman helped, throughout the writing of this book, keeping me on target. Finally, I am grateful to Robert Prior, executive editor at MIT Press, for helping me to make this book more interesting, more accessible, and more exciting.

DISSECTING GOD'S MEGAPHONE

1 DISSECTING GOD'S MEGAPHONE: THE SEARCH FOR A PAIN GENE

God shouts in our pain. It is his megaphone.

—C. S. Lewis

Each one of us, at some time during our lives, experiences physical pain. Although C. S. Lewis, in his much-cited comment, was referring to spiritual pain, physical pain can also be considered to be God's megaphone. The sensation of physical pain—"My body hurts!"—is nearly universal. When pain is transient, it can protect us, warning us to withdraw from a threatening situation. Pain can also teach us—most children rapidly learn, for example, not to touch hot objects. But pain is not always helpful. If pain persists after a painful stimulus is no longer there and becomes chronic, it can invade a life and change it.

This book tells the story of the search for a gene: a gene controlling pain. It spans forty years and 7,000 miles and describes the discovery of rare families with a fierce type of inherited pain. The search extended from Alabama to Europe, then to Beijing and then back to Alabama. Affected individuals within these families have a hyperactive mutant gene—a pain gene—which makes them feel intense burning pain. Their disease is called "inherited erythromelalgia" (pronounced a•rith•ro•mel•AL•ja). The pain is often described as excruciating, and people harboring the broken gene feel as if they are on fire. Figure 1.1, drawn by a person with erythromelalgia to depict her pain, tells the story better than words.

To explore the physiological basis for chronic pain, and ultimately to cure it, we need to understand where it comes from. Throughout our body we have specialized pain-signaling nerve cells that innervate the body surface and organs and act as sentries. These pain-signaling cells act as a protective, early-warning system. They sense the presence of threatening stimuli—dangerous heat or cold, pinch, pinprick, pressure, or chemical irritant—and evoke protective responses like pulling a threatened limb away. In response to these stimuli, these nerve cells produce nerve impulses that carry the pain signal from our body surface and organs to the spinal cord, where the message is relayed to the brain, where pain enters consciousness and takes on its unpleasant quality. In the absence of threatening external stimuli, these pain-signaling neurons are normally quiet, and we do not have a sensation of pain. But after these cells are injured by trauma or disease, they can become hyperactive, taking on a life of their own and sending pain signals to the brain even when a threatening stimulus is not there. The result is a sensation of being burned when there is no flame or hot object touching the body, or of sticking pain when there is no pointy object injuring the body. This abnormal form of pain is called neuropathic pain; it is defined by scientists as pain due to disease or dysfunction of sensory neurons within the nervous system.

Neuropathic pain is common and can erode the quality of life in people with disorders as diverse as diabetes, traumatic nerve injury, a complication of shingles called postherpetic neuralgia, and peripheral neuropathy that arises as a complication of cancer chemotherapy. A report by the Institute of Medicine of the National Academy of Sciences (Committee on Advancing Pain Research, Care, and Education,

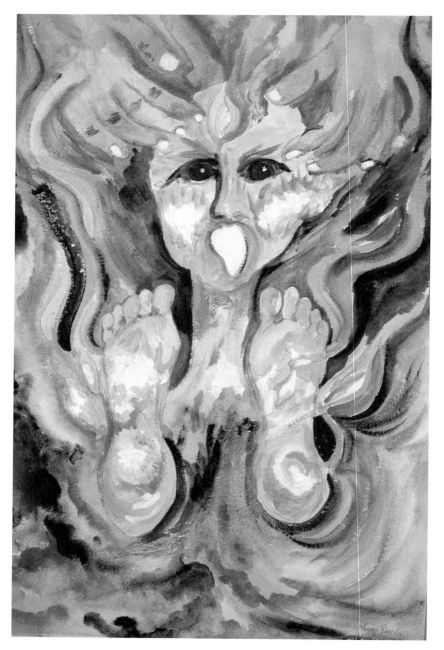

Figure 1.1
Drawing, entitled *A Constant Battle*, submitted to The Erythromelalgia Association for their 2012
art contest, depicting the pain of erythromelalgia. Reproduced with permission of Jennifer Beech
and The Erythromelalgia Association.

Institute of Medicine, National Academy of Sciences 2011) estimated that approximately 100 million adults in the United States are burdened by various types of chronic pain, at an estimated annual economic cost of more than $500 billion. Chronic pain occurs, in fact, in more patients than cancer, heart disease, and diabetes combined. Amplifying the impact, chronic pain is often unresponsive or responds only partially to treatment with existing medications. Many of these medications cause side effects that can include double vision, confusion, sleepiness, loss of balance, gastrointestinal irritation, or constipation. And some of them can cause addiction. There is a pressing need for new, more effective pain medications devoid of these side effects.

The stories of five ordinary people show just how devastating neuropathic pain can be:

• A soldier who, while on the battlefield, sustained severe burn injuries. We usually think of burns as injuring peripheral tissues such as skin and underlying muscle. But burns can singe the distal tips of sensory nerves, leading to severe neuropathic pain. The soldier cannot bear the intense discomfort triggered by even light touch on parts of the body supplied by the injured nerve fibers.

• A police officer with multiple citations for exemplary performance who sustained a gunshot wound to a nerve in his arm. Persistent numbness and weakness are present but do not debilitate him. What disables this person is unbearable pain, triggered by mild touch. Medications appeared to provide some relief but have had to be stopped because they caused double vision or confusion or made the patient sleepy. The patient receives medical care from a neurologist, a pain specialist, and a psychiatrist but is totally disabled.

• A nurse with breast cancer. Against the advice of her physicians and family, she is considering stopping her cancer chemotherapy because it is causing, as a side effect, an agonizing burning sensation in her feet, legs, and hands.

• An 82-year-old retired businessman with diabetes and diabetic nerve damage. His blood sugar is well controlled with medications. But he is racked by pain from unrestrained firing in injured nerve fibers. Opiate medications make him groggy yet do not relieve his pain.

• A 65-year-old physician with a common form of arthritis of the spine called spinal stenosis. As a result of degeneration of the spinal column and a herniated disc, a spinal nerve is compressed. None of the available medications relieve the ensuing pain. He is unable to work.

Now, consider a final and very different case history:

• A child with the "man on fire" syndrome, in which abnormal hyperactive pain-signaling nerves produce excruciating pain in response to even mild warmth. Currently available medications do not provide relief. Due to pain attacks, the child rarely plays in the park, and although she is a good student, she must frequently miss school. As often occurs in hereditary diseases, one-half of the people in her family are affected by the same disorder.

This book describes the search for a gene controlling pain. The human genome—more than 20,000 genes—contains a molecular blueprint for the body. Each of the genes contains the instructions for making a protein. And genes, in some ways, are easier to study than proteins. The chapters in this book tell the story of the hunt, within the labyrinth of genes that make up the human genome, for a gene pointing to a key protein molecule, a master switch that turns pain on or off.

No two people—except for identical twins—are exactly the same. Two patients with diabetes may both suffer from weakness and atrophy of the muscles due to injury of their nerves called peripheral neuropathy. In both, the reflexes are blunted by their nerve disease so that the neurologist's hammer cannot trigger a response. But one of these patients is debilitated by pain that almost never abates, while the other notices numbness and mild tingling but does not seek medical attention and goes dancing on the weekend. Two soldiers may both have missile wounds injuring the same nerve. One is disabled by neuropathic pain, unable to touch the injured limb because feather-light contact triggers immense discomfort, while the other notices numbness but no pain at all. Might the difference lie in their genes?

When a gene goes awry, the protein that it produces may be changed. Some alterations in genes produce especially dramatic changes in the proteins they encode. The changes in these altered genes are commonly known as "mutations." Mutations cause hereditary diseases, but, in addition to the negative connotation that we associate with them, mutations can act as guideposts for researchers.

So, why search the globe for families containing people who feel they are on fire? Certain patterns of disease, like its presence in multiple generations, suggest parent-to-child passage and heighten the likelihood that a mutation is at work. The history of modern medicine teaches us that rare families—families carrying uncommon mutations—can point to critically important genes and the proteins they produce, thereby identifying critically important molecular players in a disease. Some mutations, identified in families with rare inherited diseases, can teach us important lessons that are relevant to *common* disorders.

Families with rare inherited diseases, and the mutations that cause them, can also point us in the direction of new therapies, including new treatments for common disorders in "the rest of us." As one example, some readers of this book may take medications called statins, which control the levels of certain lipids within our blood. The introduction of statins into medical practice has substantially reduced the incidence of heart attacks and strokes. Development of the statins had its roots in genetics. A key step was the discovery of rare families in which heart disease occurred prematurely due to a genetic disorder—inherited hypercholesterolemia—in which high levels of cholesterol plug up blood vessels. This provided a basis for the identification of mutations in specific genes, and this, in turn, pointed the way to the culprit molecules. And this permitted the development of a new class of statin drugs that targeted these culprit molecules, effectively lowering the incidence of heart disease in the broad general population.

There was still another reason for the search for families with inherited pain. The development of new medications consumes the time and energy of researchers and is expensive. And it is scientifically challenging. It can take fifteen years or more—and a lot of luck—for a new molecular entity (a potential drug) to progress from early studies at the laboratory bench to the clinical marketplace. It has been estimated that the cost of developing a new medication, from early work in the laboratory until it is introduced into the clinic, is about $1 billion. Each clinical trial can cost tens of millions of dollars. A clinical trial also requires patients as "human subjects." In many cases this means that there is some other clinical trial that cannot be carried out, since these studies compete for human subjects as well as dollars. A clinical trial done to test drug A may mean that a trial for drug B cannot be completed. Given the investment of time and effort and this immense cost, there is not much room for false starts—which takes us back to this question: In developing a new medication, which of the myriad molecules within the body should be targeted?

Imagine what we could learn if researchers had, in hand, knowledge of a pain gene—a specific gene that could turn pain on or off. At a minimum that would teach us new lessons about how—in a fundamental way—pain arises. And, ultimately, it might facilitate the development of new treatments that would more effectively relieve pain.

This book is about the search for that gene.

References

Committee on Advancing Pain Research, Care, and Education, Institute of Medicine, National Academy of Sciences. 2011. *Relieving pain in America: A blueprint for transforming prevention, education and research.* Washington, DC: National Academies Press.

2   SHERRINGTON'S ENCHANTED LOOM AND HUXLEY'S SCIENCE FICTION

> When Hodgkin and I finished writing the 1952 papers, each of us moved to other lines of work. … Any idea of analyzing the channels by molecular genetics would have seemed to us to be … science fiction.
>
> —Andrew Huxley, in *The Axon*, 1995

The human nervous system—our brain, spinal cord, and nerves—is the world's most complex computer. There are more than 100 billion nerve cells in the human brain and spinal cord, greater than the number of stars within the Milky Way.

These nerve cells, called neurons by scientists, act as tiny transistors, or in some cases as integrated circuits. They send electrical impulses to and fro along nerve fibers, termed "axons" by neuroscientists, as the nervous system makes countless computations each second. In 1942, the pioneering British neuroscientist Charles S. Sherrington referred in his book *Man on His Nature* to the active brain as "an enchanted loom where millions of flashing shuttles weave a dissolving pattern, always a meaningful pattern … a shifting harmony of subpatterns" (Sherrington 1942).

As a student, I was fascinated by the brain, and as I contemplated a career in biomedical research, I wanted to understand the ways in which the activities of the billions of nerve cells within the brain lead to human thought—consciousness, reasoning, planning, understanding, and emotion. I was fascinated by the work of MIT scientists Warren McCulloch and Walter Pitts, who, in a seminal article, "A Logical Calculus of the Ideas Immanent in Nervous Activity" (McCulloch and Pitts 1943), observed in 1943 that, at any given moment, each neuron is either firing or not, and suggested that neurons could serve as "threshold logic units," a conclusion that led them to postulate that it might be possible to mimic brain activity by building a large electrical device consisting of a multitude of on-or-off switches. This suggestion, well before the word "neuroscience" had been coined, provided a basis for neural network theory and, in the opinion of some, contributed to the thinking that led to the development of modern computers.

My first forays into research as a student at Harvard focused on attempts to explain, at the level of single nerve cells, how the human brain categorizes complex external stimuli. I wanted, as my overall goal, to solve the "mind–brain" problem. But, while my interest in higher nervous function and in questions about the brain and behavior allowed me to publish my first papers, I came to the conclusion that full answers to these philosophically grand questions would not be forthcoming during my professional lifetime.

My interest in the nervous system deepened over the next few years, but refocused on the simpler and more tractable problem of how single neurons, or well-defined circuits of neurons, function in health and disease. Questions about the pathophysiology of neurological disease were to drive me for the rest of my career. What fundamental changes in the nervous system cause neurological disease? How do these changes cause the neurological signs and symptoms that bring patients to the clinic? And, as clinicians, what can we do about it? Might it be possible—using fundamental information about the cells and molecules responsible for diseases of the brain, spinal cord, and peripheral nerves—to develop new and more effective treatments for disorders of the nervous system? Three themes echoed as I thought about these questions: Axons, sodium channels, and pain. These themes converged in the search for a pain gene.

Axons

My early mentors, J. D. Robertson (professor of cell biology at Harvard and the discoverer of the molecular structure of the myelin insulation that surrounds nerve fibers) and J. Z. Young (professor at University College London and the discoverer of the squid giant axon, a model that subsequently yielded crucial lessons about sodium channels), provided encouragement that fueled my earliest research on axons. Discussions with J. D. Robertson while waterskiing at his lakeside retreat in Wayland, Massachusetts, and interchanges with J. Z. Young at teatime at University College London convinced me that axons were not just passive wires—they were elegantly architected biological machines that function with millisecond accuracy. I was fascinated by the ingenious design principles of nerve fibers, which optimized their performance and matched their architecture to the functional needs of each specialized part of the nervous system. Some axons were built to conduct impulses as quickly as possible (Waxman and Bennett 1972). Other axons acted as precisely timed "delay lines," getting the message to their recipient neurons, one synapse down the line, not as quickly as possible but in just the right amount of time (Waxman 1970), and still other axons had evolved so as to process information in highly complex ways, in some cases generating external electrical fields that could, for example, be used by fish, like sonar, to navigate (Waxman, Pappas, and Bennett 1972). I did not imagine, as I did these early studies, that they would propel me toward research on the human malady of chronic pain.

A Morse Code in the Brain

Communication between neurons can be thought of as using a form of Morse code, which, in the era of the telegraph, enabled people to communicate by sending a series of dots and dashes. In a broad-brush sense, Morse code applies to pain signaling as well as other aspects of coding within the nervous system. Neurons within the brain and spinal cord use nerve impulses, called action potentials by neuroscientists, to communicate. The action potential is about 100 millivolts or one-tenth of a volt in size, and it lasts only about 1 millisecond (one one-thousandth of a second); a representative action potential from a pain-signaling spinal neuron is shown in figure 2.1. For a given nerve cell the action potentials are always the same, just like the dots in Morse code. It is the rate and pattern of the action potentials, sent on to downstream neurons, by which that nerve cell delivers its message.

Some neurons are *excitatory* and stimulate downstream neurons that receive their message. Other neurons are *inhibitory* and have a calming effect on downstream neurons. McCulloch and Pitts argued that each individual neuron integrates its multiple excitatory and inhibitory inputs into a message which it conveys to other neurons via a series of nerve impulses or action potentials. How might a series of action potentials—the dots of Morse code but not the dashes—carry meaning? Codes based on the frequency of action potentials produced by a given neuron, the pattern of action potentials over time, or the particular neuron involved (the "labeled line" theory) have all been proposed, and each applies at some sites in the nervous system. Irrespective of which coding mechanism is involved, it would be expected that underactivity of neurons due to disease would interfere with their computational function,

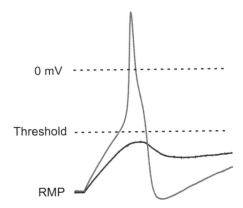

Figure 2.1
Nerve impulse (action potential) from a dorsal root ganglion (DRG) neuron, shown in green. Until it is stimulated, the neuron is quiescent and sits at resting membrane potential (RMP) with the inside of the cell negative by about –60 millivolts with respect to the outside. When the cell is depolarized by a sufficient amount, it reaches threshold, and, at that point, there is an explosive, nearly simultaneous activation of many sodium channels, producing a pulse-like depolarization of the cell membrane which actually crosses 0 millivolts, so that the inside of the cell is briefly positive before the cell repolarizes and returns to resting potential. The action potential, which always has the same configuration and time course in any given cell, lasts about 1 millisecond. $Na_V1.7$ sodium channels play a particularly important role in DRG neurons. They act within the subthreshold domain, below threshold, to amplify small depolarizing stimuli (blue). Acting in this way, $Na_V1.7$ channels determine the sensitivity, or "set the gain," on DRG neurons. Modified from Rush et al. (2007).

and that, conversely, overactivity of neurons (termed *hyperexcitability*) would also perturb their output. Extreme hyperactivity of neurons in some parts of the brain can cause epileptic seizures which can be likened to tornados of nervous system activity.

Sodium Channels: Molecular Batteries in Our Nerve Cells

As a beginning undergraduate I became aware of the seminal work of the British scientists Alan Hodgkin and Andrew Huxley. At a remarkably young age these intellectual giants, who had been research fellows at Trinity College, Cambridge, had discovered the crucial role of sodium channels in nerve impulse conduction (Huxley 1995). Their experiments capitalized on the large size—a diameter of about a millimeter—of specialized nerve fibers called "giant" axons of the squid, which allowed Hodgkin and Huxley to insert electrodes within them. This enabled them to measure the actual electrical currents underlying nerve impulses, a feat that had not been previously possible. An incisive analysis of the generation of action potentials in the squid's giant axon allowed them to formulate a set of equations—still widely referred to as the Hodgkin–Huxley equations—that explained how sodium channels within nerve cells open and close to generate nerve impulses. Working before the advent of the finely honed microelectrode that neuroscientists now use, without modern computers, and prior to the maturation of molecular biology, these pioneers presciently demonstrated the presence of sodium channels within nerve cell membranes. Acting as tiny batteries, the sodium channels open and close rapidly in response to depolarizations of the nerve cell membrane to allow small flows of sodium ions that produce the electrical current underlying nerve impulses. It was not until the 1980s that, as a result of molecular cloning, it became possible to understand the conformation of sodium channels and the ways in which they open and close within milliseconds to produce nerve impulses—an attribute that led to their being described as "some of the most conformationally versatile structures in nature" (Pascual 2016). Although Hodgkin and Huxley could not see sodium channels and had no idea of their molecular structure, they accurately predicted many of their properties (Hodgkin and Huxley 1952). Their work was honored with the 1963 Nobel Prize and still is used for understanding ion channels.

It was also during my time as an undergraduate that I was fortunate to meet Patrick Wall, considered by many as the father of modern pain research. Known for his wit as well as his incisive thinking, he worked in the Department of Biology at MIT, a mile down Commonwealth Avenue from Harvard College. As a junior, and then as a senior at Harvard, I visited Pat Wall, watched his experiments, and offered my guesses as to what to do next. In the late 1960s he moved to University College London to head up a new research center and invited me to move with him as a PhD student. London was too far from home for me, and I did not take him up on the invitation. However, several years later, as an MD–PhD student at Albert Einstein College of Medicine, I applied for a fellowship from The Epilepsy Foundation, and I worked for four months with Wall in his University College laboratory on Gower Street. At that time an investigator could achieve preeminence with a small laboratory, and I had the privilege of working one-on-one together with Wall, who, between cigarettes he rolled himself, coached me on the minutiae of electrophysiological recording. The resulting paper (Wall, Waxman, and Basbaum 1974) described the barrage of impulses generated by axons within peripheral nerves in the first few minutes immediately following traumatic injury. I didn't realize it at the time, but my experience working with one of the giants of pain research set the stage for the second half of my career. Twenty years later I returned to pain research, combining my interests in sodium channels and neuropathic pain.

The themes of axons, sodium channels, and neurological disease began to come together for me in 1975. A decade after Hodgkin and Huxley's Nobel Prize, as a new assistant professor at Harvard and MIT, I turned my attention to nerve fibers, how they work, and why they don't work properly in some disease states. Much of the previous work on which I based my studies had been carried out in lower species such as the squid or other invertebrates, where nerve fibers are larger and easier to study. I reasoned that if the axon of a squid could be interesting, the axon of a human being—especially a human being with diseased nerve fibers—could be an even more interesting topic for study.

My first research as a faculty member at Harvard and MIT focused on how the molecular architecture of axons determines their functional properties. In one of my projects I was exploring the ways in which sodium channels contribute to the pathophysiology of diseases such as multiple sclerosis. I was interested in multiple sclerosis for two reasons: First, it is the most frequent neurologic crippler of young adults in industrialized societies, usually rearing its head and producing symptoms in the third decade of life, just as people are establishing their adult trajectories. Second, multiple sclerosis was, for me, a "model disease," a disease that might hold general lessons about how the nervous system adapts to injury.

My classmates and I had been taught in medical school that following any type of injury to the brain or spinal cord, there was little if any functional recovery. We watched well-meaning professors declare that following injury to the nervous system as occurs in spinal cord injury or stroke, the outlook was hopeless. We saw our mentors make the diagnosis of these disorders, turn around, and walk away from the bedside because they had no effective treatments to offer, and we were disappointed. But multiple sclerosis did not follow this rule. People with multiple sclerosis often experience remissions in which they spontaneously regain previously lost functions. A person with multiple sclerosis loses nearly all vision in one eye and, four weeks later, is able to read the newspaper. Another person with multiple sclerosis develops paralysis of the legs and then, without any treatment, recovers the ability to walk. This exception to the rule suggested to me that multiple sclerosis might hold more general lessons about recovery of function after injury to the nervous system.

It was well established at this time that the generation and transmission of electrical impulses along axons required the activity of sodium channels. We knew from earlier work that, in model systems such as the squid giant axon, sodium channels were sprinkled in a low but relatively uniform density along the entire length of the fiber. But what about axons in higher species such as humans? Many of those axons are surrounded by myelin, a lipid-containing material that acts as an insulator, like the covering of an electrical wire. The myelin sheath is periodically punctuated by small areas devoid of myelin, called nodes of Ranvier, and physiologists had known for some time that, in myelinated fibers, the impulse did not move continuously along the axon as in the squid giant fiber, but jumped in a discontinuous or "saltatory" manner from node of Ranvier to node of Ranvier, and so on, progressing node by node along the length of the nerve fiber.

My first major observation relevant to multiple sclerosis showed that, in myelinated fibers, the sodium channels are not distributed uniformly along the length of the axons, but are rather focused in a highly nonuniform way at the nodes of Ranvier where they are highly concentrated. My studies also showed that under the myelin, where they are not needed, there were very few sodium channels (Waxman 1977, 1982). As I made these observations at Harvard and MIT, J. Murdoch Ritchie, a pharmacologist working at Yale who was to become a friend and colleague, came to a similar conclusion. It was hard not to be enamored with the elegance of the axon even as reflected by the placement of the sodium channels. Every molecule in its place, precisely where needed for optimal function, a beautiful example of purpose-driven biological architecture.

But what happens when the myelin insulation is injured? Demyelination had classically been known to be a hallmark of multiple sclerosis. Traditional dogma posited that damage to the myelin caused neurological deficits such as blindness, weakness, or incoordination because the conduction of action potentials fails along axons within the brain and spinal cord as a result of current leakage through the damaged myelin insulation: a "short circuit." This, for me, posed an enigma: Following loss of the myelin within the brain and spinal cord in multiple sclerosis, there is little remyelination. The damage to the myelin insulation was permanent. Yet remissions were common in multiple sclerosis, suggesting that some demyelinated axons had recovered the capability to conduct action potentials. How were my patients recovering the ability to see? Or to walk? For me, this raised the following more general question: How do remissions occur?

One of the challenges faced by a nerve impulse trying to invade a demyelinated part of an axon arises from the increased surface area of the denuded axon membrane. This type of problem has been termed "impedance mismatch" by electrical engineers. Working at MIT and aided immeasurably by new methods for computer simulation, developed by biophysicist John Moore and based, in part, on the Hodgkin–Huxley equations, in 1978 we showed that changes in the geometry of demyelinated nerve fibers, together with the production of new sodium channels, could provide a basis for resumption of impulse conduction along demyelinated axons (Waxman and Brill 1978). In 1980, in studies on the nerves of rats in which we induced demyelination, postdoctoral fellow Robert Foster and I showed that there is remarkable molecular plasticity in some demyelinated axons, which synthesize new sodium channels and plug them into the demyelinated, previously sodium-channel-poor membrane. The newly deployed sodium channels function like the sodium channels sprinkled along the length of the giant axon of the squid, to support restoration of impulse conduction (Foster, Whalen, and Waxman 1980). Here we had an explanation for recovery of impulse conduction along demyelinated axons. In 2004, together with colleagues Matthew Craner and Joel Black, we showed the same molecular plasticity along demyelinated axons within the human nervous system, within the brains of people with multiple sclerosis; in that study we refined our analysis so that we could precisely identify the types of sodium channels involved (Craner et al. 2004). In 2006, I was invited to give the J. Z. Young Memorial Lecture at University College London. I entitled it "From Squid to Clinic: Sodium Channels in Neurological Disease," and in it, I described this research. It is not the topic of this book, but the goal of being able to *induce* remissions in multiple sclerosis continues to drive research in some of my laboratories.

Dorsal Root Ganglion (DRG) Neurons as Generators of Pain

In the mid-1990s I turned my attention to sodium channels and neuropathic pain—chronic pain rising as a result of damage to, or dysfunction of, the nervous system. My first experiments on pain-signaling neurons were an outgrowth of my earlier discovery that neurons produce new sodium channels after injury to the myelin surrounding their axons. In these new experiments I wanted to answer the question, "Might some sodium channel genes in a neuron turn on, while others turn off, following injury to its axon?" (Waxman, Kocsis, and Black 1994).

Serving as sentinels or an early-warning system, pain-signaling dorsal root ganglion (DRG) neurons innervate our body surface, teeth, cornea, gut, bladder, and many of our organs. Trigeminal ganglion neurons serve the same function for the face. The cell bodies of DRG neurons are located within clusters called dorsal root ganglia located just outside the spinal cord; since DRG neurons are not located within the central nervous system (the brain or spinal cord), these cells are sometimes referred to as "peripheral" neurons. From the cell body of each DRG neuron, a peripheral nerve fiber or axon extends to the body surface, and a central axon extends into the spinal cord. Altogether, the DRG neuron provides a pathway for signaling via nerve impulses that originate in the periphery and propagate into the spinal cord (figure 2.2). Pain-signaling DRG neurons, sometimes called nociceptors, are sensitive to the presence of threatening mechanical stimuli such as a pinprick or a blow from a hammer, injurious thermal stimuli such as damaging levels of heat or dangerous levels of cold, and noxious chemical irritants such as acids. These "first-order" pain-sensing neurons signal the presence of threats to the body by generating nerve impulses that they send, via our peripheral nerves, to the spinal cord. Within the spinal cord, these nerve impulses excite "second-order" pain-signaling neurons, which relay the signal upward toward the brain. When the message reaches the brain, it is processed by still other circuits of neurons which elicit the experience of pain. The process of pain signaling begins in the periphery. The sites of origin of nerve impulses that encode pain—DRG neurons and trigeminal neurons—are major players in pain.

Pain can serve a protective purpose when it elicits an adaptive response such as pulling a hand away from a hot stove. It can have an instructive role during development, teaching a person, early in life, what is safe and what is not. Or pain can be *inflammatory*, signaling the presence of tissue damage.

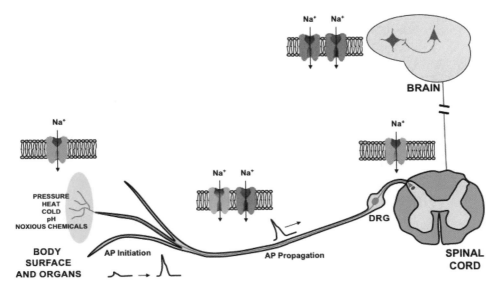

Figure 2.2
Dorsal root ganglion (DRG) neurons, with cell bodies within the dorsal root ganglia, extend an axon from the body surface and organs, all the way into the spinal cord. Sodium channels within the cell membrane of DRG neurons enable them to produce action potentials (APs). Pain-signaling DRG neurons are excited by dangerous levels of pressure, heat, cold, acidity (pH), or irritating chemicals and, in response, send action potentials to the spinal cord, which relays them to the brain. Multiple types of sodium channels, shown in orange, red, and green, participate in this signaling. $Na_V1.7$ channels (green) play a particularly crucial role, amplifying small stimuli in the periphery and thereby setting the gain on DRG neurons, and facilitating impulse transmission close to the spinal cord. Modified from Waxman and Zamponi (2014).

Inflammatory pain can also be protective, warning, for example, against overuse of an injured and healing joint. Alternatively, pain can be *neuropathic*. Neuropathic pain reflects dysfunction of the nervous system and can occur when DRG neurons take on a life of their own and generate pain signals even in the absence of a noxious stimulus or inflammation.

Like the unbridled flashing of shuttles within Sherrington's loom, neuropathic pain is the result of inappropriate firing—in the absence of a noxious stimulus or out of proportion to a noxious stimulus— by an injured or diseased nerve cell along the pain-signaling pathway. An example of this abnormal firing is shown in figure 2.3, from a paper that Jeffery Kocsis and I published in *Nature* in 1983. Here, using a tiny microelectrode carefully placed within a single axon inside the nerve of a rat that had been subjected to a nerve injury, we can see the abnormal generation of multiple repetitive nerve impulses in an injured nerve fiber—machine gun–like, staccato—in response to a small stimulus that should elicit only a single nerve impulse (Kocsis and Waxman 1983). Recordings such as this from an axon less than 10 μm (1/100th of a millimeter, much smaller than a wisp of thin hair) in diameter were not easy to achieve and are testimony to Kocsis's prowess with the microelectrode. Four years later Kocsis and I had the opportunity to record from the axons in nerves from human subjects with painful neuropathy that had been removed for diagnostic purposes (figure 2.4), and again we observed abnormal repetitive impulse activity (Kocsis and Waxman 1987). In both of the experiments the abnormal

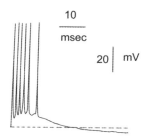

Figure 2.3
Inappropriate repetitive firing of action potentials, recorded with a microelectrode from a single axon within the sciatic nerve of a rat that had received a nerve injury one year previously. The aberrant repetitive action potentials sit upon an abnormal depolarization of the axon membrane which suggests abnormal sodium channel activity. From Kocsis and Waxman (1983).

repetitive nerve impulses were generated by a sustained depolarization of the axon membrane. Here we could see neuropathic pain in the making. Something was producing abnormal depolarizations in DRG neurons and their axons after nerves were injured. These recordings suggested to us that, if we could identify the molecules responsible for generating this depolarization, we might be able to pinpoint the drivers of neuropathic pain. Although it was not yet known that there were nine different types of sodium channels, and peripheral sodium channels had not yet been discovered, recordings of this type led us to think that sodium channels might act as generators of pain.

Peripheral Sodium Channels—A Holy Grail

Anyone who has gone to a dentist knows that nerve impulses within pain-signaling nerves can be silenced with certain medications—a nerve can be put to sleep, and pain within its territory will not be felt while it is anesthetized. In the case of dental anesthesia the nerve is infiltrated by injecting it with the local anesthetic Novocaine or a related drug that blocks sodium channels, thereby preventing the generation and transmission of electrical impulses in nerve fibers that innervate the teeth and oral cavity.

Given the remarkable efficacy of sodium channel blockers when they are injected to locally prevent pain during dental procedures, it might have been hoped that sodium channel blockers could be used more broadly, as medications taken by mouth, to alleviate chronic pain. Indeed, a number of sodium channel blocking drugs exist and some can be taken orally. However, these drugs have limited effectiveness for the treatment of pain because they block sodium channels throughout the nervous system. The unwanted block of sodium channels outside of pain-signaling neurons, particularly in neurons throughout the brain, produces dose-limiting side effects that include confusion, loss of balance, double vision, and sleepiness. Thus a major question in pain research focused on whether it might be possible to develop highly specific medications that selectively block sodium channels in pain-signaling peripheral neurons so as to put these cells to sleep while having no effect on the sodium channels within other types of neurons. This targeted approach would avoid unwanted side effects.

A sodium channel is a protein molecule, consisting of a string of around 1,800 amino acids, strung together like the beads in a necklace which then folds into a barrel-like structure. Beginning in the

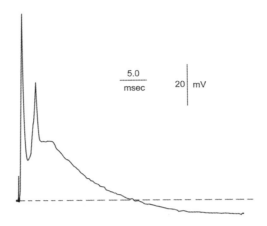

$$\frac{5.0}{msec} \qquad 20 \mid mV$$

Figure 2.4
Microelectrode recording from a single axon within the sural nerve of a patient with a painful peripheral neuropathy. The nerve was biopsied for diagnostic evaluation. Aberrant repetitive action potentials can be seen, arising from an abnormal depolarization suggesting abnormal sodium channel activity within the axon membrane. From Kocsis and Waxman (1987).

mid-1980s, it was becoming clear that the sodium channel was not a singular entity. Studies in laboratories around the world were beginning to show that there was not a single, unitary type of sodium channel. We knew, by the early 1990s, that multiple genes encoded multiple sodium channels, all sharing a similar overall molecular structure, but with slightly different amino acid sequences, and different physiological and pharmacological properties. The question of whether there might be sodium channels that play preferentially important roles in peripheral nerve cells, particularly pain-signaling DRG neurons and their axons, emerged as a major challenge in pain research. The logic was that, if these "peripheral" sodium channels existed, it might be possible to develop appropriately focused medications that would mute the activity of peripheral pain-signaling DRG neurons without having a significant effect on neurons within the brain. If this could be achieved, it would permit pain relief without side effects such as double vision, confusion, or sleepiness, and with little potential for abuse or addiction. But first, it had to be shown that peripheral sodium channels existed. Peripheral sodium channels became a "holy grail" of pain research.

Between 1996 and 1999 three different subtypes of peripheral sodium channels meeting this specification were identified by gene cloning in the DRG neurons of rodents, rats, and mice (table 2.1).

They are called $Na_V1.7$, $Na_V1.8$, and $Na_V1.9$ (Catterall, Goldin, and Waxman 2005). The $Na_V1.8$ sodium channel, initially called SNS (Sensory Neuron Specific), was discovered and characterized in 1996 by John Wood and his colleagues at University College London (Akopian, Sivilotti, and Wood 1996). The $Na_V1.9$ sodium, initially called NaN (Na-Nociceptive), was cloned and characterized in my laboratory in 1998 by Sulayman Dib-Hajj (Dib-Hajj et al. 1998). $Na_V1.9$ was subsequently described by Simon Tate and his research group at Glaxo (Tate et al. 1998), who called it SNS2. Gail Mandel

Table 2.1
Peripheral Sodium Channels

Channel	Function
Na$_V$1.7 (gene *SCN9A*)	Boosts small stimuli to initiate firing of pain-signaling peripheral neurons; facilitates neurotransmitter release at first synapse within the spinal cord; sets gain in pain-signaling DRG neurons to control their firing
Na$_V$1.8 (gene *SCN10A*)	Produces the electrical current needed for high-frequency firing of action potentials in pain-signaling DRG neurons
Na$_V$1.9 (gene *SCN11A*)	Depolarizes resting potential of pain-signaling neurons; amplifies response to small stimuli

Note. DRG, dorsal root ganglion.

and her colleagues at Stony Brook University reported that a third sodium channel, initially called PN1 and hNE—now called Na$_V$1.7—was not detectable in the brain but was present at high levels in peripheral nerve cells (Toledo-Aral et al. 1997). Our experiments also showed that this channel, not detectable within the brain, was present within DRG neurons (Felts et al. 1997). As with Na$_V$1.8 and Na$_V$1.9, it was not possible to rule out the presence of some Na$_V$1.7 channels within the brain—expression at very low levels throughout the brain, or within a small subgroup of neurons within the brain might escape detection. But the high level of expression within DRG neurons, in the context of a low level of expression, if any, in the brain, suggested a much more important role of Na$_V$1.7 within peripheral pain-signaling neurons. Even before the search for a pain gene, Na$_V$1.7 became a major focus for me and my colleagues.

Sodium channels are beautiful and complex molecules. Figure 2.5 displays the three-dimensional configuration of the folded human Na$_V$1.7 polypeptide as determined by computer modeling at a resolution of 2.7Å (one Ångstrom, Å, equals 1.0×10^{-10} or one ten-billionth of a meter—about one millionth of a diameter of a human hair). This powerful methodology allows us to infer the locations of some of the crucial atoms within the channel and permits us to make potentially important predictions about the actions of specific drugs on the channel.

The pivotal functional role of Na$_V$1.7 in controlling the firing of peripheral pain-signaling neurons began to emerge in 1997 when we examined the electrophysiological properties of this channel, which at that time was called PN1 or hNE. Our work was carried out at the Center for Neuroscience and Regeneration Research, a Yale University research center housed in a purpose-designed building erected with funds provided by the Paralyzed Veterans of America at the Veterans Affairs Medical Center in West Haven. The goal of the Center was to capitalize on the "molecular revolution" to bring a better understanding of, and ultimately new and more effective treatments for, the pain and paralysis that result from injury or disease of the nervous system.

Inscribed at the Medical Center's entrance were the words "Here you can see the price of freedom." There was no shortage of poignant illustrations of these words. Among them were men and women seeking relief from chronic pain that was an accompaniment of nerve injury, burn injury, or traumatic limb amputation, an injury which severs not only arms and legs but also the nerve fibers within them. Here one could see, loud and clear, the price of freedom. And that reminded me, daily, of the importance of unraveling pain's mysteries.

Knowing that Na$_V$1.7 channels were highly expressed in pain-signaling peripheral neurons, physiologist Ted Cummins and I used patch-clamp electrodes to study them. We found that Na$_V$1.7 channels

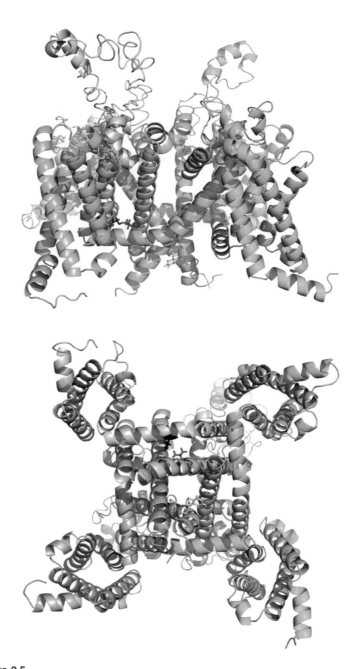

Figure 2.5
Atomic-level model of the Na$_V$1.7 sodium channel. The green, salmon, purple, and blue spirals show the course of the channel protein as it weaves in and out of the cell membrane within four different parts (domains) of the Na$_V$1.7 channel. Single amino acids can be seen in red and gold. The top diagram shows a side view of the channel, as seen by an observer within the membrane. The bottom diagram shows the channel as seen from within the cell, looking out. Just above the yellow amino acid, the pore in the center of the channel can be seen. From Yang et al. (2012).

respond to, and amplify, stimuli that are too small to activate other sodium channels (Cummins, Howe, and Waxman 1998). In response to stimulation, $Na_V1.7$ channels bring the neuron closer to the potential needed to turn on other types of sodium channels such as $Na_V1.8$, which then produce most of the electrical current underlying the nerve impulses used by pain-signaling DRG nerve cells to signal the presence of painful stimuli (Renganathan, Cummins, and Waxman 2001; Rush, Cummins, and Waxman 2007). We learned, in our early studies between 1997 and 2001, that $Na_V1.7$ plays a powerful role in setting the gain on peripheral nerve cells isolated from laboratory animals such as rats. We did not yet know, when we did these initial studies, that they would set the stage for subsequent demonstration, in humans, that $Na_V1.7$ is a gatekeeper for pain.

References

Akopian AN, Sivilotti L, Wood JN. 1996. A tetrodotoxin-resistant voltage-gated sodium channel expressed by sensory neurons. *Nature* 379(6562): 257–262.

Catterall WA, Goldin AL, Waxman SG. 2005. International Union of Pharmacology. XLVII. Nomenclature and structure-function relationships of voltage-gated sodium channels. *Pharmacol Rev* 57(4): 397–409.

Craner MJ, Newcombe J, Black JA, Hartle C, Cuzner ML, Waxman SG. 2004. Molecular changes in neurons in multiple sclerosis: Altered axonal expression of Nav1.2 and Nav1.6 sodium channels and Na+/Ca2+ exchanger. *Proc Natl Acad Sci USA* 101(21): 8168–8173.

Cummins TR, Howe JR, Waxman SG. 1998. Slow closed-state inactivation: A novel mechanism underlying ramp currents in cells expressing the hNE/PN1 sodium channel. *J Neurosci* 18(23): 9607–9619.

Dib-Hajj SD, Tyrrell L, Black JA, Waxman SG. 1998. NaN, a novel voltage-gated Na channel, is expressed preferentially in peripheral sensory neurons and down-regulated after axotomy. *Proc Natl Acad Sci USA* 95(15): 8963–8968.

Felts PA, Yokoyama S, Dib-Hajj S, Black JA, Waxman SG. 1997. Sodium channel alpha-subunit mRNAs I, II, III, NaG, Na6 and hNE (PN1): Different expression patterns in developing rat nervous system. *Brain Res Mol Brain Res* 45(1): 71–82.

Foster RE, Whalen CC, Waxman SG. 1980. Reorganization of the axon membrane in demyelinated peripheral nerve fibers: Morphological evidence. *Science* 210(4470): 661–663.

Hodgkin AL, Huxley AF. 1952. A quantitative description of membrane current and its application to conduction and excitation in nerve. *J Physiol* 117(4): 500–544.

Huxley A. (1995). Electrical activity in nerve: The background up to 1952. In S. G. Waxman, J. D. Kocsis, & P. K. Stys (Eds.), *The axon: Structure, function, and pathophysiology.* New York: Oxford University Press.

Kocsis JD, Waxman SG. 1983. Long-term regenerated nerve fibres retain sensitivity to potassium channel blocking agents. *Nature* 304(5927): 640–642.

Kocsis JD, Waxman SG. 1987. Ionic channel organization of normal and regenerating mammalian axons. *Prog Brain Res* 71: 89–101.

McCulloch W, Pitts W. 1943. A logical calculus of the ideas immanent in nervous activity. *Bull Math Biol* 7: 115–133.

Pascual JM. 2016. Understanding atomic interactions to achieve well-being. *JAMA Neurol* 73(6): 626–627.

Renganathan M, Cummins TR, Waxman SG. 2001. Contribution of Na(v)1.8 sodium channels to action potential electrogenesis in DRG neurons. *J Neurophysiol* 86(2): 629–640.

Rush AM, Cummins TR, Waxman SG. 2007. Multiple sodium channels and their roles in electrogenesis within dorsal root ganglion neurons. *J Physiol* 579(Pt 1): 1–14.

Sherrington CS. (1942). *Man on his nature.* Cambridge: Cambridge University Press.

Tate S, Benn S, Hick C, Trezise D, John V, Mannion RJ, et al. 1998. Two sodium channels contribute to the TTX-R sodium current in primary sensory neurons. *Nat Neurosci* 1(8): 653–655, doi:10.1038/3652.

Toledo-Aral JJ, Moss BL, He ZJ, Koszowski AG, Whisenand T, Levinson SR, et al. 1997. Identification of PN1, a predominant voltage-dependent sodium channel expressed principally in peripheral neurons. *Proc Natl Acad Sci USA* 94(4): 1527–1532.

Wall PD, Waxman S, Basbaum AI. 1974. Ongoing activity in peripheral nerve: Injury discharge. *Exp Neurol* 45(3): 576–589.

Waxman SG. 1970. Closely spaced nodes of Ranvier in the teleost brain. *Nature* 227(5255): 283–284.

Waxman SG. 1977. Conduction in myelinated, unmyelinated, and demyelinated fibers. *Arch Neurol* 34(10): 585–589.

Waxman SG. 1982. Membranes, myelin, and the pathophysiology of multiple sclerosis. *N Engl J Med* 306(25): 1529–1533.

Waxman SG, Bennett MV. 1972. Relative conduction velocities of small myelinated and non-myelinated fibres in the central nervous system. *Nat New Biol* 238(85): 217–219.

Waxman SG, Brill MH. 1978. Conduction through demyelinated plaques in multiple sclerosis: Computer simulations of facilitation by short internodes. *J Neurol Neurosurg Psychiatry* 41(5): 408–416.

Waxman SG, Kocsis JD, Black JA. 1994. Type III sodium channel mRNA is expressed in embryonic but not adult spinal sensory neurons, and is reexpressed following axotomy. *J Neurophysiol* 72(1): 466–470.

Waxman SG, Pappas GD, Bennett MV. 1972. Morphological correlates of functional differentiation of nodes of Ranvier along single fibers in the neurogenic electric organ of the knife fish *Sternarchus*. *J Cell Biol* 53(1): 210–224.

Waxman SG, Zamponi GW. 2014. Regulating excitability of peripheral afferents: Emerging ion channel targets. *Nat Neurosci* 17(2): 153–163.

Yang Y, Dib-Hajj SD, Zhang J, Zhang Y, Tyrrell L, Estacion M, et al. 2012. Structural modelling and mutant cycle analysis predict pharmacoresponsiveness of a Na(v)1.7 mutant channel. *Nat Commun* 3: 1186.

II ▌CHASING MEN ON FIRE: THE SEARCH

3 ALABAMA TO BEIJING … AND BACK

We all try to escape pain …
—Albert Einstein

The search for the pain gene began in an Alabama neighborhood with a group of men and women carrying groceries, talking with each other, tending to their children, or driving down the street. Ordinary, at first glance. But, many of the people did not wear regular shoes. Some wore open toed sandals. Others preferred not to wear anything on their feet, to walk barefoot on a cool tile floor, or in the cold water that collected in puddles. The children avoided the playground. They sometimes missed school days. And, if you spent time with these people, you might hear a person say, "I'm getting an attack." Then, the affected person would grimace, their feet turning bright red, as if they had been badly sunburned. If asked, they would say that their feet, and sometimes their hands, felt as if they were on fire. And, if cold water or ice were available, they might place their red feet in it.

As striking as the pain in these people was, it was also unusual in another way: The pain and redness did not occur in everybody in the neighborhood. It was present in, and only in, one large, extended family. Parents, aunts, uncles, and children suffered from this fire-like pain, but neighbors from other families did not have it. Five generations were known to have this mysterious disorder, about half of the individuals in each generation.

What was going on in this Alabama family with excruciating burning pain and red feet? Doctors were baffled and could not make a diagnosis; some even wondered whether it was a physical disorder at all, or whether it was "in the mind." But it was not imagined, and it was not a creation of the mind. We now know that this family suffered from and continues to suffer from the "man on fire" syndrome. The medical names for this disorder are erythermalgia and erythromelalgia. In this book we will call it erythromelalgia.

Erythromelalgia is incredibly rare. Most physicians will never see a case. But it is a striking disorder, and, once a physician has seen a case, it remains in his or her memory because it is so unusual. Erythromelalgia was given its name by neurologist S. Weir Mitchell in 1878. Its name, from Greek, connotes some of its main features: *erythros* ("red"), *melos* ("limb"), and *algos* ("pain"). Some still refer to this disorder of red limb pain as Mitchell's disease or Weir Mitchell disease.

People with erythromelalgia suffer from periodic attacks of excruciating burning pain. To describe their pain, they use terms like "being on fire," "being scalded," or "feeling like hot lava has been poured into my body." A picture entitled "Chained to Fire," prepared by a fourteen-year-old girl to depict her erythromelalgia, is shown in figure 3.1.

The burning pain of erythromelalgia is usually symmetrical—both sides of the body tend to be affected—most commonly the feet, sometimes the hands, and occasionally the tip of the nose or ears. Superimposed on a lower level of ongoing discomfort, the severe pain of erythromelalgia comes in bursts or attacks. These are triggered by mild warmth—such as the subtle warmth that comes from putting on shoes or socks, entering a warm room, or even mild exercise like walking. On a warm day, a walk across a parking lot can be enough to trigger severe pain. The pain attacks are accompanied by

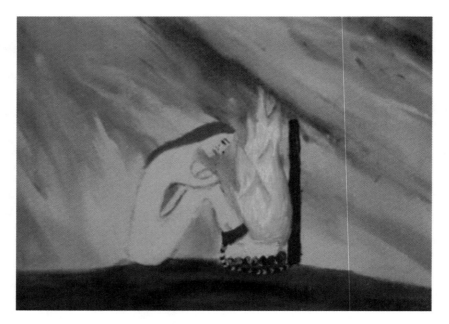

Figure 3.1
A drawing depicting the pain of erythromelalgia, entitled "Chained to Fire," prepared by Bailey
Deacon when she was fourteen years old, and submitted to an art contest sponsored by The
Erythromelalgia Association in 2012. As in many patients with erythromelalgia, the pain is most
severe in the feet. Reproduced courtesy of Bailey Deacon, Todd Deacon, and The Erythromelalgia
Association.

redness of the affected limbs. On a scale of 0 ("no pain") to 10 ("worst pain I can imagine"), people
with erythromelalgia describe their pain during attacks as a 7, 8, and too often a 9 or 10.

The pain in erythromelalgia is relieved by coolness. Characteristically, people with erythromelalgia
will seek out cold places, walking barefoot in cool weather, and immersing their burning limbs in
buckets of cold water or ice. This can lead to tissue injury, or worse, gangrene. Indeed, the literature
contains reports of people with erythromelalgia who have sustained limb amputations or gone into
septic shock as a result of infections due to skin breakdown from excessive cooling. Existing medications tend not to be helpful or are only partially helpful. Use of opiate medications is common, and
death by overdose has occurred. A few patients have requested amputation of limbs because the pain
is so severe, a maneuver that has in most cases not been helpful in the long run.

Erythromelalgia can occur in the context of other, more common disorders such as diabetes, multiple sclerosis, or disorders of the blood such as polycythemia vera in which the bone marrow produces too many blood cells. Erythromelalgia can also occur in isolation, where it is called "primary
erythromelalgia," or "primary erythermalgia." About 5% of cases of erythromelalgia are now known
to occur as an inherited disorder, as a result of mutations in a gene—these are called "inherited
erythromelalgia."

The human body is made up of cells—skin cells, muscle cells, blood cells, kidney cells, and many
other types of cells, including nerve cells. Cells, in turn, contain protein molecules. Protein molecules

are responsible for many of the activities of cells that keep them alive and allow them to perform properly in the body. Proteins are complex molecules assembled from smaller pieces called amino acids. There are twenty amino acids in humans. The amino acids line up in precise order, held together like links in a chain, to form a protein. One can also visualize the amino acids, in precise sequence, as being like a carefully designed string of multicolored beads. The identities of the amino acids—the colors of the beads, and the precise order in which they are strung together—are essential to the proper structure and function of the protein.

To form a functional protein molecule that can work properly within the body, the protein must contain the correct amino acids, in the correct order, and the string of amino acids must be folded into one particular conformation. Imagine scrunching up a string of colored beads in one's hand, so that bead number 101 lies next to bead number 148, and bead 160 touches bead 194, and so on. Within the scrunched necklace, the correct sequence of beads, which come in twenty colors, and a very precise folding configuration are necessary for the overall, three-dimensional shape of the protein to be correct, so that the protein can work properly. One bead of the wrong color—one wrong amino acid—or a missing bead, and the string may not fold into the needed three-dimensional structure. And with that incorrect configuration, the protein may not work properly. That is what happens, for example, in sickle cell anemia, where one of the 146 amino acids is substituted by another, incorrect amino acid within the β-globin component of hemoglobin, an iron-containing protein that plays an essential role, transporting oxygen within the blood. One bead of the wrong color, and hemoglobin does not work properly.

The blueprint for proteins is contained in the human genome. Each of our cells contain twenty-three pairs of chromosomes, a total of forty-six. These contain the 20,000 genes in the human genome. The gene for a particular protein encodes the amino acids, in precise sequence, that make up that protein. There are two copies of each gene, one from an individual's father, and the other from his or her mother. Genes are made of DNA (deoxyribonucleic acid) and consist of two strands, coiled around each other to form a double helix, that contain smaller molecules called nucleotides. For their discovery of the double helix configuration of DNA, James Watson, Francis Crick, and Maurice Wilkins were awarded the Nobel Prize in 1962.

There are four types of nucleotides within DNA: They are labeled A, T, G, C, and they can be considered as the letters within the alphabet of the genome. Since there are twenty amino acids which must be encoded with this alphabet, and only four letters to use, a series of three nucleotides is needed to encode each amino acid. It is as if each amino acid is identified by a code word of three letters, or three nucleotides. In 1961, at the age of 34, Marshall Nirenberg, working at the National Institutes of Health (NIH), made a stunning discovery that was a first step toward breaking the code. His experiments showed that the triplet TTT encodes the amino acid phenylalanine (Nirenberg and Matthaei 1961). He went on to a Nobel Prize, which he shared with Robert Holley and Har Gobind Khorana. Severo Ochoa (who had received a Nobel in 1959 for his work on the synthesis of RNA) went on to complete the identification of the DNA codes for all twenty amino acids.

By the mid-1960s it was clear, for example, that ATG codes for the amino acid methionine, that CCA codes for proline, and that GC, followed by any of the four nucleotides, codes for the amino acid alanine. And so forth for each amino acid. So, a stretch of a protein made up of a methionine, then a proline, and then an alanine would be encoded as follows:

ATGCCAGCT

This was the "Rosetta Stone" of genetics. By knowing the sequence of nucleotides within a gene, one could discern, amino acid by amino acid, the precise sequence of amino acids within a protein. Researchers in molecular biology laboratories were exhilarated. The genome, they hoped, would hold the key to understanding life.

Medical science moves forward in waves. Sometimes racing, sometimes crawling. And, not infrequently, multiple waves move medical research ahead on several fronts in parallel at the same time, like waves in the ocean, crashing simultaneously on different parts of a beach. This seems to have been true for the man on fire syndrome, because just as these advances in understanding DNA were occurring, physicians were beginning to recognize that this disorder had to be caused by an abnormality, hidden somewhere in the 20,000 genes that make up the human genome.

Every family has its heroes. Within the Alabama family, there was a person who recognized that, either then or sometime in the future, something might be done to help people with the man on fire syndrome.

In 1965, at the urging of a pediatrician, a mother in the Alabama family took her young daughter, with burning feet, to the Mayo Clinic in Rochester, Minnesota, a thousand miles away. It must have taken immense effort to arrange for a consultation so far away.

The visit was worth the effort.

The Mayo physicians recognized the girl's disorder as Mitchell's disease and appreciated that, in this case, it occurred as a familial or genetic disease. By the mid-1960s, the Alabama family knew that they had a very unusual disorder, and that it had a name, "familial erythromelalgia." In a brief paper in the *Journal of Laboratory and Clinical Medicine*, Mayo physician Mahlon Burbank and two colleagues noted that "we have had the opportunity to study a family in which 19 out of 51 family members, comprising 5 generations, have typical erythromelalgia. Study of this sibship indicates that the disorder in this family is inherited as a dominant trait" (Burbank, Spittel, and Fairbairn 1966). Now it was clear that the pain in this family was related to genes. The pain and redness arose in the genes, not in the mind.

Birmingham, Alabama, is fortunate to be the home of a medical school with a strong tradition of research, at the University of Alabama Birmingham. UAB was fortunate, in turn, to have on its faculty a medical geneticist, Dr. Wayne Finley. Following a period of training at the Institute for Medical Genetics at the University of Uppsala, Sweden, Finley and his wife, Dr. Sara Crews Finley, established at UAB the first medical genetics program in the southeastern United States. Over the ensuing years, the Finleys, either individually or together, published more than 250 professional abstracts, articles, and chapters on various aspects of medical genetics.

In 1986 a young girl in the Alabama family was seen at a local clinic for a urinary tract infection. The pediatrician was struck by her unusual condition and suggested that the child see Dr. Finley, who was a friend. Recognizing the girl's red, hot feet, Finley read the 1966 Burbank paper, contacted Burbank, and presciently decided to create a family tree. Finley did not have a grant to fund the work, but he persuaded the Departments of Dermatology and Pediatrics at UAB to partner with him in supporting it.

The first full-length article in the scientific literature on the Alabama family was published in 1992 by Finley and four other authors (Finley et al. 1992). Burbank was listed as the last author. The summary at the beginning of this pivotal paper notes that it "updates the family reported by Burbank 1966," although the introduction states that the initial patient studied for this paper "was different than Burbank's (and) we did not realize we were studying the same extended family." The paper carefully described the pedigree of the Alabama family—twenty-nine affected persons in five generations—and outlined their clinical features. It correctly posited that the disease "may be an autosomal dominant trait," in which a person must inherit one mutated copy of a gene from their affected parent to get the disease. Noting that "additional families must be studied," Finley and his coworkers concluded that "the mechanism for initiation of pain is not yet known." Indeed, Finley could not know—for the methods were not yet available—that mutations in one particular gene, one out of 20,000, were the cause of inherited erythromelalgia not just in this family, but in people with inherited erythromelalgia around the world.

A large family, containing multiple individuals with a rare disorder, presents an opportunity for medical researchers. Which one, out of the thousands of genes in the human genome, is responsible for their disorder? And what has gone wrong within that gene to cause disease? There was a lot of territory to cover, and a first step was to narrow the field using an assessment called "linkage analysis."

Linkage analysis takes advantage of the fact that all genes contain "single nucleotide polymorphisms" or SNPs. Each SNP is a minor variation in a gene, the substitution of a nucleotide for the one present in the majority of the population. A SNP can be thought of as a relatively inconsequential "mis-weave." SNPs do not necessarily cause disease. However, they provide markers that geneticists can use to study that gene. Polymorphisms tend to be inherited, like mutations, and polymorphisms located on the same gene as a mutation, especially polymorphisms located close to the mutation within the gene, tend to be inherited along with, or "linked" to, the mutation. It is relatively straightforward to map the pattern of polymorphisms within a family, and if the polymorphism is present in all of the affected family members and none of the nonaffected members, it suggests that that gene containing the SNP is the site of the mutation. Depending on the pattern of inheritance and the SNPs that are studied, this type of linkage analysis can point, not just to a candidate gene, but to a specific region within that gene.

Importantly, linkage analysis depends on probabilities: What is the probability that a particular gene, or a particular region within a gene, is related to a disease? If there is just a single affected family member, an apparent association of a polymorphism linked with the disease could be a random event and is not necessarily an indication of disease causation. It is only when *multiple* affected family members show the same pattern of linkage that the probability of a random association goes down, and the probability of having found the culprit gene goes up.

The Alabama family was nearly ideal for linkage analysis: a disease that is dramatic in its clinical presentation and thus easy to recognize, and a large number of affected family members in multiple generations. The Alabama family offered a good chance of pointing the way to a gene for pain. It is not surprising that medical researchers wanted to study that family.

Well before it was recognized as a genetic disorder, Joost Drenth had investigated erythromelalgia as a medical student in The Netherlands. Together with his mentor Professor Jan Michiels at the Erasmus Medical Center in Rotterdam, he had revised the diagnostic classification of various forms of erythromelalgia and described the development of erythromelalgia as a complication of treatment with certain medications (Drenth 1989; Drenth and Michiels 1990). By the mid-1990s Drenth, now trained in medical genetics in Paris, was searching for a family with erythromelalgia, the larger the better. As he worked to find a family, he discovered a pedigree of a family with erythromelalgia in a textbook on medical genetics. By 1995 he had written to American physicians, trying to find this family. His initial inquiries failed to elicit a response, and this closed the book for several years. In 1998 Drenth learned that Dr. Michiels had contacted Dr. Finley to ask for DNA from the Alabama family, and arranged for Dr. Peter Heutink at the Erasmus Medical Center, an expert on linkage studies, to attempt to do this type of analysis. The project had stalled, however, because there were inconsistencies in a few patients in the link between clinical status and genetic status.

Now working in Nijmegen, where he had been appointed professor of internal medicine, Drenth contacted Michiels in early 1999, offering to trace new families. Alternatively, he suggested, he might be able to resolve the incongruences. Later that year, Drenth's detective work paid off as he resolved the inconsistencies in Dr. Finley's family. Now the linkage analysis could move ahead. The resulting paper, which included Drenth, Finley, Michiels, and Heutink as authors, was entitled "The Primary Erythermalgia-Susceptibility Gene Is Located on Chromosome 2q31-32" (Drenth et al. 2001). The analysis showed that the gene was located on chromosome 2. Chromosome 2 is a large chromosome that contains nearly 1,500 genes. Drenth's study pointed to the gene's being located between two markers within a particular, small region of the chromosome, about 3% of its total size. The linkage analysis had narrowed the search to a specific portion of chromosome 2, termed q31–32. At that time, sodium channel genes had not yet been mapped to that region, so these investigators could not know that their results pointed toward a sodium channel gene. Nevertheless, their result was important: It had limited the search from 20,000 genes to about 50. The search for the pain gene no longer required finding a needle in a haystack. Now the search could focus on a small but still formidable tangle of hay.

The search now moved to Beijing where a young dermatologist, Yong Yang, was seeing patients within a major referral clinic at the Peking University First Hospital. Yong Yang was interested in genetic causes of dermatological disease, and he had become aware of a Chinese family containing three generations of patients with burning pain and redness in their hands and feet. The disorder began in each of the patients in early childhood. In each, reddening of the skin and severe pain were evoked by warmth and relieved by cooling.

As with the Alabama family, a first step in analyzing this Chinese family was to do a linkage analysis. And as with the Alabama family, this analysis pointed to a well-defined region within chromosome 2. By now, however, it was known that this region of chromosome 2 contained a cluster of sodium channel genes, including *SCN9A*, the gene encoding sodium channel $Na_V1.7$. Every gene within this part of chromosome 2 was a candidate as a potential culprit, but there was something special about *SCN9A*: $Na_V1.7$ is present at high levels within pain-signaling DRG neurons.

Together with colleagues at the Chinese National Human Genome Center, Yang began the task of sequencing the coding portions of the *SCN9A* gene from this family. The results, a sequence of letters— one for each nucleotide—revealed the solution to a puzzle. They showed that one nucleotide (one out of thousands making up the gene) had been changed:

AAC CTC ACC

had been changed to

AAC CAC ACC

This change, of nucleotide A for nucleotide T at position 2573 within exon 15 of the gene, indicated that there was a "missense mutation," a mutation that substitutes a histidine for a leucine at position 858, within the mutant $Na_V1.7$ channel. The same L858H change was found in other affected individuals within the family. Importantly, the L858H substitution was not present in unaffected family members. The family was not a huge one, and in the absence of information about the effect of the mutation on function of the Na$_V$1.7 channel, the analysis suggested, but did not prove, that the mutation caused the disease. Yang and his colleagues had another advantage, however: a very large population available in China for them to study. Within this large population, in another patient with a similar but sporadic pain syndrome, they found another mutation, I848T, substituting a threonine for an isoleucine, at a nearby position in precisely the same gene. Again, the mutation was not present in unaffected relatives.

Yong Yang's paper (Yang et al. 2004), entitled "Mutations in *SCN9A*, Encoding a Sodium Channel Alpha Subunit, in Patients with Primary Erythermalgia," appeared in the March 2004 issue of the *Journal of Medical Genetics*. When I saw the title of the article, I initially told my team that it was a bad day and retreated to my office. We had hoped to find families with inherited pain so we could sequence their sodium channel genes, and it appeared that we had been scooped.

It was only after a cup of black coffee and reading the article that I realized what had happened. Yong Yang and his colleagues had indeed identified two mutations in the *SCN9A* gene encoding Na$_V$1.7 in an inherited pain disorder, the man on fire syndrome. This was an important step forward. But finding the mutations did not prove that they caused these patients' pain. Appropriately, Yang el al. ended their paper with the conclusion "Mutations in *SCN9A* may cause primary erythermalgia." More work was needed to move from "may cause" to "do cause," to show that the mutations actually caused the disorder.

Yang and his colleagues were dermatologists and medical geneticists, but they were not neuroscientists. They did not ask the questions that a neuroscientist would have asked, that would establish a causal role for the mutations. Now it was time for us to ask those questions. Some mutations produce amino acid substitutions that are detrimental to channel function and cause disease. But other mutations produce amino acid substitutions that are not detrimental to channel function and do not cause disease. When a mutation of an ion channel such as a sodium channel is encountered by a neuroscientist or channel biologist, it immediately triggers these questions: Does the mutation change the functional properties of the channel, that is, does it change the manner in which the channel works? If so, in what ways? If the mutation changes the functional characteristics of the channel, does that mean that nerve cells carrying the mutant channel will function in an abnormal way? And finally, if the mutation produces changes in the function of nerve cells, can these changes explain the disease? These questions—the "functional profiling" of the mutant channels which might link them to disease— had to be asked. And we were in a position to answer those questions. What had appeared to be a bad day was, in fact, a good day. My colleagues reassembled in my office. There was a lot of work to do. The ball was now in our court.

We rapidly planned the "must do" experiments. Each of the mutations substituted a single amino acid in a part of the channel called the "S4–S5 linker." The linker acts as a hinge connecting the voltage sensor which controls the state of the channel with the channel pore, which must open to produce an electrical current. We needed, therefore, to assess the effects of the mutation on opening or gating of the channel. Serendipity now came into play. Five years earlier, we had carried out a detailed analysis of the "wild-type" or normal Na$_V$1.7 channel (Cummins, Howe, and Waxman 1998). So, we already had a high-fidelity understanding of the behavior of the normal Na$_V$1.7 channel, and we had the gene encoding it in our freezer. And we had a strong toolbox for studying sodium channels. We could insert the gene for normal Na$_V$1.7 channels into immortalized cells like HEK (human embryonic kidney) cells which do not normally contain any sodium channels, and study the gating of the channel in this quiet background. And we could do the same thing with mutant Na$_V$1.7 channels.

It took us only a few months to thaw the DNA for the wild-type Na$_V$1.7 and, using that DNA as a starting point, to create the mutant gene for the L858H and I848T mutant Na$_V$1.7 channels. The DNA was then inserted into cells in tissue culture so that electrophysiologist Ted Cummins could use a technique called "voltage clamp" to determine the effect of the mutations on the function of the Na$_V$1.7 channel. The results were dramatic. Both mutations shifted activation, or opening, of the channel in a hyperpolarizing direction. The analysis was relatively straightforward because the shifts in activation were large, 13 mV and 14 mV. One millivolt (mV) is one one-thousandth of a volt; that may not seem large, but from the point of view of a neuron, it is huge. The shifted activation made it easier to activate the channel so that the mutant channels turned on too easily. Both mutations also slowed the channel deactivation process whereby the channel closes after stimulation ceases; slowed deactivation meant that, once they were turned on or activated, the mutant channels remained activated longer then they should. Finally, both mutations enhanced the amplifying effect of the channel on small depolarizing stimuli. This was like turning the volume up on a hearing aid so that small sounds were amplified, but too much.

My colleagues and I in New Haven excitedly discussed the findings as they came in from our recording rigs using terms like "trifecta." Our experiments had established, at the channel level, the pro-excitatory effect of the L858H and I848T mutations, which made the channel hyperactive. Now we had some evidence for a causative role of the mutant channels in setting men on fire. Our experiments were beginning to show us how mutations in Na$_V$1.7 produce pain. We published our paper on these findings in late 2004 (Cummins, Dib-Hajj, and Waxman 2004).

Our knowledge that the mutant Na$_V$1.7 channels were overactive, a change that would be predicted to make pain-signaling neurons hyperactive, brought us close to proof that the mutations caused the man on fire syndrome. But to make the case conclusively, we needed more definitive evidence. We wanted to more directly answer the following question: What effect do the mutant channels have on pain-signaling DRG neurons? We knew that Na$_V$1.7 channels were present in these cells, within the dorsal root ganglia (DRG) hanging just outside the spinal cord. These primary sensory neurons send peripheral axons, within peripheral nerves, to innervate the body surface; and they send a process centrally into the spinal cord, to synapse with second-order cells within the pain pathway. The functional role of DRG neurons is to carry pain messages from the periphery, the body surface, to spinal cord second-order neurons, which in turn send impulses upward toward the brain. To determine the effect of the mutant channels on the firing of DRG neurons, we needed to insert the mutant gene into these cells, then let the cells grow in tissue culture. After the cells had been in culture long enough for the mutant gene to produce mutant Na$_V$1.7 channels, we could then record the electrical activity of these cells in response to precisely calibrated stimuli, using a technique called current clamp. This analysis would require a large number of very precise measurements. It was going to take a major effort. Thus, in planning for this study, we asked "which mutation is likely to teach us the most?" This brought us back to the Alabama family.

By now, we knew the identity of the family and where they lived. After obtaining approval from the human studies committee at Yale, we contacted them. I sent a team to Birmingham and obtained DNA from seventeen affected family members. We found a mutation in *SCN9A*, the gene for Na$_V$1.7, in all of them. This mutation had not been previously described. We also obtained DNA from five unaffected family members; none of them carried the mutation. The large number of DNA samples, twenty-two for this family, was in itself important. Genetics depends on probabilities. The presence of a mutation in a family with disease can suggest that it causes disease, but there is always the possibility that the mutation is benign and appeared in particular patients by chance. But with twenty-two DNA samples the likelihood of a "false positive" was much smaller. The large number of people in the Alabama family and the observation that the mutation "segregated with disease" provided strong evidence that the mutation was disease-causing. To be sure, however, we needed to show that the mutant channels from the Alabama family made pain-signaling neurons hyperactive.

This mutation, F1449V, replaced a phenylalanine with a valine, in another functionally important part of the channel (Dib-Hajj et al. 2005). As with the L858H and I848T mutations, voltage-clamp experiments showed us that the F1449V mutation hyperpolarized activation. This pro-excitatory change at the channel level suggested that the mutation produced pain. To make an airtight case that the mutation was disease-causing, we needed to answer the question: Does the mutation change the firing properties of pain-signaling neurons? If so, do the mutations shift the activity of these nerve cells in the appropriate direction? Two electrophysiologists and two technicians worked in tandem as we moved toward an answer. Cell by cell, they assessed the effect of the mutant channels until, finally, they had enough data. Our laboratory buzzed with conversation as they announced their findings. Our observations on DRG neurons, described in Dib-Hajj et al. (2005), provided a striking parallel to the pain described by the people in the Alabama family. The presence of mutant F1449V channels lowered the threshold for firing of DRG neurons. In other words, a smaller stimulus was needed to trigger an action potential in DRG neurons containing the mutant channels. And, at a given stimulation level, the frequency of firing was much higher in DRG neurons containing the mutant channel. So, as a result of the mutation, pain-signaling DRG neurons were more likely to fire. And when they fired, these pain-signaling neurons fired at abnormally high frequencies. We now had a convincing link of $Na_V1.7$ to pain.

From Burbank's initial observations on members of the Alabama family in 1966 and the study by Finley et al. in 1992, both of which suggested that the man on fire syndrome is a genetic disorder, it had taken until 2002 for Drenth to capitalize on linkage analysis to point to a particular part of one chromosome, containing about fifty genes. It took two more years for the story to move to Beijing where the first erythromelalgia mutations were identified, and then to New Haven where we showed how these mutations change function of the $Na_V1.7$ channel, making it hyperactive. One year later, focusing again on the Alabama family, we showed how these mutations cause DRG neurons to scream when they should be whispering, closing the loop to pain.

It had taken from 1966 to 2005, thirty-nine years, for the Alabama family's genome to reveal its secret. We had crossed the threshold into Huxley's science fiction. A gene for pain had been found and its role in disease had been uncovered. But, as exhilarating as discovery of the pain gene had been, there were even more exciting things to come.

References

Burbank MK, Spittell JA, Jr, Fairbairn JF. 1966. Familial erythromelalgia: Genetic and physiologic observations. *Journal of Laboratory and Clinical Medicine* 68(5): 861.

Cummins TR, Dib-Hajj SD, Waxman SG. 2004. Electrophysiological properties of mutant $Na_V1.7$ sodium channels in a painful inherited neuropathy. *J Neurosci* 24(38): 8232–8236.

Cummins TR, Howe JR, Waxman SG. 1998. Slow closed-state inactivation: A novel mechanism underlying ramp currents in cells expressing the hNE/PN1 sodium channel. *J Neurosci* 18(23): 9607–9619.

Dib-Hajj SD, Rush AM, Cummins TR, Hisama FM, Novella S, Tyrrell L, et al. 2005. Gain-of-function mutation in $Na_V1.7$ in familial erythromelalgia induces bursting of sensory neurons. *Brain* 128(Pt 8): 1847–1854.

Drenth JP. 1989. Erythromelalgia induced by nicardipine. *BMJ* 298(6687): 1582.

Drenth JP, Finley WH, Breedveld GJ, Testers L, Michiels JJ, Guillet G, et al. 2001. The primary erythermalgia-susceptibility gene is located on chromosome 2q31-32. *Am J Hum Genet* 68(5): 1277–1282.

Drenth JP, Michiels JJ. 1990. Three types of erythromelalgia. *BMJ* 301(6758): 985–986.

Finley WH, Lindsey JR, Jr, Fine JD, Dixon GA, Burbank MK. 1992. Autosomal dominant erythromelalgia. *Am J Med Genet* 42(3): 310–315.

Nirenberg MW, Matthaei JH. 1961. The dependence of cell-free protein synthesis in E. coli upon naturally occurring or synthetic polyribonucleotides. *Proc Natl Acad Sci USA* 47: 1588–1602.

Yang Y, Wang Y, Li S, Xu Z, Li H, Ma L, et al. 2004. Mutations in *SCN9A*, encoding a sodium channel alpha subunit, in patients with primary erythermalgia. *J Med Genet* 41(3): 171–174.

ELECTROPHYSIOLOGICAL PROPERTIES OF MUTANT Na$_V$1.7 SODIUM CHANNELS IN A PAINFUL INHERITED NEUROPATHY*

Theodore R. Cummins, Sulayman D. Dib-Hajj, and Stephen G. Waxman

Although the physiological basis of erythermalgia, an autosomal dominant painful neuropathy characterized by redness of the skin and intermittent burning sensation of extremities, is not known, two mutations of Na$_V$1.7, a sodium channel that produces a tetrodotoxin-sensitive, fast-inactivating current that is preferentially expressed in dorsal root ganglia (DRG) and sympathetic ganglia neurons, have recently been identified in patients with primary erythermalgia. Na$_V$1.7 is preferentially expressed in small-diameter DRG neurons, most of which are nociceptors, and is characterized by slow recovery from inactivation and by slow closed-state inactivation that results in relatively large responses to small, subthreshold depolarizations. Here we show that these mutations in Na$_V$1.7 produce a hyperpolarizing shift in activation and slow deactivation. We also show that these mutations cause an increase in amplitude of the current produced by Na$_V$1.7 in response to slow, small depolarizations. These observations provide the first demonstration of altered sodium channel function associated with an inherited painful neuropathy and suggest that these physiological changes, which confer hyperexcitability on peripheral sensory and sympathetic neurons, contribute to symptom production in hereditary erythermalgia.

Introduction

Sensory neurons in dorsal root ganglia (DRG) express multiple voltage-gated sodium channels including Na$_V$1.7 (Klugbauer et al., 1995; Sangameswaran et al., 1997), Na$_V$1.8 (Akopian et al., 1996; Sangameswaran et al., 1996), and Na$_V$1.9 (Dib-Hajj et al., 1998; Tate et al., 1998), which play important roles in regulating their excitability (Matzner and Devor, 1994; Cummins et al., 1998, 1999; Renganathan et al., 2001). Na$_V$1.7

* Previously published in *Journal of Neuroscience* 24: 8232–8236, 2004. Copyright © 2004 Society for Neuroscience.

is selectively expressed in DRG and sympathetic ganglia (Black et al., 1996; Toledo-Aral et al., 1997) and is abundant in small-diameter DRG neurons (Black et al., 1996, 2004), including nociceptors (Djou-hri et al., 2003a). Recombinant Na$_V$1.7 produces a fast-inactivating tetrodotoxin-sensitive (TTX-S) current (Klugbauer et al., 1995; Sangameswaran et al., 1997) and displays slow repriming and slow closed-state inactivation that poise it to respond to small, slow depolarizations (Cummins et al., 1998; Herzog et al., 2003).

It is now well established that dysregulated expression of sodium channel genes, for example Na$_V$1.3, can produce changes in sodium currents within spinal sensory neurons that contribute to neuropathic pain (Cummins and Waxman, 1997; Black et al., 1999; Hains et al., 2004). Recently, Na$_V$1.7 expression in DRG neurons has been shown to increase after carrageenan-induced inflammation of rat hindpaw (Black et al., 2004). The dynamic regulation of Na$_V$1.7 suggests that this channel contributes to neuronal hyperexcitability leading to inflammatory pain.

In contrast to dysregulated sodium channel expression, to date there have been no demonstrations of changes in sodium currents attributable to mutations associated with pain. Familial primary erythermalgia is a rare, dominantly inherited painful neuropathy that is manifested as burning pain and redness of the extremities (van Genderen et al., 1993). Layzer (2001) hypothesized that sensitized C-fibers and the axon reflex underlie these symptoms. A segment of chromosome 2, which is known to contain sodium channel genes, has been linked to primary erythermalgia (Drenth et al., 2001). Subsequently, Yang et al. (2004) showed that two independent mutations in SCN9A, which encodes $Na_V1.7$, are linked to this disorder. The two substitutions produce a change of isoleucine 848 to threonine (I848T) and leucine 858 to histidine (L858H).

We investigated the effect of the I848T and L858H mutations on the biophysical properties of $hNa_V1.7$. Both mutations cause a significant hyperpolarizing shift in the $V_{1/2}$ of activation of the mutant channel, which was accompanied by a larger ramp current. Our data are consistent with a role of $Na_V1.7$ in DRG neuron hyperexcitability in erythermalgia.

Materials and Methods

Plasmids

The plasmid carrying the human $Na_V1.7$ cDNA insert was described previously (Klugbauer et al., 1995). The TTX-S determinant residue of $Na_V1.7$, tyrosine 362, was changed by site-directed mutagenesis to a serine to render the channel resistant to TTX ($Na_V1.7_R$) (Herzog et al., 2003). The I848T and L858H were individually introduced into $Na_V1.7_R$ using the Quick Change XL site-directed mutagenesis kit (Stratagene, La Jolla, CA) with two mutagenic primers that were designed according to the manufacturer recommendations.

Transfections

The $hNa_V1.7$ channels were cotransfected with the human $\beta1$ and $\beta2$ subunits (Lossin et al., 2002) into human embryonic kidney (HEK293) cells using the calcium phosphate precipitation method. HEK293 cells were grown under standard tissue culture conditions (5% CO_2; 37°C) in DMEM supplemented with 10% fetal bovine serum. The calcium phosphate–DNA mixture was added to the cell culture medium and left for 3 hr, after which the cells were washed with fresh medium. Sodium currents were recorded 40–72 hr after transfection.

Whole-Cell Patch-Clamp Recordings

Whole-cell patch-clamp recordings were conducted at room temperature (~21°C) using an EPC-10 amplifier and the Pulse program (v 8.5; HEKA Elektronik, Lambrecht/Pfalz, Germany). Fire-polished electrodes (0.8–1.5 MΩ)

were fabricated from 1.7 mm VWR Scientific (West Chester, PA) capillary glass using a Sutter Instruments (Novato, CA) P-97 puller. Average access resistance was 1.4±0.4 MΩ (mean±SD; $n=85$). Voltage errors were minimized using 80% series resistance compensation; the capacitance artifact was canceled using computer-controlled circuitry of the patch-clamp amplifier. Linear leak subtraction was used for all voltage-clamp recordings. Recordings were always started 3 min after establishing the whole-cell configuration. Membrane currents were filtered at 5 kHz and sampled at 20 kHz. The pipette solution contained the following (in mM): 140 CsF, 1 EGTA, 10 NaCl, and 10 HEPES, pH 7.3. The standard bathing solution was the following (in mM): 140 NaCl, 3 KCl, 1 $MgCl_2$, 1 $CaCl_2$, and 10 HEPES, pH 7.3. Data were analyzed using Pulsefit (HEKA Elektronik) and Origin (Microcal Software, Northampton, MA) software. Data sets used for statistical analysis were checked for normal distributions using a Shapiro–Wilks normality test.

Unless otherwise noted, statistical significance was determined ($p < 0.05$) using an unpaired t test. Results are presented as mean±SEM and error bars in the figures represent SEs.

Results

Wild-type (WT) $hNa_V1.7_R$ and the two mutant derivative channels I848T and L858H were transiently expressed along with $h\beta$-1 and $h\beta$-2 subunits in HEK293 cells. Figure 1A shows representative whole-cell currents. Although similar peak current densities were recorded from cells expressing WT (318±43 pA/pF; $n=29$) and I848T (350±37 pA/pF; $n=27$) channels, the current densities recorded from cells expressing L858H channels were significantly smaller (174±30 pA/pF; $n=27$). The voltage dependence of activation was examined using a series of depolarizing test pulses from −100 mV. Mutant channels activated at potentials 10–15 mV more negative than WT channels (figure 1B). The midpoint of activation (estimated by fitting the data with a Boltzmann function) was significantly more negative for I848T currents (−38.4± 1.0 mV; $n = 27$) and L858H currents (−37.9±

0.9 mV; $n=27$) than for WT currents ($-24.6\pm$mV; $n=29$). Although the midpoint of activation was almost identical for I848T and L858H channels, the threshold for activation appeared to be -5 mV more negative for L858H channels than for I848T channels.

The kinetics of deactivation, which reflects the transition from the open to the closed state, of WT and mutant channels was also examined by eliciting tail currents at a range of potentials after briefly activating the channels (at -20 mV for 0.5 msec). Altered deactivation of skeletal muscle sodium channels is thought to contribute to the pathophysiology of paramyotonia congen-

ita (Featherstone et al., 1998). I848T and L858H currents exhibited slower kinetics of deactivation (figure 1C). The time constant of deactivation (measured with single exponential fits) was slower at potentials ranging from -100 mV to -40 mV for the mutant channels. Interestingly, the effect on deactivation was much greater with the L858H mutation than with the I848T mutation at all deactivation voltages tested. For example, the deactivation time constants for I848T and L858H channels at -50 mV were approximately threefold and ~10-fold, respectively, larger than that of WT channels.

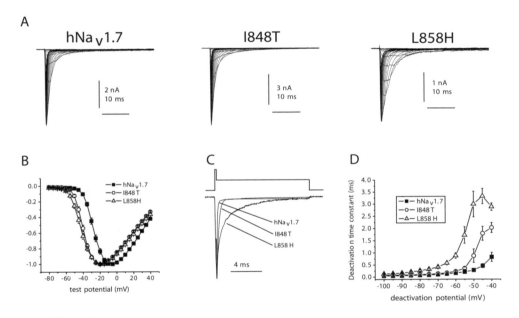

Figure 1
The I848T and L858H mutations of hNa$_V$1.7 alter activation and deactivation. (A) Current traces recorded from representative HEK293 cells expressing either wild-type hNa$_V$1.7 or mutant channels, I848T or L858H. Cells were held at -100 mV, and currents were elicited with 50 msec test pulses to potentials ranging from -80 to 40 mV. (B) Normalized peak current–voltage relationship for wild-type (filled squares; $n=29$), I848T (open circles; $n=27$), and L858H (open triangles; $n=27$) channels. (C) Representative tail currents of WT, I848T, and L858H channels. Cells were held at -100 mV and depolarized to -20 mV for 0.5 msec, followed by a repolarization to -50 mV to elicit tail currents. (D) Time constants for tail current deactivation at repolarization potentials ranging from -40 to -100 mV for wild-type (filled squares; $n=7$), I848T (open circles; $n=7$), and L858H (open triangles; $n=7$) hNa$_V$1.7 channels. Time constants were obtained with single exponential fits to the deactivation phase of the currents. Error bars represent SE.

The fast-inactivation time constant, which provides a measure of the open-to-inactivated transition, was estimated using m^3h Hodgkin and Huxley type fits to the current data. The time constants for fast inactivation between -40 and -20 mV were smaller for the mutant channels than for WT channels (figure 2A). However, the time constants of the three channels were similar at more depolarized potentials.

In contrast to the dramatic differences in the voltage dependence of activation, the voltage dependence of steady-state fast inactivation was similar for WT, I848T, and L858H (figure 2B). The midpoint of fast inactivation (measured with 500 msec prepulses) was not significantly different for WT (-73.6 ± 1.1 mV; $n=20$), I848T (-75.8 ± 1.1 mV; $n=19$), and L858H ($-76.1 \pm$ mV; $n=17$) channels. The steady-state fast-inactivation curve for L858H channels deviated from that of the other channels at negative voltages (e.g., between -120 and -80 mV). This is likely attributable to differences in slow inactivation (see below).

Defective slow inactivation of skeletal muscle sodium channels has been proposed to play a role in hyperkalemic periodic paralysis, and therefore, we also examined the voltage dependence of steady-state slow inactivation of hNa$_V$1.7 currents. Thirty second prepulses, followed by 100 msec recovery pulses to -120 mV to allow recovery from fast inactivation, preceded the test pulse (to 0 mV for 20 msec) to determine the fraction of current available. Dramatic differences were observed for slow-inactivation properties of WT, I848T, and L858H currents (figure 2C). Surprisingly, the L858H mutation substantially enhanced slow inactivation of hNa$_V$1.7. This enhancement of slow inactivation is likely to account for the enhanced inactivation of L858H currents observed at negative potentials with the steady-state fast-inactivation protocol (figure 2B). In contrast, the I848T mutations impaired slow inactivation of hNa$_V$1.7 channels. At 0 mV, only $67 \pm 6\%$ of I848T channels ($n=8$) are slow inactivated (determined from the fraction of channels available for activation as measured in figure 2C)

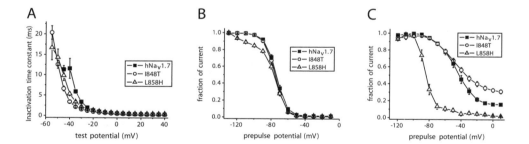

Figure 2

The I848T and L858H mutations differentially alter inactivation of hNa$_V$1.7. (A) Fast inactivation kinetics as a function of voltage for wild-type (filled squares; $n=8$), I848T (open circles; $n=8$), and L858H (open triangles; $n=8$) hNa$_V$1.7 channels. Currents elicited as described in figure 1A were fit with Hodgkin–Huxley type m^3h model to estimate the inactivation time constants. (B) Comparison of steady-state fast inactivation for wild-type (filled squares; $n=20$), I848T (open circles; $n=19$), and L858H (open triangles; $n=17$) hNa$_V$1.7 channels. Currents were elicited with test pulses to 0 mV after 500 msec inactivating prepulses. (C) Comparison of steady-state slow inactivation for wild-type hNa$_V$1.7 (filled squares; $n=9$), I848T (open circles; $n=8$), and L858H (open triangles; $n=9$) hNa$_V$1.7 channels. Slow inactivation was induced with 30 sec prepulses, followed by 100 msec pulses to -120 mV to allow recovery from fast inactivation. A test pulse to 0 mV for 20 msec was used to determine the fraction of current available. Error bars represent SE.

compared with $84\pm4\%$ of WT channels ($n=8$) and $>97\pm2\%$ of L858H channels ($n=7$). For both mutants, the percentage of channels that were slow inactivated at 0 mV was significantly different than for WT channels. Therefore, the two mutations identified in the Na$_V$1.7 channels of patients with primary erythermalgia have differential effects on slow inactivation of hNa$_V$1.7 channels.

Finally, we examined the currents induced in hNa$_V$1.7 channels by slow ramp depolarizations. Significantly larger currents were elicited with slow ramp (0.2 mV/ms) depolarizations from -100 to $+20$ mV by either I848T or L858H channels compared with WT channels (figure 3). The ramp currents (expressed as a percentage of peak current) were $1.8\pm0.2\%$ for I848T channels ($n=19$), $2.6\pm0.3\%$ for L858H channels ($n=16$), and $0.6\pm0.1\%$ for WT channels ($n=16$). The ramp currents in cells expressing I848T and L858H channels were pronounced between -70 and -40 mV (figure 3) and thus could contribute to subthreshold depolarizations and the initiation of action potentials.

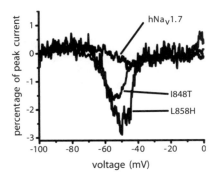

Figure 3
The I848T and L858H mutations enhance ramp currents of hNa$_V$1.7. Representative ramp currents elicited with 500 msec ramp depolarizations from -100 to 0 mV from HEK293 cells expressing wild-type, I848T, and L858H channels.

Discussion

Voltage-gated sodium channels mediate an increase in Na$^+$ permeability during depolarization of membrane potential that underlies action potential electrogenesis. Although dysregulated sodium channel expression contributes to the pathophysiology of neuropathic pain (Matzner and Devor, 1994; Waxman et al., 2000), mutations of voltage-gated sodium channel α-subunits, which underlie a number of human and animal disorders (for review, see Goldin, 2001; Keating and Sanguinetti, 2001; Meisler et al., 2001; Cannon, 2002), were not associated with painful neuropathies until Yang et al. (2004) identified two mutations in SCN9A, the gene encoding Na$_V$1.7, in patients with primary erythermalgia. In this study, we have characterized the functional consequences of these two hNa$_V$1.7 mutations, I848T and L858H. The I848T and L858H mutations are located in the S4–S5 linker region of domain II (DIIS4–S5) of the channel. Biophysical analysis of the mutant channels revealed several differences compared with wild-type hNa$_V$1.7. Both mutations significantly shifted the voltage dependence of activation in the hyperpolarizing direction. Deactivation of hNa$_V$1.7 was also slowed by both mutations, although the effect was much larger with the L858H mutation. Both mutations also significantly increased the size of ramp currents produced by hNa$_V$1.7 channels in response to slow depolarizations between -70 and -40 mV, a range that probably encompasses resting potential of sensory neurons (Harper and Lawson, 1985; Caffrey et al., 1992). These changes in the functional properties of hNa$_V$1.7 are likely to contribute to increased excitability of spinal sensory neurons that express Na$_V$1.7 and may underlie the abnormal pain sensations in patients with inherited erythermalgia.

The I848T and L858H mutations shifted the voltage dependence of activation of hNa$_V$1.7 by almost 15 mV in a hyperpolarizing direction. A shift of this magnitude is expected to decrease the threshold for action potential generation in sensory neurons and increase neuronal excitability. Both mutations also significantly slowed the rate of deactivation of hNa$_V$1.7. Impaired deactivation of skeletal muscle sodium channels (Na$_V$1.4) has been hypothesized to contribute to abnormal muscle excitability (predominantly myotonia) in patients with paramyotonia congenita (Featherstone et al., 1998). Many of the Na$_V$1.4 mutations that cause myotonia slow both the rate of fast inactivation and deactivation, and in computer simulations, this combination can induce a destabilization of repolarization after an action potential, leading to "myotonic runs" (Featherstone et al., 1998). Unlike these Na$_V$1.4 mutations, the hNa$_V$1.7-I848T and -L858H did not slow the rate of fast inactivation, and therefore the hNa$_V$1.7 mutations might not destabilize repolarization.

The mutant hNa$_V$1.7 channels produced significantly larger currents in response to slow ramp depolarizations than wild-type channels. Increased overlap between the inactivation and activation curves, resulting from the large negative shift in the voltage dependence of activation (figure 1B) and unchanged voltage dependence of steady-state inactivation (figure 2B), may underlie the larger ramp currents. Impaired deactivation, which indicates that the open-to-closed transition is altered, is also likely to contribute to the increased ramp current amplitudes. At negative potentials (less than −45 mV), the closing rate is much larger than the inactivation rate, and therefore channel openings are more likely to be terminated by deactivation than by inactivation in this voltage range (Vandenberg and Bezanilla, 1991). Vandenberg and Bezanilla (1991) suggested that the deactivation rate of sodium channels limits the ability of sodium channels to open and reopen at negative potentials. Thus, slowing the deactivation rate would be expected to increase the number of openings and open times at negative potentials, and this could contribute to increased ramp

current amplitudes. The fact that the L858H mutant exhibited the slowest deactivation kinetics and the largest ramp currents is consistent with this hypothesis. Because the ramp currents are evoked between −70 and −40 mV, close to the resting potential of DRG neurons (Harper and Lawson, 1985; Caffrey et al., 1992), the larger ramp currents in cells expressing mutant channels could amplify the response to small depolarizing inputs, increasing excitability. Na$_V$1.7 channels are expressed at high levels in small, mostly nociceptive, sensory neurons (Djouhri et al., 2003a), suggesting that changes in activation, deactivation, and ramp current amplitude contribute to pain in erythermalgia patients with the I848T and L858H mutations.

The amino acid sequence of domain II S4–S5 linker in hNa$_V$1.7 and hNa$_V$1.4 are identical (Yang et al., 2004) and are highly conserved when the sequence of all known sodium channels are aligned (data not shown). The conservation of this sequence suggests that the DIIS4–S5 linker plays a similar role in different sodium channels. The I848T mutation in erythermalgia (Yang et al., 2004) corresponds to the I693T mutation in hNa$_V$1.4 of patients with episodic muscle weakness (Cannon, 2002). The T704M mutation in hNa$_V$1.4 causes hyperkalemic periodic paralysis, another muscle disorder characterized by episodic weakness (Cannon, 2002). The L858 in hNa$_V$1.7 corresponds to L703 in hNa$_V$1.4, which is immediately adjacent to the T704 residue. Thus, DIIS4–S5 mutations in both hNa$_V$1.7 and hNa$_V$1.4 are associated with hereditary neurological and muscle disorders, which suggests that this linker contributes to the determination of biophysical properties of sodium channels including voltage dependence of activation and deactivation.

The functional consequences of the I693T and T704M mutations on hNa$_V$1.4 have been characterized after expression in HEK293 cells (Plassart-Schiess et al., 1998; Hayward et al., 1999; Bendahhou et al., 2002) and are similar to the effects of the I848T mutation on hNa$_V$1.7. All of these mutations shift the voltage dependence of activation in a hyperpolarizing direction. The Na$_V$1.4 mutations are thought to induce muscle weakness as a result of an enhanced persistent current (possibly attributable to window currents that result from the negative shift in the voltage dependence of activation) that depolarizes the muscle 5–10 mV, causing inactivation of the sodium currents and decreasing the ability of the muscle to fire action potentials (Lehmann-Horn et al., 1987; Cummins et al., 1993). The hNa$_V$1.4-I693T and hNa$_V$1.4-T704M mutations also significantly impair slow inactivation, and this impairment is thought to contribute to muscle weakness associated with these mutations (Ruff, 1994). However, whereas the I848T mutation impaired slow inactivation of hNa$_V$1.7, the L858H mutation of hNa$_V$1.7 enhanced slow inactivation. Because both mutations are associated with primary erythermalgia, this divergence might be interpreted as suggesting that slow inactivation is not important in its pathophysiology. Alternatively, there may be subtle differences in the symptoms of primary erythermalgia in patients with the I848T and L858H mutations attributable to the differential effect of the two mutations on slow inactivation.

Given that the I693T mutation in Na$_V$1.4 is associated with muscle weakness, how can the I848T mutation in Na$_V$1.7 be associated with increased pain sensations? One explanation may derive from the fact that whereas mature muscle cells express only Na$_V$1.4 channels, spinal sensory neurons express multiple sodium channel isoforms with distinct properties (Black et al., 1996). The Na$_V$1.8 channel, which is expressed at high levels in many (but not all) spinal sensory neurons, has a very depolarized voltage dependence of inactivation compared with other channels such as Na$_V$1.4 and Na$_V$1.7 (Akopian et al., 1996) and plays a critical role in action potential firing in sensory neurons (Renganathan et al., 2001). If the Na$_V$1.7-I848T muta-

tion depolarizes the sensory neurons by 5–10 mV, as the Na$_V$1.4 mutations associated with muscle weakness are thought to do in muscle (Lehmann-Horn et al., 1987; Cannon, 2002), the Na$_V$1.8 channels are likely to still be available for activation. Depolarizations of similar magnitudes might produce reduced action potential activity in muscle but could lead to enhanced excitability in neurons that also express Na$_V$1.8 because these cells would be closer to threshold for activation of Na$_V$1.8 currents. Thus, mutations of identical residues in Na$_V$1.7 and Na$_V$1.4 that have similar effects on channel properties could have differential effects on excitability and cause distinct neurological disorders because of the presence of multiple sodium channels (including Na$_V$1.8 which is not present in muscle) in spinal sensory neurons.

Non-nociceptive neurons are less likely to express Na$_V$1.8 channels than nociceptive neurons (Djouhri et al., 2003b), and thus mutant Na$_V$1.7 channels could possibly differentially alter excitability in nociceptive and non-nociceptive neurons. Moreover, although Na$_V$1.7 currents exhibit similar properties in HEK293 cells and DRG neurons (Cummins et al., 1998; Herzog et al., 2003), it is also possible that the mutant and wild-type Na$_V$1.7 channels are differentially modulated in DRG neurons, and this might contribute to the disease phenotype. For example, our studies in HEK293 cells were done with coexpression of the β1 and β2 subunits, but DRG neurons also express other β subunits such as β3 (Shah et al., 2000) that could impact the current properties. Na$_V$1.4 and Na$_V$1.7 currents exhibit distinct properties (Cummins et al., 1998) and could be differentially modulated by β subunits, and this could also contribute to the different disease phenotypes.

Our results highlight the fact that analogous mutations in sodium channels can result in dramatically different phenotypes and suggest that this difference may be attributable to the ensemble of other sodium channels (or channel subunits) that are expressed together with the mutant channel within DRG neurons.

The changes in the electrophysiological properties of mutant hNa$_V$1.7 provide the first example of altered sodium channel function in a hereditary pain syndrome and suggest that targeting of sodium channels may provide a useful therapeutic strategy for this disorder.

Acknowledgments

This work was supported in part by the Medical Research Service and Rehabilitation Research Service, Department of Veterans Affairs and by a grant from the National Multiple Sclerosis Society. The Center for Neuroscience and Regeneration Research is a collaboration of the Paralyzed Veterans of America and the United Spinal Association with Yale University. T.R.C. was supported by a Biomedical Research grant from Indiana University School of Medicine.

About the Authors

Theodore R. Cummins, Department of Pharmacology and Toxicology, Stark Neurosciences Research Institute, Indiana University School of Medicine, Indianapolis, IN

Sulayman D. Dib-Hajj, Department of Neurology and Center for Neuroscience and Regeneration Research, Yale University School of Medicine, New Haven, CT, and Rehabilitation Research Center, Veterans Administration Connecticut Healthcare System, West Haven, CT

Stephen G. Waxman, Department of Neurology and Center for Neuroscience and Regeneration Research, Yale University School of Medicine, New Haven, CT, and Rehabilitation Research Center, Veterans Administration Connecticut Healthcare System, West Haven, CT

References

Akopian AN, Sivilotti L, Wood JN. 1996. A tetrodotoxin-resistant voltage-gated sodium channel expressed by sensory neurons. *Nature* 379: 257–262.

Bendahhou S, Cummins TR, Kula RW, Fu YH, Ptacek LJ. 2002. Impairment of slow inactivation as a common mechanism for periodic paralysis in DIIS4–S5. *Neurology* 58: 1266–1272.

Black JA, Dib-Hajj S, McNabola K, Jeste S, Rizzo MA, Kocsis JD, Waxman SG. 1996. Spinal sensory neurons express multiple sodium channel alpha-subunit mRNAs. *Brain Res Mol Brain Res* 43: 117–131.

Black JA, Cummins TR, Plumpton C, Chen YH, Hormuzdiar W, Clare JJ, Waxman SG. 1999. Upregulation of a silent sodium channel after peripheral, but not central, nerve injury in DRG neurons. *J Neurophysiol* 82: 2776–2785.

Black JA, Liu S, Tanaka M, Cummins TR, Waxman SG. 2004. Changes in the expression of tetrodotoxin-sensitive sodium channels within dorsal root ganglia neurons in inflammatory pain. *Pain* 108: 237–247.

Caffrey JM, Eng DL, Black JA, Waxman SG, Kocsis JD. 1992. Three types of sodium channels in adult rat dorsal root ganglion neurons. *Brain Res* 592: 283–297.

Cannon SC. 2002. An expanding view for the molecular basis of familial periodic paralysis. *Neuromuscul Disord* 12: 533–543.

Cummins TR, Waxman SG. 1997. Downregulation of tetrodotoxin-resistant sodium currents and upregulation of a rapidly reprinting tetrodotoxin-sensitive sodium current in small spinal sensory neurons after nerve injury. *J Neurosci* 17: 3503–3514.

Cummins TR, Zhou J, Sigworth FJ, Ukomadu C, Stephan M, Ptacek LJ, Agnew WS. 1993. Functional consequences of a Na$^+$ channel mutation causing hyperkalemic periodic paralysis. *Neuron* 10: 667–678.

Cummins TR, Howe JR, Waxman SG. 1998. Slow closed-state inactivation: A novel mechanism underlying ramp currents in cells expressing the hNE/PN1 sodium channel. *J Neurosci* 18: 9607–9619.

Cummins TR, Dib-Hajj SD, Black JA, Akopian AN, Wood JN, Waxman SG. 1999. A novel persistent tetrodotoxin-resistant sodium current in SNS-null and wild-type small primary sensory neurons. *J Neurosci* 19(RC43): 1–6.

Dib-Hajj SD, Tyrrell L, Black JA, Waxman SG. 1998. NaN, a novel voltage-gated Na channel, is expressed preferentially in peripheral sensory neurons and down-regulated after axotomy. *Proc Natl Acad Sci USA* 95: 8963–8968.

Djouhri L, Newton R, Levinson SR, Berry CM, Carruthers B, Lawson SN. 2003a. Sensory and electrophysiological properties of guinea-pig sensory neurones expressing Nav1.7 (PN1) Na$^+$ channel alpha subunit protein. *J Physiol* 546: 565–576.

Djouhri L, Fang X, Okuse K, Wood JN, Berry CM, Lawson SN. 2003b. The TTX-resistant sodium channel Nav1.8 (SNS/PN3): Expression and correlation with membrane properties in rat nociceptive primary afferent neurons. *J Physiol* 550: 739–752.

Drenth JP, Finley WH, Breedveld GJ, Testers L, Michiels JJ, Guillet G, Taieb A, Kirby RL, Heutink P. 2001. The primary erythermalgia-susceptibility gene is located on chromosome 2q31–32. *Am J Hum Genet* 68: 1277–1282.

Featherstone DE, Fujimoto E, Ruben PC. 1998. A defect in skeletal muscle sodium channel deactivation exacerbates hyperexcitability in human paramyotonia congenita. *J Physiol* 506: 627–638.

Goldin A. 2001. Resurgence of sodium channel research. *Annu Rev Physiol* 63: 871–894.

Hains BC, Saab CY, Klein JP, Craner MJ, Waxman SG. 2004. Altered sodium channel expression in second-order spinal sensory neurons contributes to pain after peripheral nerve injury. *J Neurosci* 24: 4832–4839.

Harper AA, Lawson SN. 1985. Electrical properties of rat dorsal root ganglion neurones with different peripheral nerve conduction velocities. *J Physiol* 359: 47–63.

Hayward LJ, Sandoval GM, Cannon SC. 1999. Defective slow inactivation of sodium channels contributes to familial periodic paralysis. *Neurology* 52: 1447–1453.

Herzog RI, Cummins TR, Ghassemi F, Dib-Hajj SD, Waxman SG. 2003. Distinct repriming and closed-state inactivation kinetics of Nav1.6 and Nav1.7 sodium channels in mouse spinal sensory neurons. *J Physiol* 551: 741–750.

Keating MT, Sanguinetti MC. 2001. Molecular and cellular mechanisms of cardiac arrhythmias. *Cell* 104: 569–580.

Klugbauer N, Lacinova L, Flockerzi V, Hofmann F. 1995. Structure and functional expression of a new member of the tetrodotoxin-sensitive voltage-activated sodium channel family from human neuroendocrine cells. *EMBO J* 14: 1084–1090.

Layzer RB. 2001. Hot feet: Erythromelalgia and related disorders. *J Child Neurol* 16: 199–202.

Lehmann-Horn F, Kuther G, Ricker K, Grafe P, Ballanyi K, Rudel R. 1987. Adynamia episodica hereditaria with myotonia: A non-inactivating sodium current and the effect of extracellular pH. *Muscle Nerve* 10: 363–374.

Lossin C, Wang DW, Rhodes TH, Vanoye CG, George AL, Jr. 2002. Molecular basis of an inherited epilepsy. *Neuron* 34: 877–884.

Matzner O, Devor M. 1994. Hyperexcitability at sites of nerve injury depends on voltage-sensitive Na$^+$ channels. *J Neurophysiol* 72: 349–359.

Meisler MH, Kearney J, Ottman R, Escayg A. 2001. Identification of epilepsy genes in human and mouse. *Annu Rev Genet* 35: 567–588.

Plassart-Schiess E, Lhuillier L, George AL, Jr, Fontaine B, Tabti N. 1998. Functional expression of Ile693Thr Na$^+$ channel mutation associated with paramyotonia congenita in a human cell line. *J Physiol* 507: 721–727.

Renganathan M, Cummins TR, Waxman SG. 2001. Contribution of Nav1.8 sodium channels to action potential electrogenesis in DRG neurons. *J Neurophysiol* 86: 629–640.

Ruff RL. 1994. Slow Na$^+$ channel inactivation must be disrupted to evoke prolonged depolarization-induced paralysis. *Biophys J* 66: 542–545.

Sangameswaran L, Delgado SG, Fish LM, Koch BD, Jakeman LB, Stewart GR, Sze P, Hunter JC, Eglen RM, Herman RC. 1996. Structure and function of a novel voltage-gated, tetrodoxtoxin-resistant sodium channel specific to sensory neurons. *J Biol Chem* 271: 5953–5956.

Sangameswaran L, Fish LM, Koch BD, Rabert DK, Delgado SG, Ilnicka M, Jakeman LB, et al. 1997. A novel tetrodotoxin-sensitive, voltage-gated sodium channel expressed in rat and human dorsal root ganglia. *J Biol Chem* 272: 14805–14809.

Shah BS, Stevens EB, Gonzalez MI, Bramwell S, Pinnock RD, Lee K, Dixon AK. 2000. Beta3, a novel auxiliary subunit for the voltage-gated sodium channel, is expressed preferentially in sensory neurons and is upregulated in the chronic constriction injury model of neuropathic pain. *Eur J Neurosci* 12: 3985–3990.

Tate S, Benn S, Hick C, Trezise D, John V, Mannion RJ, Costigan M, et al. 1998. Two sodium channels contribute to the TTX-R sodium current in primary sensory neurons. *Nat Neurosci* 1: 653–655.

Toledo-Aral JJ, Moss BL, He ZJ, Koszowski AG, Whisenand T, Levinson SR, Wolf JJ, Silossantiago I, Halegoua S, Mandel G. 1997. Identification of PN1, a predominant voltage-dependent sodium channel expressed principally in peripheral neurons. *Proc Natl Acad Sci USA* 94: 1527–1532.

Vandenberg CA, Bezanilla F. 1991. A sodium channel gating model based on single channel, macroscopic ionic, and gating currents in the squid giant axon. *Biophys J* 60: 1511–1533.

van Genderen PJ, Michiels JJ, Drenth JP. 1993. Hereditary erythermalgia and acquired erythromelalgia. *Am J Med Genet* 45: 530–532.

Waxman SG, Dib-Hajj S, Cummins TR, Black JA. 2000. Sodium channels and their genes: Dynamic expression in the normal nervous system, dys-regulation in disease states. *Brain Res* 886: 5–14.

Yang Y, Wang Y, Li S, Xu Z, Li H, Ma L, Fan J, et al. 2004. Mutations in SCN9A, encoding a sodium channel alpha subunit, in patients with primary erythermalgia. *J Med Genet* 41: 171–174.

GAIN-OF-FUNCTION MUTATION IN Na$_V$1.7 IN FAMILIAL ERYTHROMELALGIA INDUCES BURSTING OF SENSORY NEURONS*

S. D. Dib-Hajj, A. M. Rush, T. R. Cummins, F. M. Hisama, S. Novella, L. Tyrrell, L. Marshall, and S. G. Waxman

Erythromelalgia is an autosomal dominant disorder characterized by burning pain in response to warm stimuli or moderate exercise. We describe a novel mutation in a family with erythromelalgia in SCN9A, the gene that encodes the Na$_V$1.7 sodium channel. Na$_V$1.7 produces threshold currents and is selectively expressed within sensory neurons including nociceptors. We demonstrate that this mutation, which produces a hyperpolarizing shift in activation and a depolarizing shift in steady-state inactivation, lowers thresholds for single action potentials and high frequency firing in dorsal root ganglion neurons. Erythromelalgia is the first inherited pain disorder in which it is possible to link a mutation with an abnormality in ion channel function and with altered firing of pain signalling neurons.

Introduction

Sodium channels contribute to dorsal root ganglion (DRG) neuron hyperexcitability associated with acquired pain (Waxman et al., 1999; Black et al., 2002), but their role in hereditary pain syndromes is less well understood. Primary erythromelalgia (also called primary erythermalgia) is an autosomal dominant painful neuropathy with characteristics that include burning pain of the extremities in response to warm stimuli or moderate exercise (van Genderen et al., 1993). Recently, two mutations in *SCN9A*, the gene for the human Na$_V$1.7 sodium channel, were reported in primary erythromelalgia (Yang et al., 2004). Na$_V$1.7 channels are preferentially expressed in nociceptive DRG neurons and sympathetic ganglion neurons (Sangameswaran et al., 1997; Toledo-Aral et al., 1997; Djouhri et al., 2003),

* Previously published in *Brain* 128: 1847–1854, 2005.
© The Author (2005).

and produce 'threshold currents' close to resting potential, amplifying small depolarizations such as generator potentials (Cummins et al., 1998), while other sodium channel isoforms contribute most of the current underlying all-or-none action potentials in DRG neurons (Renganathan et al., 2001; Blair and Bean, 2002). The previously described mutations of Na$_V$1.7 cause a 13–15 mV hyperpolarizing shift in activation, slow deactivation and increase the response of the channels to small ramp depolarizations (Cummins et al., 2004). We now describe a third mutation in Na$_V$1.7 which segregates with the disease phenotype in a large pedigree of primary erythromelalgia, describe its effects on channel function and show, for the first time, that a mutation in a human sodium channel can lower the threshold for single action potentials and high frequency firing of DRG neurons.

Subjects and Methods

Patients

A neurologist blinded to the genetic studies confirmed disease phenotype, based on formal clinical criteria (Drenth and Michiels, 1994), in 17 affected subjects, five unaffected subjects and three unaffected spouses after informed consent was obtained in a study approved by the Yale Medical School Human Investigation Committee. A clinical description for part of this family (Finley et al., 1992) and linkage to chromosome 2q31–q32 have been reported (Drenth et al., 2001), but detailed genetic analysis had not been carried out previously.

Exon Screening

Genomic DNA was purified from buccal swabs or venous blood from 25 family members (17 affected; eight unaffected). Human variation panel control DNA (25 males, 25 females; Caucasians) was obtained from the Coriell Institute (Camden, NJ). The genomic sequence of SCN9A (GenBank accession no. NC_000002) was used to design intron-specific primers to amplify coding and non-coding exons which produce $Na_V1.7$ cDNA. Genomic sequences were compared with the reference $Na_V1.7$ cDNA (Klugbauer et al., 1995) to identify sequence variation. Sequencing was performed at the Howard Hughes Medical Institute/Keck Biotechnology Center at Yale University. Sequence analysis used BLAST (National Library of Medicine) and Lasergene (DNAStar, Madison, WI).

Voltage-Clamp Analysis

The plasmid carrying the TTX-R version of human $Na_V1.7$ cDNA ($hNa_V1.7_R$) was described previously (Herzog et al., 2003). The F1449V mutation was introduced into $hNa_V1.7_R$ using QuickChange XL site-directed mutagenesis (Stratagene, La Jolla, CA). Wild-type or F1449V mutant $hNa_V1.7_R$ channels were co-transfected with the human b1 and b2 subunits (Lossin et al., 2002) into HEK293 cells, grown under standard culture conditions (5% CO_2, 37°C) in Dulbecco's modified Eagle's medium supplemented with 10% fetal bovine serum, by calcium phosphate precipitation (Cummins et al., 2004).

Whole-cell patch-clamp recordings were conducted at room temperature (~21°C), 40–72 h after transfection using an EPC-10 amplifier and Pulse 8.5 (HEKA, Germany) with 0.8–1.5 MΩ electrodes (access resistance 1.6±0.3 MΩ). Voltage errors were minimized using 80% series resistance compensation and linear leak subtraction; capacitance artifact was canceled using computer-controlled circuitry. Recordings were started 3.5 min after establishing whole-cell configuration. The pipette solution contained: 140 mM CsF, 1 mM EGTA, 10 mM NaCl and 10 mM HEPES (pH 7.3). The bathing solution was 140 mM NaCl, 3 mM KCl, 1 mM $MgCl_2$, 1 mM $CaCl_2$ and 10 mM HEPES (pH 7.3). Data were analyzed using Pulsefit (HEKA) and Origin (Microcal, Northampton, MA) software.

Transfection of DRG Neurons and Current-Clamp Recordings

DRG from wild-type C57/BL6 mice were treated (Rizzo et al., 1994) to obtain neurons for electroporation of sodium channel and green fluorescent protein (GFP)

constructs (Amaxa Inc., Gaithersburg, MD; see on-line Supplementary material available at *Brain* Online). Current-clamp recordings were obtained 16–24 h post-transfection. Whole-cell current-clamp recordings from small diameter DRG neurons (<30 mm) with robust GFP fluorescence were obtained at room temperature (~21°C) following transfection with either wild-type $hNa_V1.7_R$–GFP or F1449V–GFP using an Axopatch 200B amplifier (Axon Instruments, Union City, CA). Micropipettes with resistances from 1 to 2.5 MΩ were filled with a solution of 140 mM KCl, 0.5 mM EGTA, 5 mM HEPES, 3 mM Mg-ATP and 3 mM Na-GTP, pH 7.3, adjusted to 315 mOsm/l with glucose. The external solution contained 140 mM NaCl, 3 mM KCl, 2 mM $MgCl_2$, 2 mM $CaCl_2$, 10 mM HEPES, pH 7.3, adjusted to 320 mOsm/l with glucose. The pipette potential was adjusted to zero before seal formation; liquid junction potentials were not corrected. Capacity transients were canceled before switching to current-clamp mode, and series resistance (~3–6 MΩ) was compensated by ~70%. Traces were acquired from cells with stable resting potentials less than –40 mV using Clampex 8.1 software, filtered at 5 kHz and sampled at 20 kHz. When required, steady polarizing currents were applied to set a holding potential of –60 mV.

Results

Clinical Description

The pedigree of this family contains 36 members (figure 1); 16 subjects with the erythromelalgia phenotype (mean age 37 years; range 3–75) were clinically evaluated (10 women, six men). Mean age of onset of symptoms was 3 years; four patients had onset in infancy, and all had onset of symptoms by their sixth birthday. All subjects experienced symptoms typical of erythromelalgia (Drenth and Michiels, 1994), with attacks of burning pain and erythema involving both surfaces of the hands, and feet up to or slightly proximal to the ankles. Ten subjects (63%) reported involvement of other areas, including face, ears, elbows and knees; one reported involvement of the vaginal area. Eleven (69%) reported attacks one or more times per day; three (19%) reported several attacks per month. All subjects but one (94%) reported that attacks are triggered by heat and improved by cold, although one reported that extreme cold can also trigger attacks.

Mutation in Exon 23

Genomic DNA from the proband and control subjects was isolated from venous blood samples and used as template to amplify all known exons of *SCN9A* and compare the sequence with Na$_V$1.7 cDNA (Klugbauer et al., 1995). Proband and control templates produced similar amplicons which were purified and sequenced. Sequence analysis identified a T-to-G transversion in exon 23 (E23), corresponding to position 4393 of the reference sequence (see Supplementary material). This mutation substitutes phenylalanine (F) by valine (V) at position 1449 of the polypeptide, located at the N-terminus of loop 3 which joins domains III and IV. F1449 is invariant in all known mammalian sodium channels (figure 2). Restriction digestion analysis (see Supplementary material) confirmed the presence of the F1449V mutation in 17 out of 17 affected individuals, and its absence in five out of five unaffected family members, three out of three unaffected spouses and 100 ethnically matched control chromosomes. Segregation of the T4393G mutation with disease was confirmed by DNA sequencing of E23 in all family members.

Voltage-Clamp Analysis

Wild-type hNa$_V$1.7$_R$ and the mutant channel F1449V were transiently expressed along with β1 and β2 subunits (Lossin et al., 2002) in HEK293 cells (figure 3A), where Na$_V$1.7 displays biophysical properties (Cummins et al., 1998) similar to those in DRG neurons (Herzog et al., 2003). We examined the voltage dependence of activation using depolarizing test pulses from −100 mV. Mutant channels activated at potentials 5–10 mV more negative than wild-type channels (figure 3B). The midpoint of activation for F1449V (estimated by fitting with a Boltzmann function) was significantly shifted to -22.8 ± 1.3 mV ($n = 12$) compared with wild-type currents (-15.2 ± 1.3 mV, $n = 11$; $P < 0.05$), a smaller shift than for the previously described Na$_V$1.7 mutations (Cummins et al., 2004). The time course of activation, estimated using a Hodgkin–Huxley fit of currents elicited with a step depolarization to −20 mV, was not significantly different for wild-type ($\tau = 482 \pm 25$ μs) and F1449V channels ($\tau = 431 \pm 17$ μs). Deactivation kinetics, examined by eliciting tail currents at different potentials after briefly activating the channels (at −20 mV for 0.5 μs), were not altered at potentials ranging from −100 to −40 mV for the F1449V mutant channel (figure 3C), in contrast to the previously described Na$_V$1.7 mutations where deactivation was slower.

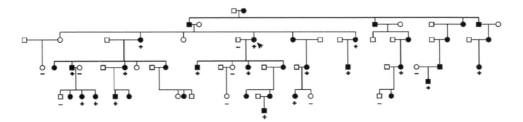

Figure 1
Family pedigree. Circles denote females; squares denote males. The proband is shown by an arrow. Blackened symbols indicate subjects affected with erythromelalgia. (+) denotes subjects heterozygous for the T4393G mutation; (−) denotes subjects without the mutation.

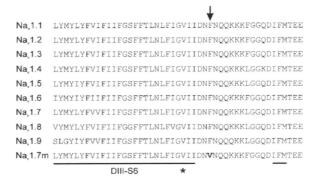

Figure 2
F1449 (arrow) is conserved within loop 3 in all known sodium channels. The lower line delineates the sequence of transmembrane segment S6 of domain III and the N-terminal half of L3 for $Na_V1.1$–$Na_V1.9$, together with the F1449V mutation ($Na_V1.7$ m). The asterisk denotes the position of V1293 which is replaced with isoleucine (I) in the skeletal muscle disorder paramyotonia congenita (Green et al., 1998). The fast inactivation tripeptide IFM is underlined.

Steady-state fast inactivation of F1449V channels (figure 4A) was shifted slightly in the depolarizing direction. The $V_{1/2}$ measured with 500 ms pre-pulses was -71.3 ± 0.8 mV for wild-type ($n=16$) and -67.0 ± 1.4 mV for F1449V ($n=16$; $P<0.05$) channels. Voltage dependence of steady-state slow inactivation was shifted in the negative direction by the F1449V mutation (figure 4B).

The time constants for open state inactivation (figure 4C) were smaller for F1449V than for wild-type currents over the entire voltage range from -50 to $+40$ mV. At -10 mV, wild-type currents inactivated with a $\tau=1.4 \pm 0.1$ ms ($n=7$) and F1449V currents inactivated with a significantly smaller ($P<0.05$) $\tau=1.0 \pm 0.2$ ms ($n=8$). Development of closed state inactivation was faster for F1449V channels, with significantly smaller ($P<0.05$) time constants for inactivation at -80, -70 and -60 mV (figure 4D). Repriming (recovery from fast inactivation) was significantly faster ($P<0.05$) for F1449V channels than for wild-type channels (figure 5A). The time constant for repriming of wild-type channels ($\tau=89 \pm 14$ ms, $n=8$) was 3-fold larger at -70 mV than for F1449V channels ($\tau=27 \pm 2$ ms, $n=8$).

Ramp currents (figure 5B), elicited with slow (0.2 mV/ms) depolarizations from -100 to $+20$ mV, were not different for F1449V channels ($0.4 \pm 0.1\%$; $n=7$) and wild-type channels ($0.4 \pm 0.1\%$; $n=12$). In contrast, the I848T and L858H $hNa_V1.7$ erythromelalgia mutations elicited significantly larger ramp currents compared with wild-type channels (Cummins et al., 2004).

Current-Clamp Analysis

Reasoning that changes in voltage dependence could lower the firing threshold, we expressed wild-type or F1449V channels in small (<30 μm) DRG neurons which include nociceptors. Resting potential was similar ($P>0.05$) in DRG neurons transfected with F1449V (-51.3 ± 1.6 mV; $n=19$) and with wild type (-49.0 ± 1.3 mV; $n=16$). To eliminate cell-to-cell variations, cells were held at -60 mV.

$Na_V1.7$ is important in early phases of electrogenesis in DRG neurons, producing graded depolarizations which may boost subthreshold inputs (Cummins et al., 1998) to bring DRG neurons to voltages at which $Na_V1.8$ [which has a more depolarized activation threshold (Akopian et al., 1996)] opens to produce all-or-none action

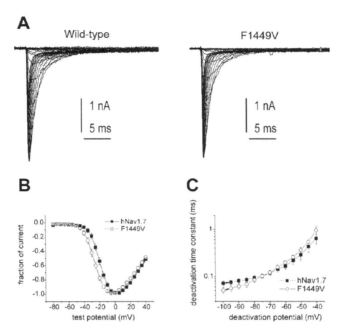

Figure 3
The F1449V mutation alters activation but not deactivation of hNa$_V$1.7. (A) Current traces recorded from representative HEK293 cells expressing either wild-type (left) or F1449V (right) channels. Cells were held at −100 mV and currents elicited with 50 ms test pulses to −80 to +40 mV. (B) Normalized peak current–voltage relationship for wild-type (filled squares, $n=11$) and F1449V (open circles, $n=12$) channels. (C) Time constants for tail current deactivation at repolarization potentials from −40 to −100 mV for wild-type (filled squares, $n=8$) and F1449V (open circles, $n=7$) channels. Time constants were obtained with single exponential fits. Error bars show standard errors.

potentials (Renganathan et al., 2001). Figure 6A, B and E shows the effect of the F1449V mutation on the firing threshold. Figure 6A shows traces from a representative DRG neuron expressing wild-type hNa$_V$1.7. Subthreshold responses, which depolarized the cell slightly but not to −19 mV where an action potential is triggered, were elicited with 50–65 pA current injections. All-or-none action potentials required stimuli of >130 pA (current threshold for this neuron). In contrast, figure 6B shows responses from a representative DRG neuron expressing F1449V, where action potentials were produced at a lower current threshold of 60 pA. Current threshold (current required to generate an all-or-

none action potential) was significantly reduced ($P<0.05$) following expression of F1449V (93.1±12.0 pA; $n=19$) compared with wild-type (124.1±7.4 pA; $n=16$) (figure 6E). However, the voltage at which takeoff occurs for an all-or-none action potential was not significantly different ($P>0.5$) in cells expressing wild-type (−21.4±0.9 mV; $n=16$) or F1449V channels (−22.5±1.4 mV; $n=19$).

Similarly to native small DRG neurons, ~50% of which fire repetitively in response to prolonged stimuli (Renganathan et al., 2001), the majority of neurons expressing wild-type Na$_V$1.7 (11 out of 16; 69%) or the F1449V channel (12 out of 19; 63%) can fire repetitively (figure 6C and

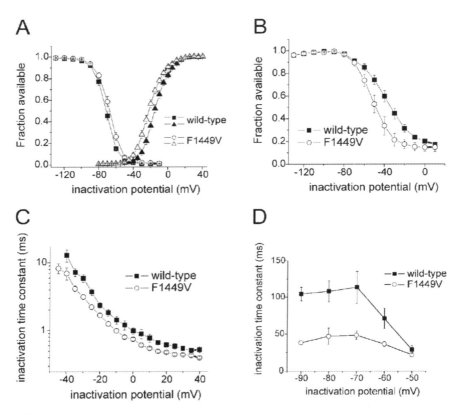

Figure 4

The F1449V mutation differentially alters fast and slow inactivation of hNa$_V$1.7. (A) Comparison of steady-state fast inactivation for wild-type (filled squares, $n=13$) and F1449V (open circles, $n=14$) channels. Currents were elicited with test pulses to 0 mV following 500 ms inactivating pre-pulses. The voltage dependence of activation, derived by fitting Boltzmann functions to the data shown in figure 3, is shown for wild-type (closed triangles) and F1449V (open triangles). (B) Comparison of steady-state slow inactivation for wild-type (filled squares, $n=4$) and F1449V (open circles, $n=4$) channels. Slow inactivation was induced with 30 s pre-pulses, followed by 100 ms pulses to −120 mV to allow recovery from fast inactivation. A 20 ms test pulse to 0 mV was used to determine the fraction of current available. (C) Fast inactivation kinetics as a function of voltage for wild-type (filled squares, $n=7$) and F1449V (open circles, $n=8$) channels. The decay phases of currents elicited as described in figure 3A were fitted with single exponentials to estimate open state inactivation time constants. (D) Time constants for development of closed state inactivation were estimated from single exponential fits to time courses measured at inactivation potentials from −90 to −50 mV for wild-type (filled squares, $n=6$) and F1449V channels (open circles, right; $n=9$), by holding cells at −100 mV, pre-pulsing to the inactivation potential for increasing durations, then stepping to 0 mV to determine the fraction of current inactivated during the pre-pulse. Development of closed state inactivation for F1449V currents is faster than for wild-type currents.

A

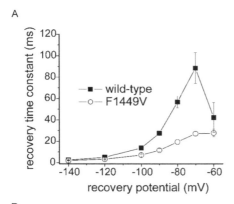

B

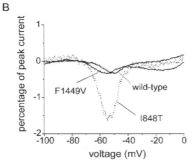

Figure 5
Recovery from inactivation kinetics is faster for F1449V
mutant channels than for wild-type channels. (A) Time
constants for recovery from inactivation of wild-type
(filled squares, $n=8$) and F1449V (open circles, $n=8$)
currents are shown as a function of voltage. Time constants
were estimated from single exponential fits to time courses
measured at recovery potentials from −140 to −60 mV, by
pre-pulsing the cell to +20 mV for 20 ms to inactivate all
of the current, then stepping back to the recovery potential
for increasing recovery durations prior to the test pulse
to 0 mV. The maximum pulse rate was 0.5 Hz. (B)
Representative ramp currents, elicited with 500 ms ramp
depolarizations from −100 to 0 mV for wild-type and
mutant F1449V. The increase in ramp current amplitude,
seen for the previously described I848T mutation
(Cummins et al., 2004), is not observed.

D). Figure 6C shows the firing of a representative neuron expressing wild-type channels, which
responded to a 950 ms stimulation of 150 pA
with two action potentials. In contrast, a neuron
expressing F1449V responds to an identical
150 pA depolarizing stimulus with high frequency
firing (figure 6D). The firing frequency evoked
with 100 pA current injections was increased
from 1.24±0.58 Hz ($n=11$) for wild-type to
5.34±1.21 Hz ($n=12$; $P<0.01$) for F1449V channels. Current injection of 150 pA evoked firing
at 3.03±0.75 Hz ($n=9$) following expression of
wild-type and 6.48±1.41 Hz ($n=12$; $P<0.05$)
following expression of F1449V channels (figure
6F). Thus, in addition to a lower current threshold for action potentials, the frequency of firing
at graded stimulus intensities was higher for cells
expressing F1449V.

Discussion

This study demonstrates, in a large family with
primary erythromelalgia, a single substitution
of phenylalanine by valine (F1449V) at codon
1449 in the sodium channel Na$_V$1.7. This single
amino acid substitution alters the biophysical
properties of hNa$_V$1.7 and reduces the threshold
for action potential firing and bursting of DRG
neurons. F1449 is located within L3, the cytoplasmic loop which joins domains III and IV,
11 amino acid residues N-terminal to the fast
inactivation IFM (isoleucine–phenylalanine–
methionine) motif (West et al., 1992). F1449V
substitution produces an ~8 mV hyperpolarizing
shift in voltage dependence of activation, smaller
than the 13–15 mV shifts in the previously
described I848T and L858H hNa$_V$1.7 erythromelalgia mutations (Cummins et al., 2004). F1449V
substitution also produces an ~4 mV depolarizing shift in fast inactivation, which is expected
to increase the fraction of channels available for
activation close to resting potential. Increased
overlap between activation and steady-state
inactivation for F1449V channels also increases

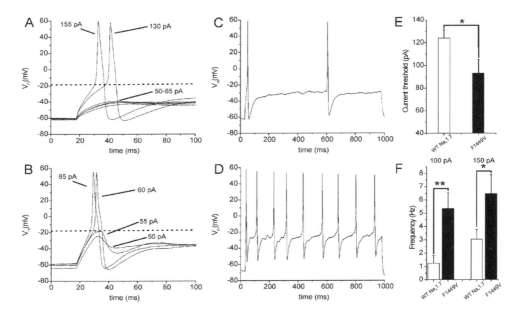

Figure 6

F1449V, expressed in small DRG neurons, lowers the current threshold for action potential generation and repetitive firing. Action potentials were evoked using depolarizing current injections from a membrane potential of –60 mV. (A) Representative traces from a cell expressing wild-type $Na_V1.7$, showing subthreshold responses to 50–65 pA current injections and subsequent all-or-none action potentials evoked by injections of 130 pA (current threshold for this neuron) and 155 pA. (B) In contrast, in a cell expressing F1449V, action potentials were evoked by a 60 pA current injection, demonstrating a lower current threshold for action potential generation. The voltage for takeoff of the all-or-none action potential (dotted line) was similar for the neurons in (A) and (B). (C and D) The frequency of firing at graded stimulus intensities was higher for cells expressing F1449V mutant channels than with wild-type channels. (C) The firing of a neuron expressing $hNa_V1.7$ (same neuron as in A), which responded to a 950 ms stimulation of 150 pA with two action potentials. In contrast, D shows that, in a neuron expressing the mutant channel F1449V (same cell as in B), an identical 150 pA depolarizing stimulus evoked high frequency firing. (E) There is a significant (*$P<0.05$) reduction in current threshold in cells expressing F1449V ($n=19$) compared with cells expressing wild-type $Na_V1.7$ ($n=16$). (F) There is a significant increase in the frequency of firing in response to 100 and 150 pA stimuli (950 ms) following expression of F1449V ($n=12$), in comparison with wild-type $Na_V1.7$ ($n=11, 9$) (**$P<0.01$; *$P<0.05$).

the predicted window current. These changes each would be expected to lower the threshold of nociceptive DRG neurons which express mutant channels. Current-clamp recordings demonstrated, in fact, a lower threshold for single action potentials and high frequency firing in response to graded stimuli in DRG neurons expressing the mutant channel.

The F1449V mutation also changed some $hNa_V1.7$ properties in ways that might decrease excitability, by enhancing slow inactivation and the rate of closed state inactivation. Because slow closed state inactivation promotes larger ramp currents, F1449V substitution would be expected to attenuate ramp currents. Indeed, in contrast to the I848T and L858H $hNa_V1.7$ erythromelalgia mutations which increased ramp currents

(Cummins et al., 2004), F1449V did not alter ramp currents compared with wild-type channels.

Domain III/S6 and the III–IV linker sequences are highly conserved among the known sodium channels. This region is crucial to fast inactivation (Patton et al., 1992), and has been implicated in other inherited disorders of excitability. Several mutations in the skeletal muscle sodium channel (Na$_V$1.4) that underlie myotonic disorders are located in this region. The Na$_V$1.4 V1293I mutation, at a position corresponding to V1444 in hNa$_V$1.7, five amino acids N-terminal to F1449, causes a mild variant of paramyotonia congenita. The functional consequences of the V1293I mutation in hNa$_V$1.4 (Green et al., 1998) are similar to those of F1449V substitution in hNa$_V$1.7. Both mutations shift activation in a hyperpolarizing direction and inactivation in a depolarizing direction, and accelerate recovery from inactivation. In a model of muscle excitability, V1293I substitution lowered the threshold for action potential generation and caused myotonia; the −6 mV shift in activation was the major factor leading to this enhanced excitability (Green et al., 1998). However, myotonia produced by the Na$_V$1.4-V1293I mutation is often precipitated by cold, whereas cooling reduces pain in most erythromelalgia patients with the F1449V mutation.

Current-clamp recordings demonstrated a lower current threshold for single action potentials and higher frequency firing in response to graded stimuli, in DRG neurons expressing mutant F1449V channels. Thus, even though F1449V displays a shift in activation that is relatively modest, deactivation that is not prolonged and ramp currents that are not enhanced in comparison with previously described mutations in Na$_V$1.7 (Cummins et al., 2004), F1449V substitution imparts a gain-of-function change on DRG neurons, consistent with the autosomal dominant inheritance of familial erythromelalgia (Drenth et al., 2001; Yang et al., 2004) and our finding that affected family members are heterozygous for the mutation. Nevertheless, the inflec-

tion in voltage recordings, at which the upstroke of the all-or-none action potentials arose (approximately −20 mV), was essentially the same in neurons expressing wild-type and F1449V channels. This probably reflects the role of Na$_V$1.7 as a 'threshold channel' which activates at more hyperpolarized potentials so as to boost small, slow depolarizing inputs below action potential threshold (Cummins et al., 1998), and the fact that Na$_V$1.8, with a threshold closer to −20 mV (Akopian et al., 1996), generates most of the current underlying the action potential upstroke in DRG neurons (Renganathan et al., 2001; Blair and Bean, 2002).

The present results demonstrate that a sodium channel mutation can reduce the firing threshold and produce abnormal repetitive firing in sensory neurons in an inherited painful syndrome, primary erythromelalgia. Two anecdotal reports describe partial relief from pain in patients with erythromelalgia treated with lidocaine and mexiletine (Kuhnert et al., 1999; Davis and Sandroni, 2002), and a study on four patients reported reduced pain lasting for at least 2 years with oral mexiletine (Legroux-Crespel et al., 2003). Identification of this mutation and its role in the pathophysiology of erythromelalgia suggest that rational treatment with sodium channel blockers may be efficacious in this disorder.

Acknowledgments

We wish to thank R. Blackman, S. Liu and X. Peng for excellent technical assistance, and the family members for participating in this study. This work was supported by the Medical Research Service and Rehabilitation Research Service, Department of Veterans Affairs and by grants from the National Multiple Sclerosis Society, the Erythromelalgia Association, the Paralyzed Veterans of America and the United Spinal Association. F.M.H. was supported by a Paul Beeson Physician Scholar Award (American Federation for Aging Research). T.R.C. was supported by a Biomedical Research Grant from Indiana University School of Medicine.

About the Authors

S. D. Dib-Hajj, Department of Neurology and Center for Neuroscience and Regeneration Research, Yale University School of Medicine, New Haven; Rehabilitation Research Center, VA Connecticut Healthcare System, West Haven, CT

A. M. Rush, Department of Neurology and Center for Neuroscience and Regeneration Research, Yale University School of Medicine, New Haven; Rehabilitation Research Center, VA Connecticut Healthcare System, West Haven, CT

T. R. Cummins, Department of Pharmacology and Toxicology, Stark Neurosciences Institute, Indiana University School of Medicine, Indianapolis, IN

F. M. Hisama, Department of Neurology, Yale University School of Medicine, New Haven

S. Novella, Department of Neurology, Yale University School of Medicine, New Haven

L. Tyrrell, Department of Neurology and Center for Neuroscience and Regeneration Research, Yale University School of Medicine, New Haven; Rehabilitation Research Center, VA Connecticut Healthcare System, West Haven, CT

L. Marshall, Department of Neurology, Yale University School of Medicine, New Haven

S. G. Waxman, Department of Neurology and Center for Neuroscience and Regeneration Research, Yale University School of Medicine, New Haven; Rehabilitation Research Center, VA Connecticut Healthcare System, West Haven, CT

References

Akopian AN, Sivilotti L, Wood JN. 1996. A tetrodotoxin-resistant voltage-gated sodium channel expressed by sensory neurons. *Nature* 379: 257–262.

Black JA, Cummins TR, Dib-Hajj SD, Waxman SG. 2002. Sodium channels and the molecular basis for pain. In: Malemberg AB, Chaplan SR, editors. *Mechanisms and mediators of neuropathic pain.* Basel: Birkhauser Verlag; p. 23–50.

Blair NT, Bean BP. 2002. Roles of tetrodotoxin (TTX)-sensitive Na$^+$ current, TTX-resistant Na$^+$ current, and Ca^{2+} current in the action potentials of nociceptive sensory neurons. *J Neurosci* 22: 10277–10290.

Cummins TR, Howe JR, Waxman SG. 1998. Slow closed-state inactivation: A novel mechanism underlying ramp currents in cells expressing the hNE/PN1 sodium channel. *J Neurosci* 18: 9607–9619.

Cummins TR, Dib-Hajj SD, Waxman SG. 2004. Electro-physiological properties of mutant Nav1.7 sodium channels in a painful inherited neuropathy. *J Neurosci* 24: 8232–8236.

Davis MD, Sandroni P. 2002. Lidocaine patch for pain of erythromelalgia. *Arch Dermatol* 138: 17–19.

Djouhri L, Newton R, Levinson SR, Berry CM, Carruthers B, Lawson SN. 2003. Sensory and electrophysiological properties of guinea-pig sensory neurones expressing Na(v)1.7 (PN1) Na$^+$ channel alphasubunit protein. *J Physiol* 546: 565–576.

Drenth JP, Finley WH, Breedveld GJ, Testers L, Michiels JJ, Guillet G, et al. 2001. The primary erythermalgia-susceptibility gene is located on chromosome 2q31–32. *Am J Hum Genet* 68: 1277–1282.

Drenth JP, Michiels JJ. 1994. Erythromelalgia and erythermalgia: Diagnostic differentiation. *Int J Dermatol* 33: 393–397.

Finley WH, Lindsey JR, Jr, Fine JD, Dixon GA, Burbank MK. 1992. Autosomal dominant erythromelalgia. *Am J Med Genet* 42: 310–315.

Green DS, George AL, Jr, Cannon SC. 1998. Human sodium channel gating defects caused by missense mutations in S6 segments associated with myotonia: S804F and V1293I. *J Physiol* 510: 685–694.

Herzog RI, Cummins TR, Ghassemi F, Dib-Hajj SD, Waxman SG. 2003. Distinct repriming and closed-state inactivation kinetics of Nav1.6 and Nav1.7 sodium channels in mouse spinal sensory neurons. *J Physiol* 551: 741–750.

Klugbauer N, Lacinova L, Flockerzi V, Hofmann F. 1995. Structure and functional expression of a new member of the tetrodotoxin-sensitive voltage-activated sodium channel family from human neuroendocrine cells. *EMBO J* 14: 1084–1090.

Kuhnert SM, Phillips WJ, Davis MD. 1999. Lidocaine and mexiletine therapy for erythromelalgia. *Arch Dermatol* 135: 1447–1449.

Legroux-Crespel E, Sassolas B, Guillet G, Kupfer I, Dupre D, Misery L. 2003. Treatment of familial erythermalgia with the association of lidocaine and mexiletine. *Ann Dermatol Venereol* 130: 429–433.

Lossin C, Wang DW, Rhodes TH, Vanoye CG, George AL, Jr. 2002. Molecular basis of an inherited epilepsy. *Neuron* 34: 877–884.

Patton DE, West JW, Catterall WA, Goldin AL. 1992. Amino acid residues required for fast Na$^+$-channel inactivation: Charge neutralizations and deletions in the III–IV linker. *Proc Natl Acad Sci USA* 89: 10905–10909.

Renganathan M, Cummins TR, Waxman SG. 2001. Contribution of Nav1.8 sodium channels to action potential electrogenesis in DRG neurons. *J Neurophysiol* 86: 629–640.

Rizzo MA, Kocsis JD, Waxman SG. 1994. Slow sodium conductances of dorsal root ganglion neurons: Intraneuronal homogeneity and interneuronal heterogeneity. *J Neurophysiol* 72: 2796–2815.

Sangameswaran L, Fish LM, Koch BD, Rabert DK, Delgado SG, Ilnicka M, et al. 1997. A novel tetrodotoxin-sensitive, voltage-gated sodium channel expressed in rat and human dorsal root ganglia. *J Biol Chem* 272: 14805–14809.

Toledo-Aral JJ, Moss BL, He ZJ, Koszowski AG, Whisenand T, Levinson SR, et al. 1997. Identification of PN1, a predominant voltage-dependent sodium channel expressed principally in peripheral neurons. *Proc Natl Acad Sci USA* 94: 1527–1532.

van Genderen PJ, Michiels JJ, Drenth JP. 1993. Hereditary erythermalgia and acquired erythromelalgia. *Am J Med Genet* 45: 530–532.

Waxman SG, Dib-Hajj S, Cummins TR, Black JA. 1999. Sodium channels and pain. *Proc Natl Acad Sci USA* 96: 7635–7639.

West JW, Patton DE, Scheuer T, Wang Y, Goldin AL, Catterall WA. 1992. A cluster of hydrophobic amino acid residues required for fast Na(+)-channel inactivation. *Proc Natl Acad Sci USA* 89: 10910–10914.

Yang Y, Wang Y, Li S, Xu Z, Li H, Ma L, et al. 2004. Mutations in SCN9A, encoding a sodium channel alpha subunit, in patients with primary erythermalgia. *J Med Genet* 41: 171–174.

4 AVALANCHE

Soon after we published the functional analysis of the first $Na_V1.7$ mutations from patients with erythromelalgia, I was deluged with an avalanche of emails, letters, and telephone calls from around the world. They were from people with chronic pain. Some of these people had erythromelalgia, and some of them had mutations of $Na_V1.7$ that we had not seen before. Here were new clues. But there also were entreaties, requests for help. Especially touching were the enquiries from parents of children in pain. In the beginning, I felt nearly helpless. I was navigating a large, complex sea.

We were looking for rare experiments of nature in which the gene for $Na_V1.7$ had gone awry, with the hope that each new genetic mistake would teach us something new. To do this, we established a network of physicians and scientists not only in North America, but also in Europe and Asia, who helped us to sift out, from an overall population of more than two billion, the most instructive cases. Investigation of each new patient took a long time, and we needed to prioritize so that we could focus on the ones we could learn from. The work-up for each mutation required months of work by teams of scientists that moved like clockwork within my laboratory. Sulayman Dib-Hajj led a team of molecular biologists that carefully re-created, in the laboratory, DNA for each mutation. Then our physiologists went to work. The 2006 paper by Han et al. (Han et al. 2006), for example, described a sporadic de novo mutation that we encountered in a child with normal parents. Undoubtedly, many mutations in $Na_V1.7$ arose in this way rather than being inherited from parents.

As researchers working in a competitive arena, my team was used to working at a "let's be first" pace. We weren't quite frenzied but, until we had completed our analysis of the first four or five mutations, we moved forward in "hurry-up" mode. Each mutation taught us something new. In 2006 our analysis of the S241T mutation taught us that the size of the substituted residue was important in determining pathogenicity of the mutation (Lampert et al. 2006). Soon after that, molecular modeling gave us a picture of the ring of four amino acids, at the cytoplasmic mouth of the channel pore, that act as a gate, stabilizing the channel in the closed state (Lampert et al. 2008). Mutations described in our papers by Cheng et al. (2008) and Han et al. (2009) taught us that the magnitude of the change in channel function caused by the mutation plays a role in determining the age of onset of pain—mutations that produced large hyperpolarizations of activation caused pain beginning in infancy, while mutations that produced smaller shifts in activation caused pain with a later onset. We found two mutations that not only cause inherited erythromelalgia, but also sensitize the $Na_V1.7$ channel to particular drugs (Choi et al. 2009; Fischer et al. 2009), a finding that pointed us toward development of personalized, genomically guided pharmacotherapy for pain (Yang et al. 2012). In 2011 we discovered a mutation which causes erythromelalgia not by substituting an incorrect amino acid for the correct one, but by deleting an amino acid (Cheng et al. 2011). We also learned that there are polymorphisms, or minor misweaves, in the gene for $Na_V1.7$ that, while not causing disease within themselves, impose increased risk for developing neuropathic pain after nerve injury (Estacion et al. 2009). Each gene variant showed us something about the disease or the channel. And, as we looked at the entire group of mutations, there was another, broader observation: In all of these cases, hyperactive $Na_V1.7$ channels caused pain but did not cause epileptic seizures, an observation that reinforced our notion of a major functional role of Na$_V$1.7 in peripheral nerves, but not in the brain.

Following our description of Na$_V$1.7 gain-of-function mutations in inherited erythromelalgia, a research group at University College London described another set of gain-of-function mutations of Na$_V$1.7 that cause a second, distinct clinical disorder, paroxysmal extreme pain disorder (PEPD) (Fertleman et al. 2006). PEPD, which had previously been called familial rectal pain disorder (Fertleman et al. 2007), presents with a clinical picture very different than that from inherited erythromelalgia. These mutations were unique in that they tended to cause disease, not by enhancing activation, but by impairing the process of channel inactivation which prevents channels from operating for a brief period after stimulation. Impaired inactivation makes more channels available for operation. In patients with PEPD, lower body stimulation, particularly stimulation close to the rectum, triggers excruciating rectal pain which, later in life, migrates to the area around the eyes and jaw. The reason for this peculiar pattern of pain is not known, but, importantly, patients with PEPD usually respond well to treatment with the sodium channel blocker carbamazepine, making the diagnosis clinically important.

We also learned that, while inherited erythromelalgia and PEPD each present striking and very different clinical features, they are part of a continuum. In 2008, we described a patient with an "overlap" syndrome and clinical features of both disorders (Estacion et al. 2008). The Na$_V$1.7 mutation in this patient had multiple effects on the function of the channel, including the enhanced activation characteristic of erythromelalgia mutations and the impaired inactivation usually seen with PEPD mutations. We subsequently described several additional mutations which caused atypical forms of erythromelalgia.

Inherited erythromelalgia and PEPD represented graphic examples of "gain-of-function mutations," with heightened function of the mutation resulting in excruciating pain. In 2006, patients with "loss-of-function" mutations of Na$_V$1.7 and "channelopathy-associated insensitivity to pain" were found. These patients failed to make functional Na$_V$1.7 channels. The affected individuals felt no pain. The first patient described was a teenager, from tribal Pakistan, who helped to support his family with "street performances" in which he would injure himself by putting blades through his limbs or walking on hot coals, feeling no pain. His family carried a mutation that impaired their ability to produce Na$_V$1.7 channels. This family was replete with individuals who had experienced painless fractures, painless burns, painless tooth extractions, and painless childbirth (Cox et al. 2006). Other, similar families were soon identified, each family carrying a "null" mutation so that they did not produce functional Na$_V$1.7 channels (Ahmad et al. 2007; Goldberg et al. 2007). What was remarkable about these families was not that there was a diminished sense of pain, but rather that they did not feel *any* pain.

These "human knock-out" mutations reminded us that, in the absence of pain, people do not learn to protect themselves by limiting their activities in the way most of us do. Individuals lacking Na$_V$1.7, with channelopathy-associated insensitivity to pain, will continue to play a game of soccer, for example, after sustaining a fracture, and accumulate multiple unhealed injuries. Na$_V$1.7 was known to be present in olfactory sensory neurons which are essential for our sense of smell, and, consistent with this, anosmia—loss of the sense of smell—was also observed in these loss-of-function patients. Aside from this, as would be predicted for a channel that does not play a major role within the brain, people with channelopathy-associated insensitivity to pain showed no other signs of brain dysfunction.

By 2006, just two years after the first Na$_V$1.7 mutations were found, we had been able to move from gene, to altered channel protein, to pain-signaling DRG neurons that scream when they should be silent. We knew that gain-of-function mutations of Na$_V$1.7 produce hyperexcitability of DRG neurons that causes excruciating pain. And we knew by 2006 that loss-of-function of Na$_V$1.7 produces inability to sense pain. We were in the unusual situation of understanding Na$_V$1.7 through both gain-of-function and loss-of-function.

References

Ahmad S, Dahllund L, Eriksson AB, Hellgren D, Karlsson U, Lund PE, Meijer IA, et al. 2007. A stop codon mutation in SCN9A causes lack of pain sensation. *Hum Mol Genet* 16(17): 2114–2121.

Cheng X, Dib-Hajj SD, Tyrrell L, Te Morsche RH, Drenth JP, Waxman SG. 2011. Deletion mutation of sodium channel Na(V)1.7 in inherited erythromelalgia: Enhanced slow inactivation modulates dorsal root ganglion neuron hyperexcitability. *Brain* 134(Pt 7): 1972–1986.

Cheng X, Dib-Hajj SD, Tyrrell L, Waxman SG. 2008. Mutation I136V alters electrophysiological properties of the Na$_V$1.7 channel in a family with erythromelalgia with onset in the second decade. *Mol Pain* 4: 1.

Choi JS, Zhang L, Dib-Hajj SD, Han C, Tyrrell L, Lin Z, Wang X, Yang Y, Waxman SG. 2009. Mexiletine-responsive erythromelalgia due to a new Na(v)1.7 mutation showing use-dependent current fall-off. *Exp Neurol* 216(2): 383–389.

Cox JJ, Reimann F, Nicholas AK, Thornton G, Roberts E, Springell K, Karbani G, et al. 2006. An SCN9A channelopathy causes congenital inability to experience pain. *Nature* 444(7121): 894–898.

Estacion M, Dib-Hajj SD, Benke PJ, Te Morsche RH, Eastman EM, Macala LJ, Drenth JP, Waxman SG. 2008. Na$_V$1.7 gain-of-function mutations as a continuum: A1632E displays physiological changes associated with erythromelalgia and paroxysmal extreme pain disorder mutations and produces symptoms of both disorders. *J Neurosci* 28(43): 11079–11088.

Estacion M, Harty TP, Choi JS, Tyrrell L, Dib-Hajj SD, Waxman SG. 2009. A sodium channel gene SCN9A polymorphism that increases nociceptor excitability. *Ann Neurol* 66(6): 862–866.

Fertleman CR, Baker MD, Parker KA, Moffatt S, Elmslie FV, Abrahamsen B, Ostman J, Klugbauer N, Wood JN, Gardiner RM, Rees M. 2006. SCN9A mutations in paroxysmal extreme pain disorder: Allelic variants underlie distinct channel defects and phenotypes. *Neuron* 52(5): 767–774.

Fertleman CR, Ferrie CD, Aicardi J, Bednarek NA, Eeg-Olofsson O, Elmslie FV, Griesemer DA, et al. 2007. Paroxysmal extreme pain disorder (previously familial rectal pain syndrome). *Neurology* 69(6): 586–595.

Fischer TZ, Gilmore ES, Estacion M, Eastman E, Taylor S, Melanson M, Dib-Hajj SD, Waxman SG. 2009. A novel Na$_V$1.7 mutation producing carbamazepine-responsive erythromelalgia. *Ann Neurol* 65(6): 733–741.

Goldberg YP, MacFarlane J, MacDonald ML, Thompson J, Dube MP, Mattice M, Fraser R, et al. 2007. Loss-of-function mutations in the Nav1.7 gene underlie congenital indifference to pain in multiple human populations. *Clin Genet* 71(4): 311–319.

Han C, Rush AM, Dib-Hajj SD, Li S, Xu Z, Wang Y, Tyrrell L, Wang X, Yang Y, Waxman SG. 2006. Sporadic onset of erythermalgia: A gain-of-function mutation in Nav1.7. *Ann Neurol* 59(3): 553–558.

Han C, Dib-Hajj SD, Lin Z, Li Y, Eastman EM, Tyrrell L, Cao X, Yang Y, Waxman SG. 2009. Early- and late-onset erythromelalgia: Genotype-phenotype correlation. *Brain* 132(Pt 7): 1711–1722.

Lampert A, Dib-Hajj SD, Tyrrell L, Waxman SG. 2006. Size matters: Erythromelalgia mutation S241T in Na$_V$1.7 alters channel gating. *J Biol Chem* 281(47): 36029–36035.

Lampert A, O'Reilly AO, Dib-Hajj SD, Tyrrell L, Wallace BA, Waxman SG. 2008. A pore-blocking hydrophobic motif at the cytoplasmic aperture of the closed-state Na$_V$1.7 channel is disrupted by the erythromelalgia-associated F1449V mutation. *J Biol Chem* 283(35): 24118–24127.

Yang Y, Dib-Hajj SD, Zhang J, Zhang Y, Tyrrell L, Estacion M, Waxman SG. 2012. Structural modelling and mutant cycle analysis predict pharmacoresponsiveness of a Na(v)1.7 mutant channel. *Nat Commun* 3: 1186.

THE Na$_V$1.7 SODIUM CHANNEL: FROM MOLECULE TO MAN*

Sulayman D. Dib-Hajj, Yang Yang, Joel A. Black, and Stephen G. Waxman

The voltage-gated sodium channel Na$_V$1.7 is preferentially expressed in peripheral somatic and visceral sensory neurons, olfactory sensory neurons and sympathetic ganglion neurons. Na$_V$1.7 accumulates at nerve fibre endings and amplifies small subthreshold depolarizations, poising it to act as a threshold channel that regulates excitability. Genetic and functional studies have added to the evidence that Na$_V$1.7 is a major contributor to pain signalling in humans, and homology modelling based on crystal structures of ion channels suggests an atomic-level structural basis for the altered gating of mutant Na$_V$1.7 that causes pain.

Voltage-gated sodium channels are essential for electrogenesis in excitable cells. Nine pore-forming α-subunits of such channels (referred to as channels hereinafter), Na$_V$1.1–Na$_V$1.9, have been identified in mammals.[1] These isoforms share a common overall structural motif (figure 1). They are each composed of a long polypeptide (1,700–2,000 amino acids) that folds into four homologous domains (DI–DIV) that are linked by three loops (L1–L3), with each domain having six transmembrane segments (S1–S6).[2] The recent determination of the crystal structure of the homotetrameric bacterial sodium channel[3] has provided insights into the atomic structure of mammalian sodium channels and the interactions between the voltage-sensing domain (VSD; encompassing S1–S4) and the pore module (PM; S5–S6) within each of the four homologous domains. Genetic, structural and functional studies have shown that Na$_V$1.7 regulates sensory neuron excitability and is a major contributor to

several sensory modalities, and have established the contribution of this sodium channel isoform to human pain disorders (figure 1).

The nine sodium channel isoforms display different kinetics and voltage-dependent properties.[1] Their differential deployment in different types of neurons endows these cells with distinct firing properties. Sodium channels associate with multiple protein partners that regulate channel trafficking and gating,[4–7] allowing sodium channel properties to be modulated in a cell-type-specific manner (for examples, see refs. 8–10), highlighting the need to study these channels within their native neuronal background whenever practicable. For example, the pathogenic G616R variant of Na$_V$1.7 displays gating abnormalities within dorsal root ganglion (DRG) neurons that are not seen when these channels are expressed in HEK 293 cells.[11] Methods are now available that allow the expression and functional profiling of sodium channels in peripheral neurons, which more closely mimic the *in vivo* environment of such channels.[12]

In humans, gain-of-function mutations in *SCN9A*, which encodes Na$_V$1.7, lead to severe **neuropathic pain**, whereas loss-of-function mutations in this gene lead to an indifference to pain.[13] Studies involving animal injury models and functional studies of neuronal excitability following expression of human mutant Na$_V$1.7 have provided mechanistic insights into the role of this channel in the pathophysiology of pain. Additional studies have linked NA$_V$1.7 to other sensory modalities, including olfaction,[14,15] the afferent limb of the cough reflex[16] and acid sensing.[17]

* Previously published in *Nature Reviews Neuroscience* 14(1): 49–62, 2013. © 2013 Macmillan Publishers Limited.

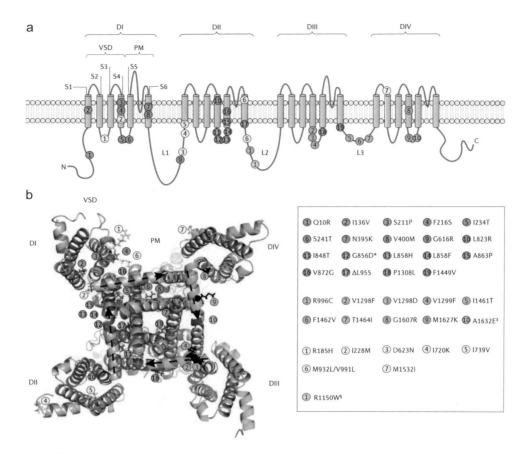

Figure 1

Domain structure of Na$_V$1.7 and locations of characterized mutations in Na$_V$1.7-related pain disorders. (a) The sodium channel α-subunit is a long polypeptide that folds into four homologous domains (DI–DIV), each of which consists of six transmembrane segments (S1–S6). The four domains are joined by three loops (L1–L3). Within each domain, S1–S4 comprise the voltage-sensing domain (VSD; S4, depicted in green, characteristically contains positively charged arginine and lysine residues), and S5–S6 and their extracellular linker comprise the pore module (PM). The linear schematic of the full-length channel shows the locations of amino acids affected by the gain-of-function *SCN9A* mutations that are linked to inherited erythromelalgia (IEM; red symbols), paroxysmal extreme pain disorder (PEPD; grey symbols), and small-fibre neuropathy (SFN; yellow symbols). (b) View of the folded Na$_V$1.7 from the intracellular side of the membrane based on the recently determined crystal structure of a bacterial sodium channel.[3] The structure shows the central ion-conducting PM and four peripheral VSDs. Conformational changes in the VSDs in response to membrane depolarization are transmitted to the PMs through the S4–S5 linkers (identified by arrows through the helices). Mutations that seem distant from each other on the linear model can in fact be in close proximity to each other in the more biologically relevant folded structure. *The patient with this mutation showed symptoms common to IEM and SFN. ‡The patient carrying this mutation showed symptoms and channel properties common to both IEM and PEPD. §This substitution is encoded by a polymorphism that was present in approximately 30% of ethnically matched Caucasian individuals of European descent in a control population.[81] Part a is modified, with permission, from ref. 37 © (2007) Elsevier Science.

In this Review, we discuss functional and modeling studies of Na$_V$1.7 that have yielded new insights into the structure–function relationship of gating mechanisms in this channel and its contribution to neuronal responses under normal and pathological conditions. We also explore strategies for targeting Na$_V$1.7 in the treatment of pain and, finally, identify unanswered questions regarding the role of Na$_V$1.7 in pain signaling.

Cellular and Subcellular Distribution

Three sodium channels—Na$_V$1.7, Na$_V$1.8 and Na$_V$1.9—are preferentially expressed in peripheral neurons. Na$_V$1.7 expression was first detected in somatosensory and sympathetic ganglion neurons,[18] and has since been reported in myenteric neurons,[19] olfactory sensory neurons (OSNs),[14,15] visceral sensory neurons[16,20] and smooth myocytes.[21–23] Na$_V$1.7 is expressed in both large and small diameter DRG neurons (figure 2), including functionally identified Aβ-fibres and C-fibres.[24] Na$_V$1.7 is also the predominant sodium channel isoform present in OSNs[14,15] (box 1) and in nodose ganglion neurons.[16] Measurable Na$_V$1.7 levels have not been detected in the CNS[18,25] (but see the discussion below on the purported role of Na$_V$1.7 in epilepsy). Na$_V$1.7 expression has also been detected within some non-excitable cells, including prostate and breast tumor cells,[26,27] human erythroid progenitor cells[28] and immune cells.[29] Na$_V$1.7 and Na$_V$1.8 are both expressed at relatively high levels within functionally identified nociceptive neurons (**nociceptors**),[24,30] in which their co-expression has important functional implications.[10] Last, Na$_V$1.7 is present peripherally within free nerve endings in the epidermis[31] and centrally within superficial lamina of the dorsal horn in the spinal cord.[32] The presence of Na$_V$1.7 at nerve endings (figure 2) is consistent with its proposed role in amplifying weak stimuli.[33]

Box 1
Na$_V$1.7 contributes most of the sodium current in OSNs

Na$_V$1.7 is the predominant sodium channel in olfactory sensory neurons (OSNs).[14,15] Although an elaborate Ca^{2+}-based and Cl$^-$-based signaling amplification system in the OSN cilia can boost odorant receptor potential,[133,134] the abundant expression of Na$_V$1.7 in these cells[14,15] and the ability of Na$_V$1.7 to boost weak depolarizations, support a role for this sodium channel in the initiation of action potential firing along the peripheral olfactory neuraxis. Mouse and rat OSNs produce a tetrodotoxin (TTX)-sensitive current[14,15,135] that is consistent with the predominant expression of Na$_V$1.7 in these cells. Interestingly, the hyperpolarized activation and inactivation properties of this TTX-sensitive current are different from those recorded from Na$_V$1.7 expressed in HEK 293 cells[33,136] or dorsal root ganglion (DRG) neurons,[11,35] and those in native rat DRG neurons.[137–139] Ahn et al.[14] reported identical sequences of the Na$_V$1.7 cDNA in mouse OSN and DRG neuron samples. Together, these data suggest that post-translational modulation of Na$_V$1.7 or interaction with OSN-specific channel partners may lead to altered gating properties of Na$_V$1.7 in OSNs compared with DRG neurons.

Biophysical Properties

Na$_V$1.7 produces a rapidly activating and inactivating, but slowly **repriming** (slow recovery from inactivation), current that is blocked by nanomolar concentrations of tetrodotoxin (TTX).[34] The slow repriming nature of Na$_V$1.7 makes it well-suited for low-frequency firing in C-fibres, but less well-suited to neurons that fire at a high frequency.[33,35] Importantly, Na$_V$1.7 is characterized by slow closed-state inactivation, allowing the channel to produce a substantial

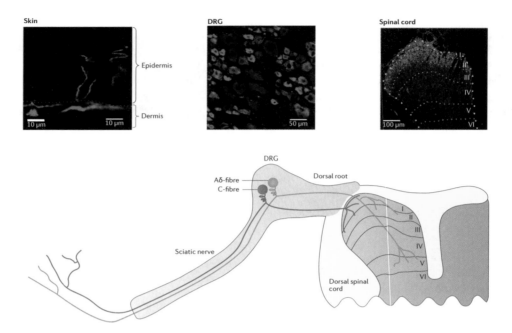

Figure 2

Pain signal transmission from peripheral terminals of DRG neurons that form synapses onto second-order neurons within the spinal cord. Dorsal root ganglion (DRG) neurons can be broadly classified into three types based on their soma size and the state of myelination of their axons: large diameter with heavily myelinated and rapidly conducting axons (Aβ-fibres; not shown here for simplicity); medium diameter with thinly myelinated and intermediate conducting axons (Aδ-fibres; cyan); and small diameter with unmyelinated and slowly conducting axons (C-fibres; red). Five voltage-gated sodium channels are reported to be expressed in DRG neurons,[13] with $Na_V1.7$ expressed in the majority of small unmyelinated neurons and in a notable population of medium and large diameter myelinated neurons (see middle panel; $Na_V1.7$ expression is shown in red in this and other panels). Signals originating from the periphery are initiated by external stimuli (for example, thermal, mechanical or chemical stimuli) or injury- and inflammation-induced mediators (for example, cytokines or trophic factors), and are transduced by specific G protein-coupled receptors or acid- and ligand-gated ion channels at peripheral termini. Membrane depolarizations evoked by the graded receptor potential are integrated by voltage-gated sodium channels; when a threshold is reached, an action potential is initiated at these terminals and centrally propagated. $Na_V1.7$ extends to the peripheral ends of these terminals (left panel) where it amplifies small depolarizing inputs. Although $Na_V1.7$ is considered a peripheral sodium channel because it is expressed in peripheral neurons, it is present in central axonal projections of DRG neurons and their presynaptic terminals within the dorsal horn (right panel) where it may facilitate impulse invasion or evoked release of neurotransmitters that may include substance P, calcitonin-gene related peptide and glutamate.

ramp current in response to small, slow depolarizations.[33,35] The ability of $Na_V1.7$ to boost subthreshold stimuli increases the probability of neurons reaching their threshold for firing action potentials. Thus, $Na_V1.7$ is considered to be a threshold channel.[36,37] $Na_V1.7$ produces resurgent currents in DRG neurons,[38,39] which are triggered by repolarization following a strong depolarization. Resurgent currents support burst firing in, for example, cerebellar Purkinje neurons.[40,41] Production of a resurgent current by a given sodium channel isoform crucially depends on cell background; the same sodium channel that produces a robust resurgent current in one neuronal type may not generate such a current in a different neuronal type.[40–42] Thus, it is not surprising that Na$_V$1.7 produces a resurgent current only in a subset of DRG neurons.

Roles in Multiple Sensory Modalities

Pain

As stated above, Na$_V$1.7 is expressed in both large and small diameter DRG neurons,[13] including 85% of functionally identified nociceptors.[24] These observations, together with its properties as a threshold channel, suggested that Na$_V$1.7 contributes to pain signaling. The recent discovery of gain-of-function *SCN9A* mutations in human pain disorders solidified the status of Na$_V$1.7 as having a central role in pain signaling,[13] and its involvement in pathological pain signaling is discussed below.

Olfaction

The initial discovery that global knockout of *Scn9a* in mice is neonatally lethal, probably because the newborn mice do not feed,[43] and the subsequent discovery that humans with homozygous *SCN9A*-null mutations are anosmic[44,45] suggested that Na$_V$1.7 is important in olfaction. Nassar et al.[43] noted the absence of milk in the stomach of *Scn9a$^{-/-}$* pups. As no hand-feeding was attempted to rescue these mice, the most parsimonious explanation for the observed neonatal lethality is anosmia, leading to a loss in the ability to suckle. In agreement with this observation, Na$_V$1.7 is the predominant sodium channel isoform present in presynaptic OSNs in rodents.[14,15] Knockout of *Scn9a* in OSNs in mice blocks odorant-induced synaptic transmission to mitral cells in the olfactory glomeruli and leads to weight loss in mice,[15] providing compelling evidence that Na$_V$1.7 has a central role in the sense of smell.

Cough Reflex

Two types of coughs involve the vagus nerve: aspiration-induced cough and irritating, itchy urge-to-cough. Aspiration-induced cough is mediated by the stimulation of touch-sensitive Aδ-fibres and occurs even in unconscious subjects, whereas irritating, itchy urge-to-cough is mediated by C-fibre stimulants, including acidic compounds, and occurs only in conscious animals.[46] Nodose ganglion neurons produce both TTX-sensitive and TTX-resistant currents,[47] but action potentials in the vagus nerves of rats or guinea pigs are completely blocked with 1 μM TTX,[16,48] suggesting a crucial role for TTX-sensitive channels in the cough reflex. Recent data suggest that Na$_V$1.7 produces almost all of the TTX-sensitive current in the majority of nodose ganglion neurons in guinea pigs, and adeno-associated virus (AAV)-mediated short hairpin RNA (shRNA) knockdown of Na$_V$1.7 expression in these neurons markedly increases the rheobase and attenuates the firing of both Aδ-fibres and C-fibres.[16] In agreement with this finding, selective knockdown of Na$_V$1.7 expression in nodose ganglion neurons suppresses citric acid-induced coughing in guinea pigs, without having any effect on the rate of aspiration.[16] Whether knocking down Na$_V$1.7 expression has a similar effect on aspiration-induced cough remains untested.

Acid Sensing

Naked mole rats do not develop pain-related behaviors when they are exposed to acid or capsaicin, despite the presence of transient receptor potential vanilloid subfamily member 1 (TRPV1) channels in their nociceptors.[49] This mystery has recently been resolved by the identification of a variant amino acid sequence in the outer vestibule of their Na$_V$1.7 channels.[17] In almost all mammalian orthologs of Na$_V$1.7, the extracellular linker between S5 and S6 in DIV includes a KKV tripeptide sequence. This tripeptide sequence is replaced by EKE in the naked mole rat and by EKD in the microbat, which also lacks acid-induced pain-related behaviors. Interestingly, these two species live in large colonies in which high concentrations of CO_2 can be generated. Such high levels of CO_2 can cause tissue acidification and acid-induced pain in other animals. The EKE substitution in human $Na_V1.7$ enhances acid-induced blockade of this channel, consistent with a failure to induce firing of action potentials in naked mole rat nociceptors.[17] The corresponding tripeptide sequence in human $Na_V1.6$, the other TTX-sensitive channel in adult nociceptors, is DKE, suggesting that it might be more sensitive to acidic conditions than $Na_V1.7$.

Putative Role in Epilepsy

One study reported the presence of *SCN9A* variants in patients with seizures, including those with Dravet syndrome (Online Mendelian Inheritance in Man (OMIM) database #607208); these variants were present in the control population used in the study at >1% allele frequency.[50] However, the function of $Na_V1.7$ in CNS neurons and its role, if any, in the pathophysiology of seizures has not been established, although a knock-in mouse expressing one of these variants was reported to exhibit seizures. Importantly, neither patients with small-fibre neuropathy (SFN)[39] carrying the same $Na_V1.7$ variants reported by Singh et al.,[50] nor patients with other gain-of-function *SCN9A* mutations associated with inherited erythromelalgia (IEM; also known as familial erythromelalgia and primary erythermalgia; OMIM #133020)[13,51] have reported seizures. Thus, the contribution of *SCN9A* mutations, if any, to epilepsy remains incompletely understood.

Roles in Pain States

Na_V1.7 in Acquired Pain Conditions

$Na_V1.7$ has an important role in pain signaling.[13,51] Axotomy of peripheral axons can

produce a **neuroma** in which ectopic impulses arise, causing spontaneous pain.[52] Application of TTX at concentrations that block only TTX-sensitive channels ameliorates neuropathic pain behavior in a rat axotomy model,[53] suggesting that these channels contribute to spontaneous pain. Although the TTX-sensitive sodium channel $Na_V1.3$ has been implicated in ectopic firing and spontaneous pain,[13] $Na_V1.7$ accumulates at nerve endings within neuromas together with activated mitogen-activated protein kinase 1 (MAPK1; also known as ERK2) and MAPK3 (also known as ERK1) in humans[54] and in rats.[31] MAPK1 and MAPK3 phosphorylate $Na_V1.7$ at four sites within L1, producing a graded hyperpolarizing shift of channel activation. The extent of graded hyperpolarizing shift in $Na_V1.7$ activation depends on the number of phosphorylated residues.[55] Together with the finding that MAPK1 and MAPK3 exert a pro-excitatory effect on DRG neurons,[55] these data suggest that $Na_V1.7$ can contribute to injury-mediated DRG neuron excitability.

$Na_V1.7$ expression levels and TTX-sensitive current density are increased in DRG neurons in response to inflammation.[56] The increase in $Na_V1.7$ expression levels is more robust than that of $Na_V1.3$—the other TTX-sensitive channel that is upregulated under these conditions.[56,57] $Na_V1.7$ levels in DRG neurons are also increased in diabetic rats,[58,59] a change that is predicted to contribute to hyperexcitability associated with pain. A direct contribution of $Na_V1.7$ to pathological DRG neuronal hyperexcitability is further supported by knockdown and knockout studies in rodents. Knockdown of $Na_V1.7$ attenuates complete Freund's adjuvant-induced thermal hyperalgesia[60] and diabetic pain.[61] Conditional knockout of $Na_V1.7$ expression in mouse DRG neurons, where $Na_V1.8$ is expressed, abrogates inflammation-induced and burn injury-induced thermal hyperalgesia, but does not impair mechanical allodynia or hyperalgesia (neuropathic pain).[43,62,63] However, a recent report[62] provided evidence suggesting that knocking out

Na$_V$1.7 expression in both DRG and sympathetic neurons abrogated neuropathic pain (box 2).

Na$_V$1.7 in Inherited Pain Disorders

The co-segregation of a familial mutation and disease symptoms in more than one generation provides a compelling case for a direct link between a target gene and a disease. Recently, mutations in *SCN9A* that alter the functional properties of Na$_V$1.7 in a pro-excitatory manner have been shown to produce familial pain disorders that follow a Mendelian inheritance pattern (**inherited sodium channelopathies**). These findings provided a causative link in these pain disorders and confirmed that Na$_V$1.7 has a central role in pain signaling in humans. Dominantly inherited gain-of-function missense mutations in *SCN9A* are found in individuals with IEM[64] and paroxysmal extreme pain disorder (PEPD; previously known as familial rectal pain; OMIM #167400).[65] By contrast, recessively inherited loss-of-function mutations in *SCN9A* are linked to complete insensitivity (indifference) to pain (CIP; OMIM #243000).[66] Functional characterization of these gain-of-function mutations has elucidated the patho-physiological basis for DRG neuron excitability in these disorders, establishing a mechanistic link to pain.

Pain in IEM is localized to the feet and hands, and symptoms of this condition usually appear in early childhood.[13,51] Multiple families with IEM carry mutations in *SCN9A* that segregate with disease in affected individuals, providing strong genetic evidence for the pathogenicity of these mutations (figure 1). The familial IEM mutations in *SCN9A* that have been characterized to date all shift the voltage-dependence of Na$_V$1.7 activation in a hyperpolarized direction (figure 3a), increase ramp current (figure 3b) and slow deactivation. IEM-linked *SCN9A* mutations can impair slow inactivation (figure 3c), thus enhancing DRG neuron hyperexcitability,[67] whereas other IEM mutations enhance slow inactivation and therefore attenuate DRG neuron excitability.[68]

Box 2
Na$_V$1.7 in sympathetic neurons and pain signaling

The contribution of Na$_V$1.7 to electrogenesis in sympathetic neurons and the contribution of these neurons to pain are not well understood. Although Na$_V$1.7 is normally expressed in sympathetic neurons,[18] individuals with Na$_V$1.7-related complete insensitivity to pain (CIP) do not report sympathetic deficits,[66] suggesting that the role of Na$_V$1.7 in these neurons might be redundant. Gain-of-function mutant Na$_V$1.7 in patients with severe pain can depolarize the resting membrane potential of dorsal root ganglion (DRG) neurons and sympathetic neurons. The resulting effect renders DRG neurons hyperexcitable and sympathetic neurons hypoexcitable,[10] suggesting that severe pain may still occur even when sympathetic neuron excitability is reduced. However, studies in mice suggest that functional features of both sensory and sympathetic neurons, which are dependent on Na$_V$1.7, contribute to the manifestation of pain symptoms.[43,62] Minett et al.[62] reported that knocking out *Scn9a* (the gene encoding Na$_V$1.7) in DRG neurons alone does not cause a total loss of pain, whereas knocking out the expression of this channel in both sensory and sympathetic neurons recapitulates features of human CIP. Future studies are needed to investigate the role of Na$_V$1.7 in sympathetic neurons and pain signaling.

Another distinct set of mutations in *SCN9A* underlies PEPD, in which severe perirectal pain typically starts in infancy.[65] The rectal pain is accompanied with skin flushing of the lower or upper body or face and can present in a harlequin pattern,[69] which can alternate between the left and right sides of the body during different pain episodes.[70] PEPD-linked *SCN9A* mutations produce different effects on Na$_V$1.7 gating compared with IEM-associated mutations.[13,65] PEPD-linked *SCN9A* mutations shift the voltage-dependence of steady-state fast inactivation toward a depolarizing direction (figure 3d) and, depending upon the specific mutation, make channel inactivation incomplete, which results in a persistent current (figure 3d,e). PEPD, but not IEM, mutant Na$_V$1.7 manifests increased resurgent currents[38] (figure 3f).

The IEM-linked *SCN9A* mutations studied to date[13] lower the threshold for single action potentials (figure 4a–c) and increase the frequency of firing in DRG neurons (figure 4d–f), with many IEM-linked *SCN9A* mutations causing a depolarizing shift in resting potential.[13] At the cellular level, PEPD mutant Na$_V$1.7 lowers the threshold for single action potentials and increases the frequency of firing in DRG neurons, without altering the resting potential.[71–73] Importantly, these functional profiles have been obtained by recordings from the somas of DRG neurons. It will be important, in the future, to assess the properties of these mutant channels and their effect on excitability near nerve terminals where Na$_V$1.7

is thought to exert its influence as a threshold channel. A recent study from our group[74] has begun to address this point, demonstrating a resting potential for DRG neurites close to −60 mV, a potential at which Na$_V$1.7 channels are not strongly inactivated and are available for activation in fine diameter axons of DRG neurons. This study also demonstrated that action potential electrogenesis in DRG neurites in culture is driven by the sequential activation of TTX-sensitive and then TTX-resistant sodium currents.

De novo mutations in *SCN9A* in individuals with IEM, but without a family history of this disorder, produce similar functional changes in mutant Na$_V$1.7 to those produced by familial mutations and render DRG neurons hyperexcitable, which is consistent with the pathogenicity of these mutant variants.[75,76] However, the molecular genetic basis of delayed onset of pain in adult-onset IEM is not yet understood. As in IEM, *de novo* mutations in *SCN9A* in individuals with PEPD and no family history of this disorder

---

Figure 3

Biophysical properties of wild-type and mutant Na$_V$1.7 channels. (a) Inherited erythromelalgia (IEM)-related *SCN9A* mutations shift the activation of Na$_V$1.7 in a hyperpolarized direction, allowing the mutant channels to open in response to a weaker depolarization than open wild-type (WT) channels. A comparison of the activation of WT and P1308L mutant Na$_V$1.7 channels[73] shows that the latter exhibits a hyperpolarizing shift (−9.6 mV) in activation. (b) Activation of Na$_V$1.7 boosts small, slow depolarizations, producing ramp currents. The ramp currents produced by the IEM I136V mutant Na$_V$1.7 channel,[140] normalized to maximal peak currents elicited by step depolarizations, are markedly increased compared with the ramp currents for WT Na$_V$1.7 channels. (c) The slow-inactivated state of Na$_V$1.7 makes these channels unavailable for further opening after they have been activated by sustained (>10 s) membrane depolarization. Mutations in *SCN9A* that impair slow inactivation (such as N395K and I739V) increase the firing rate of dorsal root ganglion (DRG) neurons.[67,141] Error bars represent standard error of the mean. (d) Fast inactivation is a process that transiently makes Na$_V$1.7 unavailable for further opening after it has been activated by relatively short (100–500 ms) depolarizations. A hallmark of paroxysmal extreme pain disorder (PEPD)-related *SCN9A* mutations is that they cause a depolarizing shift in fast inactivation that results in fewer inactivated channels at any given potential, and resistance of a subpopulation of channels to inactivation. The PEPD G1607R mutant Na$_V$1.7 channel[70] shows a −30 mV depolarizing shift in fast inactivation, and the presence of a subpopulation of channels that resist inactivation (represented by orange shading in the graph). Error bars represent standard error of the mean. (e) Normalized current traces for WT and G1607R Na$_V$1.7 evoked by a depolarizing pulse to 0 mV show the transient current (I$_{Na-trans}$) and that the mutant channels retain a persistent current (I$_{Na-per}$) at the end of a 100 ms depolarizing pulse (represented by orange shading in the graph). (f) Resurgent currents (I$_{Na-res}$) are triggered by repolarization following a strong depolarization, and support burst firing. Note the increase in resurgent current recorded from DRG neurons expressing the M932L/V991L Na$_V$1.7 variant from a patient with small-fibre neuropathy.[39] Impaired fast- and slow-inactivation and resurgent currents are manifested by PEPD and SFN channel variants, as indicated in the main text, and the panels in this figure should be regarded as examples of these changes. Part a is modified from ref. 73. Part b is modified from ref. 140. Part c is modified, with permission, from ref. 67 © (2007) The Physiological Society. Parts d and e are modified, with permission, from ref. 70 © (2011) Macmillan Publishers Limited. All rights reserved. Part f is modified, with permission, from ref. 39 © (2012) American Neurological Association.

have been identified; the effects of these *de novo* mutations on Na$_V$1.7 gating is similar to those in familial PEPD, which is consistent with the pathogenicity of these mutations.[70]

The distinct and focal patterns of pain in IEM and PEPD are remarkable, considering that Na$_V$1.7 is expressed in most DRG neurons (figure 2) and trigeminal neurons. An individual with a mixed phenotype that included symptoms of IEM and PEPD symptoms was found to carry the *SCN9A* mutation A1632E, which hyperpolarizes activation and depolarizes steady-state fast inactivation.[71] Thus, Na$_V$1.7-associated IEM and PEPD might be considered to be part of a clinical

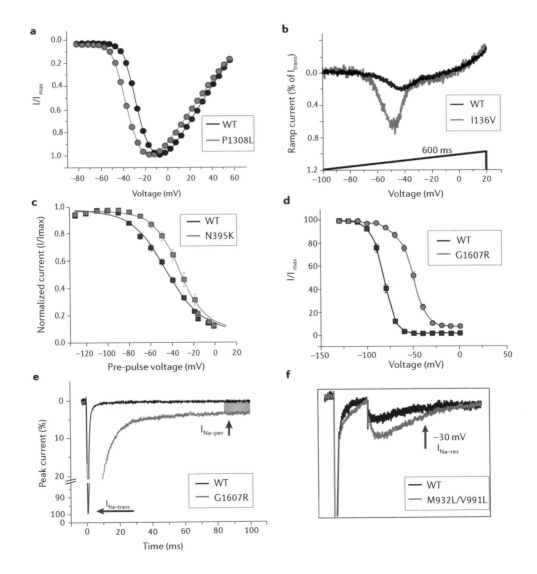

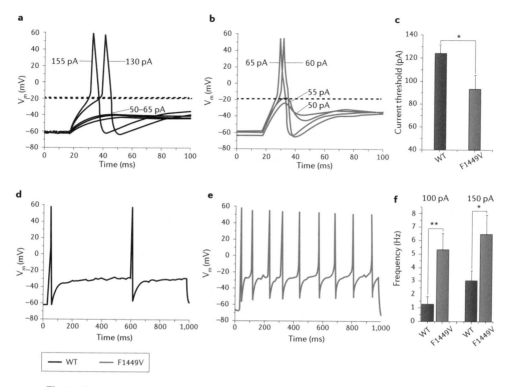

Figure 4

The F1449V mutation in Na$_V$1.7 makes DRG neurons hyperexcitable. (a,b) Representative traces from small (<30 μm) dorsal root ganglion (DRG) neurons expressing wild-type (WT) Na$_V$1.7 or Na$_V$1.7 with the F1449V mutation (the variant linked to inherited erythromelalgia). These traces show that neurons expressing the mutant channel have a lower current threshold for action potential generation. (c) The average current threshold is notably reduced in cells expressing F1449V compared with cells expressing WT channels (*P <0.05). (d,e) A neuron expressing WT Na$_V$1.7 responds to a 950 ms stimulation of 150 pA with a lower number of action potentials than does the neuron expressing the F1449V mutant (same cells as in panels a and b). (f) There is a sizeable increase in the frequency of firing of action potentials in response to 100 pA and 150 pA stimuli (950 ms) with expression of F1449V versus expression of WT Na$_V$1.7 (*P <0.05; **P <0.01). Figure is reproduced, with permission, from ref. 94 © (2005) Oxford University Press.

and physiological continuum that can produce IEM, PEPD and disorders that have characteristics of both of these conditions.

Recessively inherited *SCN9A* nonsense or splicing-defective mutations have been linked to Na$_V$1.7-related CIP.[66] Heterozygous parent carriers of these mutations are asymptomatic, indicating that the loss of one *SCN9A* allele does not lead to clinically manifested haploinsufficiency.

Truncated Na$_V$1.7 CIP fragments do not assemble into functional channels[66,77] and do not act as dominant negative proteins,[77] which reflects the normal pain experienced in the heterozygous carrier parents of patients with CIP. Although the first cases of Na$_V$1.7-related CIP were from consanguineous families,[66] later cases were identified in non-consanguineous marriages,[44,45] indicating that there is a higher incidence of carriers of non-functional *SCN9A* alleles in the general population than was predicted from the initial reports. However, neither homozygous nonsense mutations nor compound heterozygous null mutations have been reported in healthy individuals. Patients with Na$_V$1.7-related CIP do not experience any form of pain. Notably, they do not display motor, cognitive, sympathetic or gastrointestinal deficits, and have intact sensory modalities.[66,77] An exception to this is that several patients have reported that they have an impaired sense of smell,[44,45] although a recent study has described several members of a family with a non-sense *SCN9A* mutation, CIP and normal sense of smell.[78]

Although the expression of wild-type Na$_V$1.7 at 50% of the normal protein level (that is, there is one functional allele) is sufficient for a normal pain phenotype (that is, there is no haploinsufficiency), the minimum level of functional Na$_V$1.7 required to maintain the capacity to experience normal pain is not known. Interestingly, an individual with incomplete CIP (the patient retained some pain sensation) was found to carry compound heterozygous mutations in *SCN9A*, including a missense mutation (C1719R) affecting the S5–S6 extracurricular linker in DIV, and a one base-pair deletion in the 5′ splice donor site of exon 17 of *SCN9A*.[79] Impaired splice donor sites, like most splice-site mutations, may cause exclusion of exon 17 and therefore lead to non-functional channels, which is consistent with the phenotype of impaired sensing. The reporting of some pain experience in this individual suggests that successful but inefficient exon 17 inclusion and production of functional Na$_V$1.7 have occurred, but at levels that do not support full manifestation of pain.

Positive symptoms (pain) or negative symptoms (loss of pain sensing and anosmia) of patients with *SCN9A*-linked conditions can be explained by the effects of *SCN9A* gain-of-function and loss-of-function mutations, respectively, on nociceptors. The lack of an effect of

SCN9A mutations on other sensory modalities is, however, not well understood. Although Na$_V$1.7 is expressed in more than 50% of Aβ low-threshold mechanoreceptors,[24] individuals with CIP have normal nerve conduction, tactile sense and vibration sense,[66,77] suggesting that Na$_V$1.7 function is redundant in these neurons. By contrast, normal proprioception in patients with CIP is consistent with the absence of Na$_{V1}$.7 in muscle afferents.[24] It is not fully understood why *SCN9A* gain-of-function mutations do not cause positive symptoms in carriers; for example, causing them to become 'hyper-smellers'.

Functional Variants as Risk Factors

In agreement with the 'common disease, common variant' hypothesis,[80] the R1150W variant of Na$_V$1.7 has been associated with enhanced pain sensation.[81,82] Estacion et al.[81] demonstrated that the W1150 minor allele was present in 30% of people in an ethnically matched control population of Caucasian individuals of European descent. The W1150 variant of Na$_V$1.7 induces hyperexcitability of DRG neurons, suggesting that carriers of this polymorphism might be predisposed to hyperalgesia. Indeed, a genome-wide association study found that the R1150W polymorphism is associated with an increased pain perception in patients with osteoarthritis, phantom limb pain or lumbar root pain, and that the effect is most strongly associated with C-fibre activation.[82]

About 30% of individuals with idiopathic SFN express functional mutant Na$_V$1.7 channels arising from gain-of-function *SCN9A* missense variants,[39] which may not be fully penetrant when found in families.[83] People carrying these gain-of-function Na$_V$1.7 variants are hypersensitive to pain, which reflects the expression of this channel in DRG neurons. These individuals also manifest profound autonomic dysfunction, which reflects the expression of Na$_V$1.7 in sympathetic neurons.[10,18] Gain-of-function attributes of Na$_V$1.7 variants in SFN include depolarized fast inactivation (figure 3d) and/or slow inactivation (figure 3c), or an increase in the fraction of cells that produce resurgent currents (figure 3f). Surprisingly, however, individuals with *SCN9A*-null mutations do not manifest autonomic system deficits,[66] suggesting that there is a redundant function for this channel in sympathetic neurons.

Does Na$_V$1.7 Play a Role in the Dorsal Horn?

Based on studies in HEK 293 cells and DRG neuron somata, and on computer simulations, Na$_V$1.7 is thought to act as a threshold channel that activates at relatively hyperpolarized potentials, thus amplifying small, slow depolarizations at potentials negative to an action potential threshold.[36,84] This role, however, does not explain the total lack of pain sensation in patients with Na$_V$1.7-related CIP even in response to the most intense stimulation, such as dental work or child-bearing labor. One possible theory is that Na$_V$1.7 at central termini of primary afferents (figure 2) may play a part in synaptic transmission of pain signals.

Consistent with this hypothesis, Minett et al.[62] showed that evoked release of substance P into the spinal cord in response to sciatic nerve stimulation, and synaptic potentiation of wide dynamic range neurons receiving input from primary afferents are attenuated in mice that had Na$_V$1.7 knocked out in DRG neurons. Na$_V$1.7 may have a role in facilitating the invasion of incoming action potentials from peripheral nociceptors into central pre-terminal exon branches or into terminals within the spinal cord. Alternatively, Na$_V$1.7 may be involved within the terminals in the process of neurotransmitter release onto second-order dorsal horn neurons. Thus, we speculate that Na$_V$1.7, deployed near presynaptic terminals in the dorsal horn,[32] is important for release of neurotransmitters such as substance P. If this speculation is correct, then Na$_V$1.7 inhibitors that act on both peripheral and central compartments might be needed for clinical efficacy.

Structural Features of Na$_V$1.7

Our ability to understand the mechanistic bases of pathogenic *SCN9A* mutations and to develop rationally designed small-molecule inhibitors for the treatment of hyperexcitability disorders is limited by the lack of a high-resolution crystal structure of a eukaryotic sodium channel. High-resolution crystal structures of ion channels are necessary for a comprehensive understanding of the links between voltage-sensing and channel activation and inactivation, ion selectivity, and drug interactions. Our current understanding of these channel properties was derived from comparative sequence analysis, and from functional assays that measured ion conductance or fluorescence emission of tagged channels.[2] **Atomic structural modeling** following the determination of high-resolution crystal structures of potassium channels[85–87] and, more recently, a bacterial sodium channel[3] has advanced our understanding of the structure–function relationship of human *SCN9A* mutations, which is discussed below.

Lessons Learned from Potassium and Bacterial Sodium Channels

Crystallographic studies of potassium channels provided the first direct evidence for the structural basis for ion selectivity, pore gating and coupling of a voltage sensor to the pore components.[85–87] These studies also yielded valuable insights into kinetics and sequence determinants of different gating mechanisms. Identification of the homotetramer bacterial voltage-gated sodium channel,[88] with the monomer possessing the six transmembrane segment architecture of the homologous domains in the eukaryotic channels, facilitated the production of sufficient channel protein for crystallization and high-resolution structural studies. Intriguingly, bacterial voltage-gated sodium channels are most similar to DIII of human sodium channels.[89] The first high-resolution crystal structure (resolved at 2.7 Å) of a pre-open conformation of the voltage-gated sodium channel from the bacterium *Arcobacter butzleri* (Na$_V$Ab)[3] suggested that the S4 segments are in the activated position, but that the activation gate at the cytoplasmic end of the pore domain is closed. This study provided structural evidence for several of the gating steps of sodium channels and demonstrated a possible route for access of small hydrophobic pore-blocking molecules.

Because of the nature of eukaryotic sodium channels as four-domain polypeptides, which are linked by cytoplasmic loops with divergent lengths and sequences in the different members of the sodium channel family, there may be subtle yet important structural differences between these channels and the bacterial homotetrameric channels. Thus, caution is warranted in extrapolating from high-resolution crystal structures of a symmetrical homotetrameric bacterial sodium channel to eukaryotic single polypeptide multi-domain sodium channel isoforms. Moreover, individual channel mutations should optimally be assessed in their native isoform. For example, the S241L mutation within the DI S4–S5 linker of Na$_V$1.7 produces a marked hyperpolarizing shift in its activation, steady-state fast and slow inactivation, compared with wild-type channels.[90] By contrast, substitution of the corresponding residue in Na$_V$1.4, S246L, hyperpolarizes steady-state fast and slow inactivation of the channel but, unlike S241L in Na$_V$1.7, S246L had no effect on Na$_V$1.4 activation,[91] thus providing an example of an isoform-specific effect of conserved residues.

Atomic Structural Modeling of the Putative Activation Gate

From a homology model of the Na$_V$1.7 pore components, based on the crystal structure of the *Streptomyces lividans* potassium channel KcsA,[85] we were able to identify a putative activation gate.[92] This modeling approach identified an aromatic residue within the cytoplasm-proximal portion of each of the pore-lining S6 helices (DI Y405, DII F960, DIII F1449 and DIV F1752) that were

predicted to form a hydrophobic ring at the cytoplasmic end of the pore that stabilizes the channel's pre-open state. These aromatic residues in the four S6 helices form an energetically stable assembly due to extensive van der Waals bonds between their side chains, which is further strengthened by additional edge-face interaction with the adjacent aromatic residues.[93] The hydrophobic ring is predicted to raise the energy barrier for the movement of S6, which is necessary to open the channel's pore, thus stabilizing the closed or pre-open state of the channel. Although the activation gate at the narrow cytoplasmic vestibule of the channel in the Na$_V$Ab crystal structure consists of four methionine 221 residues (one from each monomer),[3] modeling of Na$_V$1.7 based on the Na$_V$Ab crystal structure recapitulates the activation gate that was previously identified based on the KcsA structure (figure 5).

Evidence for the formation of this hydrophobic block is provided by functional studies of the F1449V mutation in Na$_V$1.7 that is found in patients with IEM. This mutation lowers the threshold for Na$_V$1.7 activation.[94] The F1449V substitution is predicted to destabilize interactions with the adjacent aromatic residues, thus reducing the energetic barrier for DIII S6 helix movement and facilitating bending motions associated with pore opening. The increased propensity of the DIII S6 helix to move would be expected to hasten channel activation. Support for this model of activation comes from studies of inwardly rectifying potassium (Kir) channels, which form a similar quadruple phenylalanine hydrophobic ring.[95] Substitution of F168 in Kir6.2 (which is analogous to F1449 in Na$_V$1.7) with smaller residues favors the channel's open-state, whereas substitution of F168 with the aromatic amino acid tryptophan retains wild-type-like function.[95]

There are limitations on the use of the crystal structure of a homotetrameric voltage-gated ion channels (bacterial sodium channel and various potassium channels) for modeling the multi-domain mammalian Na$_V$1.7, and our functional studies of the effect of F1449V on the activation gate provide an instructive example of such a limitation. Although the model suggested that phenylalanine or tyrosine residues at the carboxyl termini of the S6 segments in Na$_V$1.7 stabilize the channel's closed or pre-open state, functional analysis showed that these residues have different effects. Specifically, DII F960V and DIII F1449V markedly hyperpolarize channel activation, whereas DI Y405V and DIV F1752V do not alter channel activation.[92] This may reflect the functional specialization of the four homologous, yet not identical, domains of eukaryotic sodium channels.

Dependence on Neuronal Background

Gating of wild-type or mutant sodium channels can be modulated in a cell-type-dependent manner,

and this phenomenon can have important clinical implications. For example, resurgent sodium currents can be recorded from only a subset of small diameter DRG neurons transfected with Na$_V$1.6 (ref. 42) or Na$_V$1.7 (ref. 38), and Na$_V$1.8 channels exhibit slow-inactivation properties that are differentially regulated in different subpopulations of (peptidergic and non-peptidergic) small diameter DRG neurons.[9] For example, a single mutation in *SCN9A*, leading to L858H[10] or I739V,[96] renders DRG neurons hyperexcitable but superior cervical ganglion (SCG) neurons hypoexcitable. The latter phenomenon is related to the depolarization of the resting potential in both DRG and SCG neurons by the mutant Na$_V$1.7, which leads to resting inactivation of all of the sodium channel isoforms in SCG neurons and hypoexcitability. The presence of Na$_V$1.8, which is relatively resistant to inactivation by depolarization,[97–99] in DRG neurons renders these neurons hyperexcitable in response to depolarization.[10] These data demonstrate that sodium

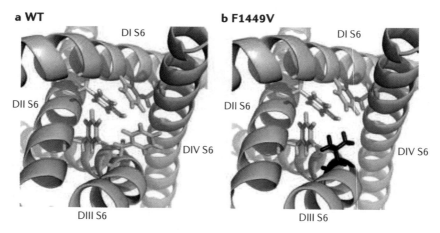

a WT
DI S6
DII S6
DIV S6
DIII S6

b F1449V
DI S6
DII S6
DIV S6
DIII S6

Figure 5
A model of the putative activation gate of Na$_V$1.7. The folded structure of the two S6 transmembrane segments presented here were based on the crystal structure of a bacterial sodium channel.[3] The carboxy-terminal aromatic residue of each S6 is shown in stick representation for wild-type (WT; a) Na$_V$1.7 and Na$_V$1.7 with the F1449V mutation (b). The assembly of aromatic residues at the cytoplasmic C terminus of each of the S6 segments forms the putative activation gate of Na$_V$1.7. The F1449V mutation in the homologous domain III (DIII) disrupts the hydrophobic ring and destabilizes the pre-open state of the channel.

channel mutations can have a range of cell-background-dependent effects in different types of neurons.

Targeting Na$_V$1.7 for Pain Treatment

The clear involvement of Na$_V$1.7 in human pain, and the lack of serious cognitive, cardiac and adverse motor effects with a total loss of Na$_V$1.7, as demonstrated in individuals with CIP, have fuelled intense efforts to develop Na$_V$1.7-specific inhibitors or modulators for the treatment of pain. Despite these intensive efforts, progress has been slow.[100] Nonetheless, the occasional reports of patients with IEM who respond to monotherapy using pan-sodium channel blockers,[101,102] and the responsiveness of patients with PEPD to carbamazepine, suggest that small molecules may be developed to either inhibit or modulate Na$_V$1.7 in a manner that can reduce excitability of DRG neurons and provide pain relief. Using the IEM Na$_V$1.7 V400M carbamazepine-responsive mutation[102] as a 'seed' for an atomic-level modeling and thermodynamic analysis, Yang et al.[103] were able to predict carbamazepine-responsiveness of a second IEM mutation, Na$_V$1.7 S241T, suggesting that, in the future, pharmacogenomic guided therapy may be possible. Alternative strategies may include the development of isoform-specific blockers or modulators of gating states of sodium channels that are differentially altered under pathological conditions; the development of compounds that weakly cross the blood–brain barrier to minimize CNS-related adverse effects; and gene therapy.

Small-Molecule Blockers

Several purportedly selective small-molecule inhibitors of Na$_V$1.7 have been described and have shown efficacy in animal models of pain.[104–107] These reports, however, lack documentation for selectivity against human sodium channel isoforms in a native neuronal environment. Reports

detailing the efficacies of these compounds in animal models of pain should therefore be interpreted with caution, as these results could be due to inhibition of any of the neuronal sodium channel isoforms. A small-molecule blocker with robust selectivity for human Na$_V$1.7 was recently developed.[108] This orally bioavailable compound bound preferentially to the slow-inactivated state of the channel, and showed notable selectivity for Na$_V$1.7 over other voltage-gated sodium channel isoforms (by 10-fold to 900-fold). The compound also showed 1,000-fold selectivity for Na$_V$1.7 over potassium and calcium channels. These favorable properties suggest that this small-molecule blocker holds promise for future clinical studies.

State-Dependent Blockers

Local anesthetics, anticonvulsants and tricyclic compounds block sodium channels, mostly in a use-dependent fashion, and are among the first-line treatments that are currently available for neuropathic pain.[109,110] However, these agents are not isoform-specific and only provide partial pain relief due in part to their limited therapeutic window that results from CNS-related adverse effects, such as dizziness or sedation.[111,112] Despite these limitations, lidocaine derivatives and carbamazepine are effective in patients carrying certain *SCN9A* mutations that render Na$_V$1.7 pharmacoresponsive,[65,101,102] suggesting that personalized, genomically based therapeutics for pain is possible.

Patients with PEPD harbouring *SCN9A* mutations respond favorably to treatment with carbamazepine, which acts to counterbalance impaired fast inactivation of the mutant channel and hence reduces the persistent current caused by these mutations.[65] Although most patients with Na$_V$1.7-linked IEM do not respond to pharmacotherapy, a few have reported control of pain symptoms with lidocaine, mexiletine or carbamazepine. Successful lidocaine or mexiletine monotherapy was reported in a patient carrying the $Na_V1.7$ V872G mutation, possibly resulting from enhanced lidocaine use-dependent block of the mutant channels.[101] Three members of a family with IEM, carrying the mutation $Na_V1.7$ V400M, reported control of their pain symptoms with carbamazepine.[102] Preincubation of V400M channels with clinically relevant concentrations of carbamazepine induced a depolarizing shift in activation, which returned to wild-type voltages.[102] This normalization of activation suggests that carbamazepine acts in an allosteric manner on the mutant $Na_V1.7$ channel and induces a wild-type-like pre-open state.

Computer simulation studies[67] and functional characterization of the $Na_V1.7$ delL955 mutation[68] suggest that enhancing the slow inactivation of $Na_V1.7$ may allow an alternative approach to the treatment of pain. Lacosamide, a functionalized amino acid with sodium channel-blocking activity, showed beneficial effects in animal studies and clinical trials of epilepsy, in animal models of acute, inflammatory and neuropathic pain,[113–116] and in initial clinical trials for diabetic neuropathic pain.[117,118] Lacosamide's blocking activity is unusual in that it involves selective enhancement of the slow inactivation of voltage-gated sodium channels, including $Na_V1.3$, $Na_V1.7$ and $Na_V1.8$ (ref. 119). Interestingly, lacosamide induces substantially greater inhibition of $Na_V1.3$, $Na_V1.7$ and $Na_V1.8$ when these channels are in an inactivated state.[119] This feature of lacosamide might mean it would exhibit a better safety profile and greater tolerability than state-independent voltage-gated sodium channel blockers, as it might preferentially target injured depolarized neurons with hyperactive sodium channels.[120] Although lacosamide has not been approved for the treatment of human neuropathic pain,[121] targeting of the $Na_V1.7$ slow-inactivated state might provide a viable drug-development option.

Natural Toxins

Natural peptide toxins might provide a source of isoform-specific inhibitors of sodium channels, because binding of these toxins to channels is regulated by multiple contact points, and minor sequence changes in the channel could have a profound effect on the affinity of the channel–toxin interaction. Venoms of a variety of snails are reservoirs of peptide toxins, and some of these have demonstrated sodium channel isoform selectivity.[122–124] However, $Na_V1.7$ is among the channels that are only weakly blocked by the conotoxins identified to date.[122,123] By contrast, peptide toxins from tarantulas manifest preferential effect on $Na_V1.7$. For example, ProTx-II is ~50-fold more selective for $Na_V1.7$ than $Na_V1.5$ (refs. 125,126). Huwentoxin-I and huwentoxin-IV are potent inhibitors of $Na_V1.7$ and other neuronal TTX-sensitive channels, but are not effective against $Na_V1.4$ (refs. 127,128). The exchange of two residues in the DII S3–S4 linker of $Na_V1.7$ and $Na_V1.4$ reverses the affinity of huwentoxins to these channels.[128] Additionally, a charge-conserving substitution in KIIIA, a member of the μ-conotoxin subfamily, enhances the selectivity for $Na_V1.7$ over $Na_V1.2$ and $Na_V1.4$ (ref. 129). It may therefore be possible to engineer peptide toxins with the desirable $Na_V1.7$ isoform specificity.

Peptide toxins, however, have poor oral bioavailability and it is difficult to deliver them to nerve endings, implying that their use as therapeutic agents remains limited. However, modification of conotoxins by cyclization can enhance their stability *in vivo* without compromising their biological activity,[130] and it may be possible to develop cyclized $Na_V1.7$-specific peptide toxins when such molecules become available.

Gene Therapy

Advances in virus-mediated gene therapy have led to the initiation of Phase I trials for pain involving a herpes simplex virus (HSV) platform to transfer human preproencephalin (*PENK*) to DRG neurons.[131] Local delivery of a gene product within the projection zone of an injured or diseased nerve associated with a focal pain syndrome (as in post-herpetic neuralgia or peripheral nerve injury) could be used to treat pain in a topologically defined manner, reducing systemic adverse effects. Animal studies have provided the proof-of-principle for this approach, showing that anti-Na$_V$1.7 antisense constructs, delivered by a HSV virion, can attenuate pain behavior in mice following peripheral inflammation[60] and in diabetic rats.[61] We have recently succeeded in targeting another sodium channel, Na$_V$1.3, in DRG neurons using RNA interference molecules (shRNA for gene knockdown) delivered using the non-virulent AAV platform,[132] which is less immunogenic than other viral delivery platforms, suggesting that a similar strategy for targeting Na$_V$1.7 using AAV-mediated delivery of shRNA may be successful.

Summary and Future Directions

Na$_V$1.7 has proven to be a key player at the organismal level in human pain, at the cellular level as a major regulator of neuronal excitability and at the molecular level as a platform for discovering the contribution of specific residues to gating mechanisms. Studies of the rare monogenic disorders IEM, PEPD and CIP definitively show that Na$_V$1.7 is critically important for human pain, and studies on SFN demonstrate a role for this channel in more common pain disorders. In addition to insights into the pathophysiology of pain gleaned from studying mutant Na$_V$1.7 in its native neuron, modeling of mutant channels, based upon the crystal structures of the bacterial sodium channel and other ion channels, has led to identification of the putative activation gate of Na$_V$1.7, and allows predictions of the dynamic interaction of the voltage-sensor and pore segments within the same domain and between different domains. Assessment of naturally occurring mutations in

these studies could be especially informative, as they are already known to have large effects on gating properties of the channel. Finally, the relatively restricted expression pattern of Na$_V$1.7, its central role in pain signaling in humans, and the minimal cognitive, cardiac, motor and sensory deficits in people totally lacking Na$_V$1.7 have shown that this channel is a valid and indeed attractive target for drug development, and support the view that single target engagement for pain treatment might have therapeutic potential.

Nevertheless, despite progress in our understanding of NaV1.7 and its contribution to diverse sensory modalities, crucial questions remain unanswered. For example, why do patients with IEM or PEPD mutations manifest different pain topography despite the ubiquitous expression of NaV1.7 in sensory neurons? Why does skin flushing in some patients with PEPD alternate from side to side of the body? Why does the age-of-onset of IEM symptoms vary from infancy to adulthood? Why is there no evidence for compensatory changes that rescue nociception in CIP? In addition to missense or nonsense substitutions or loss-of-function mutations of splice sites in *SCN9A*, do synonymous or intronic insertions–deletions affect splicing efficiency or RNA stability and cause disease? What is the relative contribution of Na$_V$1.7 to signal integration and transmission at peripheral and central termini of sensory and sympathetic neurons? Finally, why are the gating properties of the TTX-sensitive current in OSNs, which are mostly carried by Na$_V$1.7, markedly different from those in HEK 293 cells and DRG neurons? These questions, and other related questions, will undoubtedly be answered in the near future.

Acknowledgments

The authors thank the members of their group for valuable discussions. Work in the authors' laboratory is supported in part by grants from the Rehabilitation Research and Development Service and Medical Research Service, US

Department of Veterans Affairs, and from the Erythromelalgia Association. The Center for Neuroscience and Regeneration Research is a collaboration between the Paralyzed Veterans of America and Yale University, Connecticut, USA.

About the Authors

Sulayman D. Dib-Hajj, Department of Neurology, and Center for Neuroscience and Regeneration Research, Yale University School of Medicine, New Haven, CT; Rehabilitation Research Center, Veterans Affairs Connecticut Healthcare System, West Haven, CT.

Yang Yang, Department of Neurology, and Center for Neuroscience and Regeneration Research, Yale University School of Medicine, New Haven, CT; Rehabilitation Research Center, Veterans Affairs Connecticut Healthcare System, West Haven, CT.

Joel A. Black, Department of Neurology, and Center for Neuroscience and Regeneration Research, Yale University School of Medicine, New Haven, CT; Rehabilitation Research Center, Veterans Affairs Connecticut Healthcare System, West Haven, CT.

Stephen G. Waxman, Department of Neurology, and Center for Neuroscience and Regeneration Research, Yale University School of Medicine, New Haven, CT; Rehabilitation Research Center, Veterans Affairs Connecticut Healthcare System, West Haven, CT.

Competing Interests Statement

The authors declare *competing financial interests*. See Web version for details.

Databases

Online Mendelian Inheritance in Man (OMIM): http://www.ncbi.nlm.nih.gov/omim

Further Information

Center for Neuroscience and Regeneration Research, Yale School of Medicine: http://medicine.yale.edu/cnrr

Glossary

atomic structural modeling Construction of a model of a folded protein based on the atom coordinates of a related member of the family whose high-resolution crystal structure is determined and additional constraints derived from studies of distant members of the superfamily.

inherited sodium channelopathies Pathologies linked to mutations or functional variants in sodium channels that can be transmitted to progeny.

neuroma A collection of demyelinated and dysmyelinated axon sprouts and connective tissue that result from abortive regeneration of transected axons.

neuropathic pain Pain resulting from lesions or diseases of the somatosensory system.

nociceptors Pain-sensing or damage-sensing neurons.

ramp current Inward current due to transient channel activation in response to the small, slow depolarization of cell membranes.

repriming Refolding of a channel after opening and inactivating to restore a closed, but available channel. The channel is refractory to additional stimulations during repriming.

Notes

1. Catterall WA, Goldin AL, Waxman SG. 2005. International Union of Pharmacology. XLVII. Nomenclature and structure–function relationships of voltage-gated sodium channels. *Pharmacol Rev* 57: 397–409. [A general review on the sodium channel subfamily of voltage-gated ion channels.]

2. Catterall WA. 2000. From ionic currents to molecular mechanisms: The structure and function of voltage-gated sodium channels. *Neuron* 26: 13–25.

3. Payandeh J, Scheuer T, Zheng N, Catterall WA. 2011. The crystal structure of a voltage-gated sodium channel. *Nature* 475: 353–358. [The first description of a high-resolution crystal structure of a homotetrameric bacterial voltage-gated sodium channel.]

4. Catterall WA. 2010. Signaling complexes of voltage-gated sodium and calcium channels. *Neurosci Lett* 486: 107–116.

5. Dib-Hajj SD, Waxman SG. 2010. Isoform-specific and pan-channel partners regulate trafficking and plasma membrane stability; and alter sodium channel gating properties. *Neurosci Lett* 486: 84–91.

6. Leterrier C, Brachet A, Fache MP, Dargent B. 2010. Voltage-gated sodium channel organization in neurons: Protein interactions and trafficking pathways. *Neurosci Lett* 486: 92–100.

7. Patino GA, Isom LL. 2010. Electrophysiology and beyond: Multiple roles of Na$^+$ channel β subunits in development and disease. *Neurosci Lett* 486: 53–59.

8. Cummins TR, et al. 2001. Na$_V$1.3 sodium channels: Rapid repriming and slow closed-state inactivation display quantitative differences after expression in a mammalian cell line and in spinal sensory neurons. *J Neurosci* 21: 5952–5961. [This study documents the effect of cell background on the biophysical properties of voltage-gated sodium channels and highlights the need to study these channels in their native cell types.]

9. Choi JS, Dib-Hajj SD, Waxman S. 2007. Differential slow inactivation and use-dependent inhibition of Na$_V$1.8 channels contribute to distinct firing properties in IB4$^+$ and IB4$^-$ DRG neurons. *J Neurophysiol* 97: 1258–1265.

10. Rush AM, et al. 2006. A single sodium channel mutation produces hyper- or hypoexcitability in different types of neurons. *Proc Natl Acad Sci USA* 103: 8245–8250. [This study demonstrates that the distinct cellular responses of DRG neurons to expression of mutant Na$_{V1}$.7 channel depends on the presence or absence of another sodium channel, Na$_V$1.8.]

11. Choi JS, et al. 2010. Alternative splicing may contribute to time-dependent manifestation of inherited erythromelalgia. *Brain* 133: 1823–1835.

12. Dib-Hajj SD, et al. 2009. Transfection of rat or mouse neurons by biolistics or electroporation. *Nat Protoc* 4: 1118–1126.

13. Dib-Hajj SD, Cummins TR, Black JA, Waxman SG. 2010. Sodium channels in normal and pathological pain. *Annu Rev Neurosci* 33: 325–347.

14. Ahn HS, et al. 2011. Na$_V$1.7 is the predominant sodium channel in rodent olfactory sensory neurons. *Mol Pain* 7: 32.

15. Weiss J, et al. 2011. Loss-of-function mutations in sodium channel Na$_V$1.7 cause anosmia. *Nature* 472: 186–190.

16. Muroi Y, et al. 2011. Selective silencing of Na$_V$1.7 decreases excitability and conduction in vagal sensory neurons. *J Physiol* 589: 5663–5676.

17. Smith S, et al. 2011. The molecular basis of acid insensitivity in the African naked mole-rat. *Science* 334: 1557–1560.

18. Toledo-Aral JJ, et al. 1997. Identification of PN1, a predominant voltage-dependent sodium channel expressed principally in peripheral neurons. *Proc Natl Acad Sci USA* 94: 1527–1532. [The first study to report the major cellular distribution of Na$_V$1.7.]

19. Sage D, et al. 2007. Na$_V$1.7 and Na$_V$1.3 are the only tetrodotoxin-sensitive sodium channels expressed by the adult guinea pig enteric nervous system. *J Comp Neurol* 504: 363–378.

20. Kwong K, et al. 2008. Voltage-gated sodium channels in nociceptive versus non-nociceptive nodose vagal sensory neurons innervating guinea pig lungs. *J Physiol* 586: 1321–1336.

21. Holm AN, et al. 2002. Sodium current in human jejunal circular smooth muscle cells. *Gastroenterology* 122: 178–187.

22. Jo T, et al. 2004. Voltage-gated sodium channel expressed in cultured human smooth muscle cells: Involvement of *SCN9A*. *FEBS Lett* 567: 339–343.

23. Saleh S, Yeung SY, Prestwich S, Pucovsky V, Greenwood IA. 2005. Electrophysiological and molecular identification of voltage-gated sodium channels in murine vascular myocytes. *J Physiol* 568: 155–169.

24. Djouhri L, et al. 2003. Sensory and electrophysiological properties of guinea-pig sensory neurones expressing Na$_V$1.7 (PN1) Na$^+$ channel α-subunit protein. *J Physiol* 546: 565–576. [This study demonstrates the presence of Na$_V$1.7 in functionally identified nociceptors.]

25. Felts PA, Yokoyama S, Dib-Hajj S, Black JA, Waxman SG. 1997. Sodium channel α-subunit mRNAs I, II, III, NaG, Na6 and HNE (PN1) — different expression patterns in developing rat nervous system. *Brain Res Mol Brain Res* 45: 71–82.

26. Diss JK, et al. 2005. A potential novel marker for human prostate cancer: Voltage-gated sodium channel expression *in vivo*. *Prostate Cancer Prostatic Dis* 8: 266–273.

27. Fraser SP, et al. 2005. Voltage-gated sodium channel expression and potentiation of human breast cancer metastasis. *Clin Cancer Res* 11: 5381–5389.

28. Hoffman JF, Dodson A, Wickrema A, Dib-Hajj SD. 2004. Tetrodotoxin-sensitive Na$^+$ channels and muscarinic and purinergic receptors identified in human erythroid progenitor cells and red blood cell ghosts. *Proc Natl Acad Sci USA* 101: 12370–12374.

29. Kis-Toth K, et al. 2011. Voltage-gated sodium channel Na$_V$1.7 maintains the membrane potential and regulates the activation and chemokine-induced migration of a monocyte-derived dendritic cell subset. *J Immunol* 187: 1273–1280.

30. Djouhri L, et al. 2003. The TTX-resistant sodium channel Na$_V$1.8 (SNS/PN3): Expression and correlation with membrane properties in rat nociceptive primary afferent neurons. *J Physiol* 550: 739–752.

31. Persson AK, Gasser A, Black JA, Waxman SG. 2011. Na$_V$1.7 accumulates and co-localizes with phosphorylated ERK1/2 within transected axons in early experimental neuromas. *Exp Neurol* 230: 273–279.

32. Black JA, Frezel N, Dib-Hajj SD, Waxman SG. 2012. Expression of $Na_V1.7$ in DRG neurons extends from peripheral terminals in the skin to central preterminal branches and terminals in the dorsal horn. *Mol Pain* 8: 82.

33. Cummins TR, Howe JR, Waxman SG. 1998. Slow closed-state inactivation: A novel mechanism underlying ramp currents in cells expressing the hNE/PN1 sodium channel. *J Neurosci* 18: 9607–9619. [This study shows that $Na_V1.7$ can produce a robust ramp current, suggesting that $Na_V1.7$ can amplify subthreshold depolarizations and act as a threshold channel.]

34. Klugbauer N, Lacinova L, Flockerzi V, Hofmann F. 1995. Structure and functional expression of a new member of the tetrodotoxin-sensitive voltage-activated sodium channel family from human neuroendocrine cells. *EMBO J* 14: 1084–1090. [The first report of the isolation and characterization of $Na_V1.7$ as a TTX-sensitive sodium channel.]

35. Herzog RI, Cummins TR, Ghassemi F, Dib-Hajj SD, Waxman SG. 2003. Distinct repriming and closed-state inactivation kinetics of $Na_V1.6$ and $Na_V1.7$ sodium channels in mouse spinal sensory neurons. *J Physiol* 551: 741–750.

36. Rush AM, Cummins TR, Waxman SG. 2007. Multiple sodium channels and their roles in electrogenesis within dorsal root ganglion neurons. *J Physiol* 579: 1–14.

37. Dib-Hajj SD, Cummins TR, Black JA, Waxman SG. 2007. From genes to pain: $Na_V1.7$ and human pain disorders. *Trends Neurosci* 30: 555–563.

38. Jarecki BW, Piekarz AD, Jackson JO, 2nd, Cummins TR. 2010. Human voltage-gated sodium channel mutations that cause inherited neuronal and muscle channelopathies increase resurgent sodium currents. *J Clin Invest* 120: 369–378.

39. Faber CG, et al. 2012. Gain of function $Na_V1.7$ mutations in idiopathic small fiber neuropathy. *Ann Neurol* 71: 26–39. [This study was the first to show that patients with idiopathic SFN can harbour $Na_V1.7$ variants; it also shows that these variants cause hyperexcitability of DRG neurons.]

40. Raman IM, Bean BP. 1997. Resurgent sodium current and action potential formation in dissociated cerebellar Purkinje neurons. *J Neurosci* 17: 4517–4526. [This study documents a state of open channel block, which permits the passing of a current upon hyperpolarization of the cell membrane to negative potentials immediately following a strong depolarizing pulse that fully activates and inactivates the channel.]

41. Raman IM, Sprunger LK, Meisler MH, Bean BP. 1997. Altered subthreshold sodium currents and disrupted firing patterns in Purkinje neurons of *Scn8a* mutant mice. *Neuron* 19: 881–891.

42. Cummins TR, Dib-Hajj SD, Herzog RI, Waxman SG. 2005. $Na_V1.6$ channels generate resurgent sodium currents in spinal sensory neurons. *FEBS Lett* 579: 2166–2170.

43. Nassar MA, et al. 2004. Nociceptor-specific gene deletion reveals a major role for $Na_V1.7$ (PN1) in acute and inflammatory pain. *Proc Natl Acad Sci USA* 101: 12706–12711. [The first report showing that knockout of $Na_V1.7$ in DRG neurons impairs acute and inflammatory pain.]

44. Goldberg Y, et al. 2007. Loss-of-function mutations in the $Na_V1.7$ gene underlie congenital indifference to pain in multiple human populations. *Clin Genet* 71: 311–319.

45. Nilsen KB, et al. 2009. Two novel *SCN9A* mutations causing insensitivity to pain. *Pain* 143: 155–158.

46. Undem BJ, Carr MJ. 2010. Targeting primary afferent nerves for novel antitussive therapy. *Chest* 137: 177–184.

47. Schild JH, Kunze DL. 1997. Experimental and modeling study of Na^+ current heterogeneity in rat nodose neurons and its impact on neuronal discharge. *J Neurophysiol* 78: 3198–3209.

48. Farrag KJ, Costa SK, Docherty RJ. 2002. Differential sensitivity to tetrodotoxin and lack of effect of prostaglandin E on the pharmacology and physiology of propagated action potentials. *Br J Pharmacol* 135: 1449–1456.

49. Park TJ, et al. 2008. Selective inflammatory pain insensitivity in the African naked mole-rat (*Heterocephalus glaber*). *PLoS Biol* 6: e13.

50. Singh NA, et al. 2009. A role of *SCN9A* in human epilepsy, as a cause of febrile seizures and as a potential modifier of Dravet syndrome. *PLoS Genet* 5: e1000649.

51. Drenth JP, Waxman SG. 2007. Mutations in sodium-channel gene *SCN9A* cause a spectrum of human genetic pain disorders. *J Clin Invest* 117: 3603–3609.

52. Devor M. 2006. Sodium channels and mechanisms of neuropathic pain. *J Pain* 7: S3–S12.

53. Lyu YS, Park SK, Chung K, Chung JM. 2000. Low dose of tetrodotoxin reduces neuropathic pain behaviors in an animal model. *Brain Res* 871: 98–103.

54. Black JA, Nikolajsen L, Kroner K, Jensen TS, Waxman SG. 2008. Multiple sodium channel isoforms and mitogen-activated protein kinases are present in painful human neuromas. *Ann Neurol* 64: 644–653. [This study demonstrates the presence of sodium channels $Na_V1.3$, $Na_V1.7$ and $Na_V1.8$, and activated MAPK1, MAPK3 and MAPK12 within blind axon terminals of painful human neuromas.]

55. Stamboulian S, et al. 2010. ERK1/2 mitogen-activated protein kinase phosphorylates sodium channel $Na_V1.7$ and alters its gating properties. *J Neurosci* 30: 1637–1647.

56. Black JA, Liu S, Tanaka M, Cummins TR, Waxman SG. 2004. Changes in the expression of tetrodotoxin-sensitive sodium channels within dorsal root ganglia neurons in inflammatory pain. *Pain* 108: 237–247.

57. Gould HJ, et al. 2004. Ibuprofen blocks changes in Na$_V$1.7 and 1.8 sodium channels associated with complete Freund's adjuvant-induced inflammation in rat. *J Pain* 5: 270–280.

58. Chattopadhyay M, Mata M, Fink DJ. 2008. Continuous δ-opioid receptor activation reduces neuronal voltage-gated sodium channel (Na$_V$1.7) levels through activation of protein kinase C in painful diabetic neuropathy. *J Neurosci* 28: 6652–6658.

59. Chattopadhyay M, Mata M, Fink DJ. 2011. Vector-mediated release of GABA attenuates pain-related behaviors and reduces Na$_V$1.7 in DRG neurons. *Eur J Pain* 15: 913–920.

60. Yeomans DC, et al. 2005. Decrease in inflammatory hyperalgesia by Herpes vector-mediated knockdown of Na$_V$1.7 sodium channels in primary afferents. *Hum Gene Ther* 16: 271–277.

61. Chattopadhyay M, Zhou Z, Hao S, Mata M, Fink DJ. 2012. Reduction of voltage gated sodium channel protein in DRG by vector mediated miRNA reduces pain in rats with painful diabetic neuropathy. *Mol Pain* 8: 17.

62. Minett MS et al. 2012. Distinct Na$_V$1.7-dependent pain sensations require different sets of sensory and sympathetic neurons. *Nature Commun* 3: 791. [This study suggests that knockout of Na$_V$1.7 in neurons from DRG and sympathetic ganglia is needed to attenuate neuropathic pain.]

63. Shields SD, et al. 2012. Sodium channel Na$_V$1.7 is essential for lowering heat pain threshold after burn injury. *J Neurosci* 32: 10819–10832.

64. Yang Y, et al. 2004. Mutations in *SCN9A*, encoding a sodium channel α subunit, in patients with primary erythermalgia. *J Med Genet* 41: 171–174. [This report identifies gain-of-function mutations in SCN9A in patients with IEM.]

65. Fertleman CR, et al. 2006. *SCN9A* mutations in paroxysmal extreme pain disorder: Allelic variants underlie distinct channel defects and phenotypes. *Neuron* 52: 767–774. [This study identifies and characterizes gain-of-function mutations in SCN9A in patients with PEPD.]

66. Cox JJ, et al. 2006. An *SCN9A* channelopathy causes congenital inability to experience pain. *Nature* 444: 894–898. [This study identifies and characterizes loss-of-function mutations in SCN9A that underlie CIP.]

67. Sheets PL, Jackson Ii JO, Waxman SG, Dib-Hajj S, Cummins TRA. 2007. Na$_V$1.7 channel mutation associated with hereditary erythromelalgia contributes to neuronal hyperexcitability and displays reduced lidocaine sensitivity. *J Physiol* 581: 1019–1031.

68. Cheng X, et al. 2011. Deletion mutation of sodium channel Na$_V$1.7 in inherited erythromelalgia: Enhanced slow inactivation modulates dorsal root ganglion neuron hyperexcitability. *Brain* 134: 1972–1986.

69. Fertleman CR, et al. 2007. Paroxysmal extreme pain disorder (previously familial rectal pain syndrome). *Neurology* 69: 586–595.

70. Choi JS, et al. 2011. Paroxysmal extreme pain disorder: A molecular lesion of peripheral neurons. *Nat Rev Neurol* 7: 51–55.

71. Estacion M, et al. 2008. Na$_V$1.7 gain-of-function mutations as a continuum: A1632E displays physiological changes associated with erythromelalgia and paroxysmal extreme pain disorder mutations and produces symptoms of both disorders. *J Neurosci* 28: 11079–11088.

72. Dib-Hajj SD, et al. 2008. Paroxysmal extreme pain disorder M1627K mutation in human Na$_V$1.7 renders DRG neurons hyperexcitable. *Mol Pain* 4: 37.

73. Cheng X, et al. 2010. Mutations at opposite ends of the DIII/S4–S5 linker of sodium channel Na$_V$1.7 produce distinct pain disorders. *Mol Pain* 6: 24.

74. Vasylyev DV, Waxman SG. 2012. Membrane properties and electrogenesis in the distal axons of small dorsal root ganglion neurons *in vitro*. *J Neurophysiol* 108: 729–740.

75. Han C, et al. 2009. Early- and late-onset inherited erythromelalgia: Genotype–phenotype correlation. *Brain* 132: 1711–1722.

76. Harty TP, et al. 2006. Na$_V$1.7 mutant A863P in erythromelalgia: Effects of altered activation and steady-state inactivation on excitability of nociceptive dorsal root ganglion neurons. *J Neurosci* 26: 12566–12575.

77. Ahmad S, et al. 2007. A stop codon mutation in *SCN9A* causes lack of pain sensation. *Hum Mol Genet* 16: 2114–2121.

78. Kurban M, Wajid M, Shimomura Y, Christiano AM. 2010. A nonsense mutation in the *SCN9A* gene in congenital insensitivity to pain. *Dermatology* 221: 179–183.

79. Staud R, et al. 2011. Two novel mutations of *SCN9A* (Na$_V$1.7) are associated with partial congenital insensitivity to pain. *Eur J Pain* 15: 223–230.

80. Reich DE, Lander ES. 2001. On the allelic spectrum of human disease. *Trends Genet* 17: 502–510.

81. Estacion M, et al. 2009. A sodium channel gene *SCN9A* polymorphism that increases nociceptor excitability. *Ann Neurol* 66: 862–866. [This report identifies and

characterizes a common variant of SCN9A that is associated with pain.]

82. Reimann F, et al. 2010. Pain perception is altered by a nucleotide polymorphism in SCN9A. Proc Natl Acad Sci USA 107: 5148–5153.

83. Estacion M, et al. 2011. Intra- and interfamily phenotypic diversity in pain syndromes associated with a gain-of-function variant of $Na_V1.7$. Mol Pain 7: 92.

84. Choi JS, Waxman SG. 2011. Physiological interactions between $Na_V1.7$ and $Na_V1.8$ sodium channels: A computer simulation study. J Neurophysiol 106: 3173–3184.

85. Doyle DA, et al. 1998. The structure of the potassium channel: Molecular basis of K^+ conduction and selectivity. Science 280: 69–77.

86. Jiang Y, et al. 2002. The open pore conformation of potassium channels. Nature 417: 523–526.

87. Long SB, Campbell EB, Mackinnon R. 2005. Crystal structure of a mammalian voltage-dependent Shaker family K^+ channel. Science 309: 897–903.

88. Ren D, et al. 2001. A prokaryotic voltage-gated sodium channel. Science 294: 2372–2375.

89. Charalambous K, Wallace BA. 2011. NaChBac: The long lost sodium channel ancestor. Biochemistry 50: 6742–6752.

90. Lampert A, Dib-Hajj SD, Tyrrell L, Waxman SG. 2006. Size matters: Erythromelalgia mutation S241T in $Na_V1.7$ alters channel gating. J Biol Chem 281: 36029–36035.

91. Tsujino A, et al. 2003. Myasthenic syndrome caused by mutation of the SCN4A sodium channel. Proc Natl Acad Sci USA 100: 7377–7382.

92. Lampert A, et al. 2008. A pore-blocking hydrophobic motif at the cytoplasmic aperture of the closed-state $Na_V1.7$ channel is disrupted by the erythromelalgia-associated F1449V mutation. J Biol Chem 283: 24118–24127. [An atomic structural modelling of $Na_V1.7$ based on the potassium channel KcsA crystal structure identifies a putative activation gate.]

93. Burley SK, Petsko GA. 1985. Aromatic–aromatic interaction: A mechanism of protein structure stabilization. Science 229: 23–28.

94. Dib-Hajj SD, et al. 2005. Gain-of-function mutation in $Na_V1.7$ in familial erythromelalgia induces bursting of sensory neurons. Brain 128: 1847–1854. [The first demonstration that a gain-of-function familial mutation in SCN9A renders DRG neurons hyperexcitable, thus providing the pathophysiological basis for pain in these patients.]

95. Rojas A, Wu J, Wang R, Jiang C. 2007. Gating of the ATP-sensitive K^+ channel by a pore-lining phenylalanine residue. Biochim Biophys Acta 1768: 39–51.

96. Han C, et al. 2012. Functional profiles of SCN9A variants in dorsal root ganglion neurons and superior cervical ganglion neurons correlate with autonomic symptoms in small fibre neuropathy. Brain 135: 2613–2628.

97. Akopian AN, Sivilotti L, Wood JN. 1996. A tetrodotoxin-resistant voltage-gated sodium channel expressed by sensory neurons. Nature 379: 257–262.

98. Akopian AN, et al. 1999. The tetrodotoxin-resistant sodium channel SNS has a specialized function in pain pathways. Nature Neurosci 2: 541–548. [Together with reference 97, these studies were the first to identify and characterize $Na_V1.8$ from DRG neurons and demonstrates a role for this channel in pain.]

99. Sangameswaran L, et al. 1996. Structure and function of a novel voltage-gated, tetrodoxtoxin-resistant sodium channel specific to sensory neurons. J Biol Chem 271: 5953–5956.

100. England S, de Groot MJ. 2009. Subtype-selective targeting of voltage-gated sodium channels. Br J Pharmacol 158: 1413–1425.

101. Choi JS, et al. 2009. Mexiletine-responsive erythromelalgia due to a new $Na_V1.7$ mutation showing use-dependent current fall-off. Exp Neurol 216: 383–389.

102. Fischer TZ, et al. 2009. A novel $Na_V1.7$ mutation producing carbamazepine-responsive erythromelalgia. Ann Neurol 65: 733–741. [This study identifies the SCN9A mutation V400M in patients who responded to treatment with carbamazepine, and demonstrates that this mutation increases responsiveness to carbamazepine without altering the affinity of the channel to the drug.]

103. Yang Y, et al. 2012. Structural modelling and mutant cycle analysis predict pharmacoresponsiveness of a $Na_V1.7$ mutant channel. Nature Commun 3: 1186. [Using V400M as a 'seed' SCN9A mutation, this atomic structural modelling and thermodynamic coupling analysis predicts and then confirms that a second SCN9A mutation, S241T, is responsive to carbamazepine.]

104. Williams BS, et al. 2007. Characterization of a new class of potent inhibitors of the voltage-gated sodium channel $Na_V1.7$. Biochemistry 46: 14693–14703.

105. London C, et al. 2008. Imidazopyridines: A novel class of $hNa_V1.7$ channel blockers. Bioorg Med Chem Lett 18: 1696–1701.

106. Bregman H, et al. 2011. Identification of a potent, state-dependent inhibitor of $Na_V1.7$ with oral efficacy in the formalin model of persistent pain. J Med Chem 54: 4427–4445.

107. Chowdhury S, et al. 2011. Discovery of XEN907, a spirooxindole blocker of Na$_V$1.7 for the treatment of pain. *Bioorg Med Chem Lett* 21: 3676–3681.

108. Chapman ML, et al. 2012. Characterization of a novel subtype-selective inhibitor of human Na$_V$1.7 voltage-dependent sodium channels (PT 418). *IASP 14th World Congress on Pain [online]*, http://www.abstracts2view.com/iasp/sessionindex.php.

109. Rice AS, Hill RG. 2006. New treatments for neuropathic pain. *Annu Rev Med* 57: 535–551.

110. Dworkin RH, et al. 2007. Pharmacologic management of neuropathic pain: Evidence-based recommendations. *Pain* 132: 237–251.

111. Sindrup SH, Jensen TS. 2007. Are sodium channel blockers useless in peripheral neuropathic pain? *Pain* 128: 6–7.

112. Gerner P, Strichartz GR. 2008. Sensory and motor complications of local anesthetics. *Muscle Nerve* 37: 421–425.

113. Beyreuther B, Callizot N, Stohr T. 2006. Antinociceptive efficacy of lacosamide in a rat model for painful diabetic neuropathy. *Eur J Pharmacol* 539: 64–70.

114. Beyreuther BK, et al. 2007. Antinociceptive efficacy of lacosamide in rat models for tumor- and chemotherapy-induced cancer pain. *Eur J Pharmacol* 565: 98–104.

115. Hao JX, Stohr T, Selve N, Wiesenfeld-Hallin Z, Xu XJ. 2006. Lacosamide, a new anti-epileptic, alleviates neuropathic pain-like behaviors in rat models of spinal cord or trigeminal nerve injury. *Eur J Pharmacol* 553: 135–140.

116. Stohr T, et al. 2007. Lacosamide, a novel anticonvulsant drug, shows efficacy with a wide safety margin in rodent models for epilepsy. *Epilepsy Res* 74: 147–154.

117. Doty P, Rudd GD, Stoehr T, Thomas D. 2007. Lacosamide. *Neurotherapeutics* 4: 145–148.

118. Rauck RL, Shaibani A, Biton V, Simpson J, Koch B. 2007. Lacosamide in painful diabetic peripheral neuropathy: A phase 2 double-blind placebo-controlled study. *Clin J Pain* 23: 150–158.

119. Sheets PL, Heers C, Stoehr T, Cummins TR. 2008. Differential block of sensory neuronal voltage-gated sodium channels by lacosamide [(2R)-2-(acetylamino)-N-benzyl-3-methoxypropanamide], lidocaine, and carbamazepine. *J Pharmacol Exp Ther* 326: 89–99.

120. Xu GY, Zhao ZQ. 2001. Change in excitability and phenotype of substance P and its receptor in cat Aβ sensory neurons following peripheral inflammation. *Brain Res* 923: 112–119.

121. Dworkin RH, et al. 2010. Recommendations for the pharmacological management of neuropathic pain: An overview and literature update. *Mayo Clin Proc* 85: S3–S14.

122. Wilson MJ, et al. 2011. μ-Conotoxins that differentially block sodium channels Na$_V$1.1 through 1.8 identify those responsible for action potentials in sciatic nerve. *Proc Natl Acad Sci USA* 108: 10302–10307.

123. Lewis RJ, Dutertre S, Vetter I, Christie MJ. 2012. Conus venom peptide pharmacology. *Pharmacol Rev* 64: 259–298.

124. Dib-Hajj SD, et al. 2009. Voltage-gated sodium channels in pain states: Role in pathophysiology and targets for treatment. *Brain Res Brain Res Rev* 60: 65–83.

125. Middleton RE, et al. 2002. Two tarantula peptides inhibit activation of multiple sodium channels. *Biochemistry* 41: 14734–14747.

126. Smith JJ, Cummins TR, Alphy S, Blumenthal KM. 2007. Molecular interactions of the gating modifier toxin ProTx-II with Na$_V$1.5: Implied existence of a novel toxin binding site coupled to activation. *J Biol Chem* 282: 12687–12697.

127. Peng K, Shu Q, Liu Z, Liang S. 2002. Function and solution structure of huwentoxin-IV, a potent neuronal tetrodotoxin (TTX)-sensitive sodium channel antagonist from Chinese bird spider *Selenocosmia huwena*. *J Biol Chem* 277: 47564–47571.

128. Xiao Y, et al. 2008. Tarantula huwentoxin-IV inhibits neuronal sodium channels by binding to receptor site 4 and trapping the domain II voltage sensor in the closed configuration. *J Biol Chem* 283: 27300–27313.

129. McArthur JR, et al. 2011. Interactions of key charged residues contributing to selective block of neuronal sodium channels by μ-conotoxin KIIIA. *Mol Pharmacol* 80: 573–584.

130. Clark RJ, Akcan M, Kaas Q, Daly NL, Craik DJ. 2012. Cyclization of conotoxins to improve their biopharmaceutical properties. *Toxicon* 59: 446–455.

131. Fink DJ, et al. 2012. Gene therapy for pain: Results of a phase I clinical trial. *Ann Neurol* 70: 207–212.

132. Samad OA, et al. 2012. Virus-mediated shRNA knockdown of Na$_V$1.3 in rat dorsal root ganglion attenuates nerve injury-induced neuropathic pain. *Mol Ther* 21: doi:10.1038/mt.2012.169.

133. Firestein S. 2001. How the olfactory system makes sense of scents. *Nature* 413: 211–218.

134. Kaupp UB. 2010. Olfactory signalling in vertebrates and insects: Differences and commonalities. *Nat Rev Neurosci* 11: 188–200.

135. Rajendra S, Lynch JW, Barry PH. 1992. An analysis of Na$^+$ currents in rat olfactory receptor neurons. *Pflugers Arch* 420: 342–346.

136. Cummins TR, Dib-Hajj SD, Waxman SG. 2004. Electrophysiological properties of mutant Na$_V$1.7 sodium channels in a painful inherited neuropathy. *J Neurosci* 24: 8232–8236. [The first demonstration that mutations in SCN9A from patients with IEM manifest gain-of-function attributes.]

137. Blair NT, Bean BP. 2002. Roles of tetrodotoxin (TTX)-sensitive Na$^+$ current, TTX-resistant Na$^+$ current, and Ca^{2+} current in the action potentials of nociceptive sensory neurons. *J Neurosci* 22: 10277–10290.

138. Cummins TR, Waxman SG. 1997. Downregulation of tetrodotoxin-resistant sodium currents and upregulation of a rapidly repriming tetrodotoxin-sensitive sodium current in small spinal sensory neurons after nerve injury. *J Neurosci* 17: 3503–3514.

139. Elliott AA, Elliott JR. 1993. Characterization of TTX-sensitive and TTX-resistant sodium currents in small cells from adult rat dorsal root ganglia. *J Physiol* 463: 39–56.

140. Cheng X, Dib-Hajj SD, Tyrrell L, Waxman SG. 2008. Mutation I136V alters electrophysiological properties of the Na$_V$1.7 channel in a family with onset of erythromelalgia in the second decade. *Mol Pain* 4: 1.

141. Han C, et al. 2012. Na$_V$1.7-related small fiber neuropathy: Impaired slow-inactivation and DRG neuron hyperexcitability. *Neurology* 78: 1635–1643.

5 TWO SIDES OF ONE COIN

A mutation—a change in a single gene—is termed "pathogenic" when it alters the gene product in a way that causes disease. Within the human genome, there are more than 20,000 genes. Each one of the cells within our body contains all of these 20,000 genes. Yet many mutations selectively impact some tissues or cell types, leaving others unaffected. An example is provided by sickle cell anemia. In this hereditary disorder, a mutation of the *HBB* gene results in production of an abnormal form of β-globin which is a component of hemoglobin, the iron-containing protein that carries oxygen within the blood from the lungs to other tissues throughout the body. Hemoglobin is present only in red blood cells, and these cells are profoundly affected by the *HBB* mutation, taking on a sickle shape and failing in their oxygen-carrying duty, while other types of cells within the body are unaffected. There are other genes, however, that are expressed in multiple cell types, and when these genes are mutated, each of these cell types is at risk. The paper that follows (Rush et al. 2006) illustrates an interesting complexity of biology: *A single mutation can have different effects in different cell types.* This phenomenon is, in part, a result of differences in "cell background." The mutant protein may interact with one set of protein partners in cell type A, while interacting with a different set of protein partners in cell type B, or may be subject to one set of biological processes in cell type A while being subject to a different set of biological processes in cell type B.

The $Na_V1.7$ sodium channel is present at high levels in two types of peripheral neurons: DRG sensory neurons that innervate the body, including pain-signaling neurons; and sympathetic ganglion neurons, located on either side of the spinal column as the most distal outposts of the sympathetic component of the autonomic nervous system. Sympathetic ganglion neurons participate in the regulation of many homeostatic mechanisms within the body including the control of blood vessel diameter.

Without even entering the laboratory, a skilled observer might conclude that autonomic function is affected in erythromelalgia, since the pain attacks in this disorder are accompanied by dramatic reddening of the skin. Although there was no evidence at the molecular level, this aspect of erythromelalgia had been attributed by others (Mork, Kalgaard, and Kvernebo 2002; Davis et al. 2003) to an abnormality of blood vessels or disturbed vasomotor control, i.e., an abnormality of neurons such as sympathetic ganglion neurons that control the width of blood vessels that irrigate the skin. Indeed, some patients who do not carry mutations of $Na_V1.7$ develop "secondary" erythromelalgia as a result of having disorders of the blood that interfere with blood flow, such as abnormalities of the platelets that interfere with circulation, and these patients respond well to treatment with aspirin, which inhibits the action of platelets (Drenth, van Genderen, and Michiels 1994).

We addressed this issue in a paper by Rush et al. (Rush et al. 2006) by assessing the effect of a $Na_V1.7$ mutation that had been identified in a patient with painful inherited erythromelalgia within both DRG neurons and neurons from a sympathetic ganglion (the superior cervical sympathetic ganglion). We expected from our previous studies that the mutation would produce hyperexcitability within DRG neurons, but in the absence of any prior experimental results we did not know what to expect in sympathetic ganglion neurons. In the initial part of this study, we expressed the $Na_V1.7$ mutant channel in

DRG neurons, and then in sympathetic ganglion neurons. In DRG neurons, we found that the mutant channels depolarized the resting membrane potential, which we had expected because the mutation hyperpolarizes channel activation. The shift in activation increases the overlap between activation and inactivation so as to produce an enhanced persistent current called, by electrophysiologists, a "window" current. Consistent with the idea that inappropriate firing of pain-signaling neurons underlies the pain experienced by this patient, we found that the mutation produces hyperexcitability of DRG neurons, manifested by a decrease in threshold (the amount of current needed to produce a single action potential) and an increase in the firing rate in response to graded suprathreshold stimulation.

The results in sympathetic ganglion neurons were strikingly different. We found that, as expected, the mutation depolarizes the resting potential of sympathetic ganglion neurons. To our surprise, however, we observed that, rather than rendering these cells hyperexcitable, the mutant channels had the opposite effect, reducing the excitability of sympathetic ganglion neurons, by increasing their threshold and decreasing their firing rate in response to graded suprathreshold stimulation. Repeating our experiments several times, we again and again observed that a $Na_V1.7$ mutant channel could have different functional effects in different types of cells. Indeed, the $Na_V1.7$ mutant channels produced opposite effects in the two types of neurons that express $Na_V1.7$, *hyper*excitability in pain-signaling sensory neurons and *hypo*excitability in sympathetic ganglion neurons.

We had expected that the mutant channels might have different effects on the behavior of sensory and sympathetic ganglion neurons, but we had not anticipated the dramatic result of the experiment, with a single mutation having totally opposite effects in two different types of neurons. When a scientist makes an unexpected observation, one next step is to ask "why?" Reasoning that the effect of the mutant channel within each specific cell type would be shaped not just by the presence of the $Na_V1.7$ mutant channel, but also by the presence of the mutant channel within a specific cell background—which reflects the entire ensemble of ion channels present in each type of neuron—we measured mRNA and protein for various types of sodium channels in the two types of cells. This analysis showed us that DRG neurons express five types of sodium channels, $Na_V1.1$, $Na_V1.6$, $Na_V1.7$, $Na_V1.8$, and $Na_V1.9$, while sympathetic ganglion neurons express a different ensemble of sodium channels, $Na_V1.3$, $Na_V1.6$, and $Na_V1.7$.

This is a very important difference, especially since the mutant $Na_V1.7$ depolarizes cells. Most sodium channels are "inactivated" or put to sleep so they are not available for operation, by prolonged depolarization. The $Na_V1.8$ sodium channel, which was originally called SNS because it is sensory neurons specific, is different. $Na_V1.8$ is present in DRG neurons but not in sympathetic ganglion neurons. And $Na_V1.8$ is remarkable in that, unlike other sodium channels which are silenced by depolarization, $Na_V1.8$ is relatively resistant to inactivation (Akopian, Sivilotti, and Wood 1996; Cummins and Waxman 1997). We had shown a few years earlier that a major functional role of $Na_V1.8$ is to support high-frequency firing in response to sustained depolarization in cells to which it is present (Renganathan, Cummins, and Waxman 2001). These earlier results suggested that the presence of $Na_V1.8$ in DRG neurons, and its absence in sympathetic ganglion neurons, could have accounted for the different effects of the $Na_V1.7$ mutation in these two types of cells. We set out to test the hypothesis, illustrated in figure 5.1, whereby (1) the $Na_V1.7$ mutant channel depolarizes both sympathetic ganglion neurons and pain-signaling DRG neurons; (2) as a result of this depolarization, the sodium channels within sympathetic ganglion neurons are inactivated and it is harder for these cells to generate action potentials so that they become hypoexcitable; but (3) because $Na_V1.8$ channels are present within pain-signaling DRG neurons, and are not inactivated by depolarization, these cells do not become hypoexcitable but, on the contrary, become hyperexcitable, because the depolarization brings the membrane potential closer to threshold for activation of the Na$_V$1.8 channels. According to this hypothesis, the presence or absence of a single type of molecule, the Na$_V$1.8 sodium channel, was critically important in determining whether a neuron would become hyperexcitable or hypoexcitable as a result of expression of Na$_V$1.7 mutant channels within it.

We tested this hypothesis in the experiment shown in figure 5 in Rush et al. (2006). In this experiment we asked whether we could convert a sympathetic ganglion neuron into a cell with properties similar to those of a DRG neuron, by inserting Na$_V$1.8 channels within it. Insertion of the gene for Na$_V$1.8 alongside the gene for the mutant Na$_V$1.7 channel within sympathetic ganglion neurons was not easy, but Sulayman Dib-Hajj and our molecular biology team were successful in this effort, and the newly inserted genes produced their channels within their new host cells. Remarkably, we found that, indeed, it is possible to flip a sympathetic ganglion neuron expressing a mutant Na$_V$1.7 channel from hypoexcitability, to hyperexcitability, by inserting Na$_V$1.8 channels within it. We had essentially isolated a single molecule—Na$_V$1.8—that was responsible for the opposing effects of Na$_V$1.7 mutant channels within the two cell-types where Na$_V$1.7 is present. These experiments taught us two lessons: first, that a single mutation can have dramatically different effects on the firing properties of different types of neurons; and second, that Na$_V$1.8 acts as a molecular switch, with its presence or absence determining whether Na$_V$1.7 mutations produce hyper- or hypoexcitability.

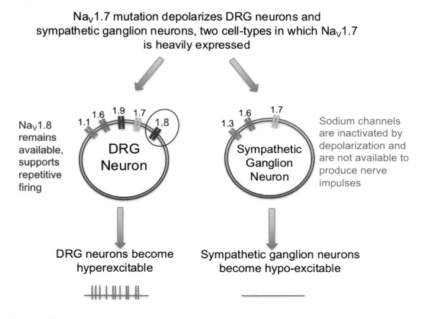

Figure 5.1
Scheme by which Na$_V$1.7 mutations, which depolarize resting membrane potential, produce hyperexcitability in dorsal root ganglion (DRG) neurons and hypoexcitability in sympathetic ganglion neurons. Note the enhanced action potential activity below the DRG neuron expressing the Na$_V$1.7 mutation, in contrast to the electrical silence of the sympathetic ganglion neuron.

There was even more to the story. In subsequent studies, carried out together with Frank Rice, an expert on skin, we showed that Na$_V$1.7 is also present within vascular myocytes, the muscle cells that form the walls of blood vessels within the skin (Rice et al. 2015). In these muscle cells, Na$_V$1.8 is not present. We hypothesized that Na$_V$1.7 mutations that depolarize resting potential produce hypoexcitability within these vascular muscle cells, thereby perturbing blood flow within the skin. We are currently testing this hypothesis, which would introduce another factor that contributes to the abnormal reddening of the limbs in people with erythromelalgia.

It is not often that one gets to see, in precise detail, how molecules like ion channels interact with each other. The Rush et al. (2006) paper provides an example of how a team effort—in this case combining ion channel biophysics, cellular electrophysiology, and molecular biology—allowed us to dissect, molecule by molecule, how a mutant ion channel interacts with other ion channels in its cellular environment.

References

Akopian AN, Sivilotti L, Wood JN. 1996. A tetrodotoxin-resistant voltage-gated sodium channel expressed by sensory neurons. *Nature* 379(6562): 257–262.

Cummins TR, Waxman SG. 1997. Downregulation of tetrodotoxin-resistant sodium currents and upregulation of a rapidly repriming tetrodotoxin-sensitive sodium current in small spinal sensory neurons after nerve injury. *J Neurosci* 17(10): 3503–3514.

Davis MD, Sandroni P, Rooke TW, Low PA. 2003. Erythromelalgia: Vasculopathy, neuropathy, or both? A prospective study of vascular and neurophysiologic studies in erythromelalgia. *Arch Dermatol* 139(10): 1337–1343.

Drenth JP, van Genderen PJ, Michiels JJ. 1994. Thrombocythemic erythromelalgia, primary erythermalgia, and secondary erythermalgia: Three distinct clinicopathologic entities. *Angiology* 45(6): 451–453.

Mork C, Kalgaard OM, Kvernebo K. 2002. Impaired neurogenic control of skin perfusion in erythromelalgia. *J Invest Dermatol* 118(4): 699–703.

Renganathan M, Cummins TR, Waxman SG. 2001. Contribution of Na(v)1.8 sodium channels to action potential electrogenesis in DRG neurons. *J Neurophysiol* 86(2): 629–640.

Rice FL, Albrecht PJ, Wymer JP, Black JA, Merkies IS, Faber CG, Waxman SG. 2015. Sodium channel Na$_V$1.7 in vascular myocytes, endothelium, and innervating axons in human skin. *Mol Pain* 11: 26.

Rush AM, Dib-Hajj SD, Liu S, Cummins TR, Black JA, Waxman SG. 2006. A single sodium channel mutation produces hyper- or hypoexcitability in different types of neurons. *Proc Natl Acad Sci USA* 103(21): 8245–8250.

A SINGLE SODIUM CHANNEL MUTATION PRODUCES HYPER- OR HYPOEXCITABILITY IN DIFFERENT TYPES OF NEURONS*

Anthony M. Rush, Sulayman D. Dib-Hajj, Shujun Liu, Theodore R. Cummins, Joel A. Black, and Stephen G. Waxman

Disease-producing mutations of ion channels are usually characterized as producing hyperexcitability or hypoexcitability. We show here that a single mutation can produce hyperexcitability in one neuronal cell type and hypoexcitability in another neuronal cell type. We studied the functional effects of a mutation of sodium channel $Na_V1.7$ associated with a neuropathic pain syndrome, erythermalgia, within sensory and sympathetic ganglion neurons, two cell types where $Na_V1.7$ is normally expressed. Although this mutation depolarizes resting membrane potential in both types of neurons, it renders sensory neurons hyperexcitable and sympathetic neurons hypoexcitable. The selective presence, in sensory but not sympathetic neurons, of the $Na_V1.8$ channel, which remains available for activation at depolarized membrane potentials, is a major determinant of these opposing effects. These results provide a molecular basis for the sympathetic dysfunction that has been observed in erythermalgia. Moreover, these findings show that a single ion channel mutation can produce opposing phenotypes (hyperexcitability or hypoexcitability) in the different cell types in which the channel is expressed.

Mutations in voltage-gated sodium channels have been associated with a number of neurological disorders including inherited epilepsy, muscle disorders, and primary erythermalgia, an autosomal dominant neuropathy characterized by pain of the extremities in response to mild warmth. Recent studies have demonstrated mutations in primary erythermalgia in $Na_V1.7$ (ref. 1), a sodium channel that is preferentially expressed within primary sensory [such as nociceptive dorsal root ganglion (DRG)] and sympathetic

* Previously published in *Proceedings of the National Academy of Sciences of the* United States of America 103: 8245–8250, 2006. © 2006 by The National Academy of Sciences of the USA.

ganglion [e.g., superior cervical ganglion (SCG)] neurons.[2–6] The $Na_V1.7$ mutations characterized to date produce changes in channel physiology that include hyperpolarizing shifts in activation, depolarizing shifts in steady-state inactivation, slowing of deactivation, and an increase in the "ramp" current evoked by slow, small depolarizations, all augmenting the response of $Na_V1.7$ channels to small stimuli.[3,6,7] One of these mutations, F1449V, has been assessed at the level of cell function within DRG neurons, where it produces hyperexcitability.[3] However, the effects on cell function of $Na_V1.7$ mutations have not been assessed in sympathetic ganglion neurons, where $Na_V1.7$ is also present.

Because different ensembles of channels are present within DRG and SCG neurons, we hypothesized that the same sodium channel mutation might have different effects on excitability in these two neuronal types. Here we test this hypothesis for one of the first $Na_V1.7$ erythermalgia mutations to be characterized, L858H.[2,7] We show that although the L858H mutation produces a depolarizing shift in resting membrane potential (RMP) in both cell types, it renders DRG neurons hyperexcitable and SCG neurons hypoexcitable. We demonstrate that the opposing functional effects of this mutation are a result of the selective presence of another sodium channel, $Na_V1.8$, in DRG, but not SCG, neurons. These results suggest a contribution of $Na_V1.7$ mutant channels to the sympathetic dysfunction that has been reported in erythermalgia. More generally, these observations show that a single mutation can cause functionally opposing changes in the different types of neurons in which the gene is expressed.

Results

L858H Mutation Produces Depolarization of RMP and Decreases Action Potential Threshold in DRG Neurons

Figure 1 shows the effect of the $Na_V1.7$/L858H mutation (L858H) on firing threshold in DRG neurons, a cell type that is known to express $Na_V1.7$ (refs. 8, 9). DRG neurons expressing wild-type (WT) $Na_V1.7$ produced robust overshooting action potentials in response to stepwise current inputs. The representative cell shown in figure 1A, with a RMP of approximately –51 mV, produced subthreshold responses to 50- to 130-pA current injections and required a $\geq$135-pA input to elicit an all-or-none action potential that arose at a voltage threshold of approximately –15 mV.

In contrast, the RMP is approximately –46 mV, i.e., is depolarized by $\approx$5 mV, in a representative DRG neuron expressing L858H mutant channels, and this cell required a much lower current input of only 60 pA for firing (figure 1B). For the entire population of cells studied, the average RMP of DRG cells expressing L858H was significantly more depolarized (–44.9 $\pm$ 1.1 mV, n = 25) than that of cells expressing WT $Na_V1.7$ (–50.1 $\pm$ 0.9 mV, n = 20) (P < 0.001; figure 1C). The current threshold was significantly decreased, by >40% (P < 0.01), in cells expressing L858H channels (69.2 $\pm$ 9.8 pA, n = 25) compared with WT $Na_V1.7$ (120.6 $\pm$ 23.9 pA, n = 20) (figure 1D). Despite the depolarized RMP and changes in current threshold, action potential overshoot was not significantly different in cells expressing WT $Na_V1.7$ (67.8 $\pm$ 3.0 mV, n = 20) or L858H channels (64.4 $\pm$ 2.6 mV, n = 20) (P > 0.05; figure 1E).

L858H Mutation Produces Depolarization of RMP but Increases Action Potential Threshold in SCG Neurons

We next investigated the functional effects of L858H mutant channels in SCG neurons, which are also known to express $Na_V1.7$ (refs. 8, 9). Figure 2A shows subthreshold responses evoked by 15- to 20-pA current injections from a representative SCG neuron expressing WT $Na_V1.7$ channels, which required current injections of $\geq$25 pA to reach the threshold of approximately –20 mV and fire all-or-none action potentials, from the RMP of –47 mV.

SCG neurons expressing L858H channels showed a depolarization of the RMP by $\approx$5 mV, similarly to DRG neurons, but the effects of L858H on excitability were markedly different. Figure 2B shows a representative SCG neuron where only subthreshold responses were seen with a <70-pA current injection, inputs that produced action potentials with WT $Na_V1.7$ channel expression. When the threshold was reached (approximately –16 mV) with a 70-pA input, the neuron generated an action potential, but it was attenuated, with substantially reduced overshoot. The average RMP of SCG neurons expressing L858H channels was significantly more depolarized (–41.6 $\pm$ 0.8 mV, n = 17) than that of cells expressing WT $Na_V1.7$ channels (–46.3 $\pm$ 0.8 mV, n = 15) (P < 0.001; figure 2C). For the entire population of SCG cells studied, current threshold was significantly increased by $\approx$88% (P < 0.01) in cells expressing L858H (42.9 $\pm$ 6.3 pA, n = 17) compared with WT $Na_V1.7$ channels (22.7 $\pm$ 3.6 pA, n = 15) (figure 2D). In contrast to DRG neurons where action potential overshoot was maintained after expression of L858H, action potential overshoot was significantly reduced by $\approx$50% (P < 0.001) in SCG neurons expressing L858H (23.8 $\pm$ 4.7 mV, n = 20) compared with WT channels (47.8 $\pm$ 3.4 mV, n = 15) (figure 2E). Thus, in contrast to DRG neurons where L858H mutant channels reduce threshold for single action potentials, expression of L858H in SCG neurons has an opposite effect, increasing threshold.

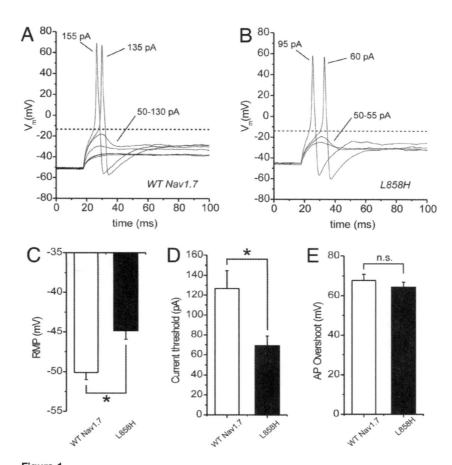

Figure 1

L858H renders DRG neurons hyperexcitable. (A and B) Action potentials were evoked from small (≤ 25 μm in diameter) DRG neurons by using depolarizing current injections from the RMP. V_m, membrane potential. (A) Representative traces from a cell expressing WT Na$_V$1.7 show subthreshold responses to 50- to 130-pA current injections and subsequent all-or-none action potentials evoked by injections of 135 pA (current threshold for this neuron) and 155 pA. (B) In contrast, in a cell expressing L858H, action potentials were evoked by a 60-pA current injection. The voltage for take-off of the all-or-none action potential (approximately –14.5 mV, dashed line) was similar for the neurons in A and B. (C) L858H causes a depolarizing shift in the RMP of DRG neurons. DRG neurons expressing WT Na$_V$1.7 had an average RMP of –50.1 $\pm$ 0.9 mV ($n = 20$), whereas those expressing L858H mutant channels had a significantly (*, $P < 0.001$) depolarized RMP of –44.9 $\pm$ 1.1 ($n = 25$). (D) The average current threshold for action potential firing of DRG neurons expressing WT Na$_V$1.7 channels was 120.6 $\pm$ 23.9 pA ($n = 20$), whereas that of neurons expressing L858H mutant channels was significantly (*, $P < 0.01$) reduced to 69.2 $\pm$ 9.8 pA ($n = 25$). (E) Action potential overshoot in cells expressing WT Na$_V$1.7 channels (67.8 $\pm$ 3.0 mV, $n = 20$) was not significantly different from that in cells expressing L858H mutant channels (64.4 $\pm$ 2.6 mV, $n = 20$; $P > 0.05$). The voltage of action potential take-off was unchanged (WT, –14.5 $\pm$ 1.2 mV, $n = 20$; L858H, –14.5 $\pm$ 1.3 mV, $n = 25$; $P > 0.05$). n.s., not significant.

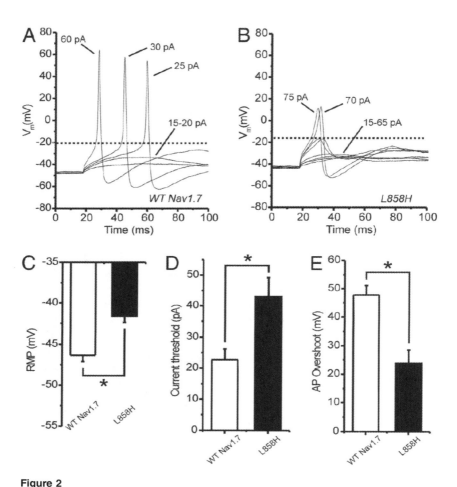

Figure 2

L858H renders SCG neurons hypoexcitable. (A and B) Action potentials were evoked by using depolarizing current injections from resting potential. (A) Representative traces from a cell expressing the WT channel show subthreshold responses to 15- to 20-pA current injections and subsequent all-or-none action potentials evoked by injections of $\geq$25 pA. (B) In contrast, in a cell expressing the L858H channel, action potentials required a $\geq$70-pA current injection. The voltage for take-off (dashed line) of the all-or-none action potential was unchanged. (C) L858H channels caused a depolarizing shift in the RMP of SCG neurons. SCG neurons expressing WT channels had an average RMP of -46.3 ± 0.8 mV ($n = 15$), whereas those expressing L858H had a significantly ($P < 0.001$) depolarized RMP of -41.6 ± 0.8 ($n = 17$). (D) The average current threshold for action potential firing of SCG neurons expressing WT channels was 22.7 ± 3.6 pA ($n = 15$), whereas that of neurons expressing L858H channels was significantly (*, $P < 0.01$) increased to $42.9 \pm$ pA ($n = 17$). (E) Action potential overshoot in cells expressing WT channels (47.8 ± 3.4 mV, $n = 15$) was significantly larger (*, $P < 0.001$) than that in cells expressing L858H (23.8 ± 4.7 mV, $n = 20$). The voltage of action potential take-off was unchanged (WT, -23.1 ± 1.2 mV, $n = 15$; L858H, -19.8 ± 1.3 mV, $n = 17$; *, $P > 0.05$).

L858H Mutation Enhances Repetitive Firing in DRG Neurons

Previous studies have shown that ≈50% of DRG neurons fire repetitively in response to sustained depolarizing stimuli.[3,10–13] In this study, 65% (13 of 20) of DRG neurons expressing WT $Na_V1.7$ fired two or more action potentials in response to prolonged stimulation. Figure 3A shows a representative DRG neuron that fired one action potential in response to a 950-ms input of 100 pA but was capable of firing multiple action potentials with a higher current injection of 250 pA (figure 3, *inset*). With expression of L858H, a higher proportion of DRG neurons (88%, or 21 of 24) fired two or more action potentials in response to 950-ms current injections. Figure 3B shows a representative DRG neuron expressing L858H, which responded to a 100-pA input with five action potentials, i.e., a higher frequency than for WT $Na_V1.7$ channels. For the entire population of DRG neurons studied, the firing frequency evoked with 50- and 100-pA inputs was increased by ≈550% ($P < 0.05$) and ≈280% ($P < 0.05$), respectively, in neurons with L858H compared with WT $Na_V1.7$ channels (figure 3C).

L858H Mutation Attenuates Repetitive Firing in SCG Neurons

SCG neurons also fired repetitively in response to prolonged stimuli, but, as with threshold, the effect of the L858H mutation was opposite to that in DRG neurons. Ninety-three percent (13 of 14) of SCG neurons expressing WT $Na_V1.7$ channels produced multiple action potentials in response to prolonged stimulation. Figure 3D shows a representative SCG neuron expressing WT $Na_V1.7$, where six action potentials were produced in response to a 950-ms current injection of 40 pA. In contrast, an identical stimulus in a SCG neuron expressing L858H evoked only two action potentials, with substantially reduced overshoot (figure 3E). Interestingly, when this cell was held at –60 mV (a maneuver that

reversed the depolarization induced by L858H), multiple overshooting action potentials could be evoked (figure 3E, *inset*); thus, the intrinsic ability of this neuron to fire repetitive and full-scale action potentials was not impaired. Compared with SCG neurons expressing WT $Na_V1.7$, a decreased proportion (53%, or 8 of 15) of SCG neurons expressing L858H produced two or more action potentials in response to prolonged stimulation. The firing frequency of SCG neurons with L858H channels in response to 950-ms inputs of 30 and 40 pA was substantially reduced by 88% ($P < 0.02$) and 72% ($P < 0.03$), respectively, compared with SCG neurons with WT $Na_V1.7$ channels (figure 3F). Attenuated repetitive firing appeared to be caused by the depolarization of RMP by L858H because, in 91% (10 of 11) of the cells tested, multiple action potential firing could be restored by hyperpolarizing to a holding potential of –60 mV.

SCG Neurons Express $Na_V1.7$ but Not $Na_V1.8$

DRG neurons express $Na_V1.8$ as well as $Na_V1.7$ sodium channels,[8,9,14–16] and action potential generation in these cells involves sequential activation of $Na_V1.7$ and then $Na_V1.8$ (refs. 10, 17, 18). SCG neurons normally express $Na_V1.7$ (refs. 8, 9), but the full complement of sodium channel isoforms within SCG neurons has not been previously defined. We therefore identified the sodium channel isoforms present in SCG neurons and compared them with DRG neurons using multiplex PCR and restriction enzyme polymorphism analysis.[19] Restriction analysis of DRG (figure 4A, lanes 1–9) demonstrated $Na_V1.1$ (lane 2), $Na_V1.6$ (lane 6), $Na_V1.7$ (lane 7), $Na_V1.8$ (lane 8), and $Na_V1.9$ (lane 9) in the cDNA pool, in agreement with previous results.[19] In contrast, profiling of the SCG products (figure 4A, lanes 10–18) demonstrated $Na_V1.3$ (lane 13), $Na_V1.6$ (lane 15), and $Na_V1.7$ (lane 16). We confirmed the presence of $Na_V1.7$ (figure 4Ba) and $Na_V1.8$ (figure 4Bb) protein in adult rat DRG and postnatal day

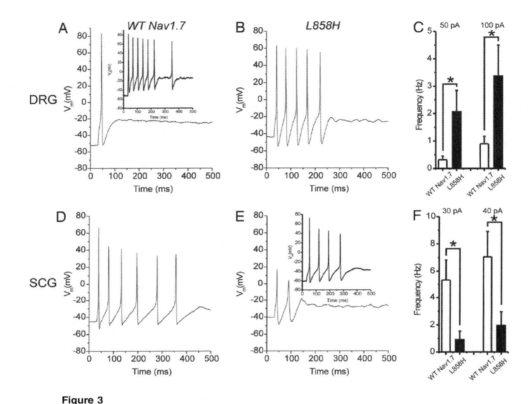

Figure 3

The L858H mutation increases firing frequency in DRG and decreases firing frequency in SCG neurons. (A) Representative DRG neuron expressing WT Na$_V$1.7 fires a single action potential in response to a 950-ms input of 100 pA from the RMP of this neuron (approximately –50 mV). (*Inset*) The same neuron fires multiple action potentials in response to a 250-pA stimulus. (B) Representative DRG neuron expressing L858H fires five action potentials in response to a 100-pA current injection from the RMP of this neuron (approximately –42 mV). (C) For the entire population of DRG neurons studied, the firing frequency evoked by 50-pA current stimuli was 0.32 ± 0.13 Hz after transfection with WT channels (*n* = 20) and 2.06 ± 0.79 Hz after transfection with L858H (*n* = 24; *, *P* < 0.05), and the firing frequency evoked by 100-pA stimuli was 0.89 ± 0.28 Hz after transfection with WT and 3.37 ± 1.13 Hz after transfection with L858H (*, *P* < 0.05). (D) Representative SCG neuron expressing WT Na$_V$1.7 fires six action potentials in response to a 950-ms input of 40 pA from the RMP (approximately –45 mV). (E) Representative SCG neuron expressing L858H fires only two action potentials in response to a 100-pA current injection from the RMP (approximately –40 mV). (*Inset*) When the cell was held at –60 mV to overcome the depolarization of the RMP caused by L858H, it produced four action potentials with an identical stimulus. (F) For the entire population of SCG neurons studied, the firing frequency evoked by 30-pA stimuli was 5.33 ± 1.5 Hz after transfection with WT channels (*n* = 14) and 0.63 ± 0.01 Hz after transfection with L858H channels (*n* = 15; *P* < 0.05). The firing frequency evoked by 40-pA stimuli was 7.05 ± 1.86 Hz after transfection with WT and 1.96 ± 1.0 Hz after transfection with L858H channels (*, *P* < 0.05).

2 (P2) rat DRG neurons in culture (figure 4Bc and d) by immunocytochemistry using isoform-specific antibodies. Consistent with published studies on sodium currents in SCG neurons,[20–22] we observed that adult rat SCG neurons express $Na_V1.7$ (figure 4Ca), but not $Na_V1.8$ (figure 4Cb), in native tissue and that $Na_V1.8$ expression is not induced in P2 rat SCG neurons under culture conditions (figure 4Cc and d).

Selective Presence of $Na_V1.8$ within DRG, but Not SCG, Neurons Contributes to Opposing Effects of the L858H Mutation in These Two Cell Types

Having demonstrated that L858H produces hyperexcitability in DRG neurons and hypo-excitability in SCG neurons, we hypothesized that this difference was caused, at least in part,

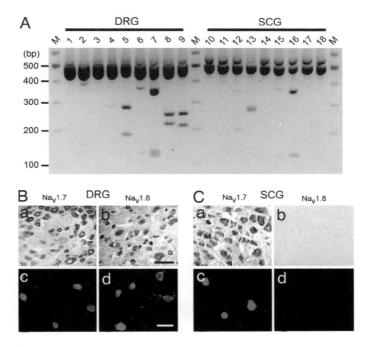

Figure 4
DRG neurons express $Na_V1.7$ and $Na_V1.8$; SCG neurons express $Na_V1.7$ but not $Na_V1.8$. (A) Restriction analysis of multiplex PCR amplification products from sodium channel domain 1 from adult DRG (lanes 1–9) and SCG (lanes 10–18). M, 100-bp ladder marker (Promega). Lanes 1 and 10 contain amplification products from DRG and SCG, respectively. Lanes 2–9 and 11–18 show results of cutting this DNA with EcoRV, EcoNI, AvaI, AccI, SphI, BamHI, AflII, and EcoRI, which are specific to subunits $Na_V1.1$, $Na_V1.2$, $Na_V1.3$, $Na_V1.5/1.9$, $Na_V1.6$, $Na_V1.7/1.8$, $Na_V1.8$, and $Na_V1.9$ (details can be found in table 1, which is published as supporting information on the PNAS web site). Restriction products in lanes 2 and 5–9 show the presence of $Na_V1.1$, $Na_V1.6$, $Na_V1.7$, $Na_V1.8$, and $Na_V1.9$ in DRG, in agreement with previous results.[19] Restriction products in lanes 13, 15, and 16 show the presence of $Na_V1.3$, $Na_V1.6$, and $Na_V1.7$ in SCG. (B and C) Immunostaining of $Na_V1.7$ and $Na_V1.8$ channels in DRG and SCG neurons *in vivo* and in cultured neurons. (B) $Na_V1.7$ (*a*) and $Na_V1.8$ (*b*) proteins are present in adult DRG neurons *in vivo*; $Na_V1.7$ (*c*) and $Na_V1.8$ (*d*) proteins are present in cultured DRG neurons from postnatal day 2 (P2) rat pups. (C) $Na_V1.7$ (*a*), but not $Na_V1.8$ (*b*), protein is present in adult SCG neurons *in vivo*; $Na_V1.7$ (*c*), but not $Na_V1.8$ (*d*), protein is present in cultured SCG neurons from P2 rat pups. (Scale bars, 50 μm.)

by the presence of $Na_V1.8$ in DRG neurons[14–16] and its absence in SCG neurons. $Na_V1.8$ channels have depolarized voltage-dependence of activation and inactivation[14,15,23,24] and thus allow DRG neurons to fire action potentials even when depolarized.[10] We tested this hypothesis by coexpressing $Na_V1.8$ together with L858H in SCG neurons and examining the effects on firing behavior. Figure 5A shows representative suprathreshold action potentials from SCG cells expressing WT $Na_V1.7$ (blue), L858H (red), and L858H plus $Na_V1.8$ (green). As before, expression of L858H channels depolarized the RMP and reduced action potential overshoot. However, when $Na_V1.8$ was coexpressed with L858H, action potential overshoot was restored, even though the depolarization of the RMP induced by L858H persisted. For the population of cells studied, the depolarization of the RMP by $\approx$5mV (-41.6 ± 0.76 mV, $n = 17$ with L858H) was maintained with coexpression of $Na_V1.8$ (-40.5 ± 1.01 mV, $n = 17$) ($P > 0.05$; figure 5B). However, current threshold for firing was reduced when $Na_V1.8$ was coexpressed with L858H ($P < 0.05$; figure 5C). In addition, action potential overshoot was restored when $Na_V1.8$ was coexpressed with L858H ($P < 0.05$; figure 5D). These results show that the presence or absence of $Na_V1.8$ is a major determinant of the functional effects of this mutation.

Discussion

The L858H erythermalgia mutation results in a single amino acid substitution in the domain II S4–S5 linker within $Na_V1.7$ (refs. 2, 7), a sodium channel that is preferentially expressed in DRG and sympathetic ganglia neurons.[8,9,16,25] Our experiments show that L858H produces hyperexcitability (decreased threshold and enhanced repetitive firing) within DRG neurons and hypoexcitability (increased threshold and attenuated repetitive firing) within sympathetic ganglion neurons. The latter observation provides a molec-

ular basis for the sympathetic dysfunction that has been reported[26,27] in erythermalgia. Moreover, this observation suggests the more general hypothesis that other ion channel mutations may have differing physiological effects in different cell types in which the channel is normally expressed. Although opposing functional effects of the same mutation in different types of neurons may at first seem paradoxical, we demonstrate that it is caused by different cell backgrounds, including different repertoires of other ion channels within the two types of neurons.

The L858H mutation produces a hyperpolarizing shift in activation, slows deactivation, and increases the ramp response of $Na_V1.7$ to small stimuli.[7] We observed that L858H produces a depolarization, of $\approx$5 mV, in the RMP of both DRG and SCG neurons. A similar depolarization has been observed with a mutation of the adjacent residue in the $Na_V1.4$ muscle sodium channel that is associated with muscle weakness.[28,29] The depolarization may be a result of increased window currents predicted from voltage-clamp analysis of L858H to be present between -80 and -35 mV and largest between -60 and -45 mV, close to resting potential[7] because of the hyperpolarizing shift in activation, as for the $Na_V1.4$ mutation.[28,29]

We hypothesized that L858H produces hyperexcitability in DRG neurons and hypoexcitability in SCG neurons because of the selective expression of $Na_V1.8$ sodium channels in DRG and its absence in SCG neurons. The majority of nociceptive DRG neurons express $Na_V1.8$ (refs. 14, 30), which contributes most of the current underlying the action potential upstroke.[10,18] Because it has depolarized voltage-dependence of activation [$V_{1/2} = -16$ to -21 mV (refs. 14, 15, 23, 24)] and inactivation [$V_{1/2} = -30$ mV (refs. 14, 15, 23, 24)] compared with other sodium channels, $Na_V1.8$ permits DRG neurons to generate action potentials and sustain repetitive firing when depolarized.[10,12] This finding led us to predict that $Na_V1.7$ mutations can produce hyperexcitability of DRG

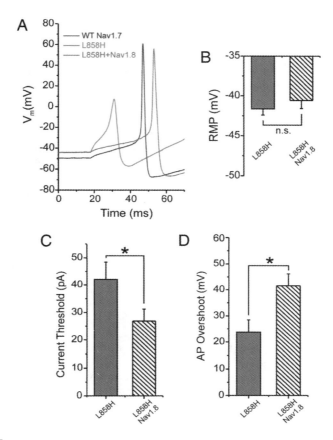

Figure 5

Coexpression of L858H and Na$_V$1.8 channels rescues electrogenic properties in SCG neurons. When Na$_V$1.8 was coexpressed with L858H, current threshold and action potential overshoot were restored, although the depolarization of the RMP induced by L858H persisted. (A) Suprathreshold action potentials recorded from representative SCG neurons transfected with WT (blue), L858H (red), and L858H plus Na$_V$1.8 (green) channels. (B) Depolarized RMP in cells with L858H channels (-41.6 ± 0.76 mV, $n = 17$) was maintained with coexpression of Na$_V$1.8 (-40.5 ± 1.01 mV, $n = 17$; $P > 0.05$). n.s., not significant. (C) Current threshold for action potential firing was reduced from 42.9 ± 6.3 pA ($n = 17$) for L858H to 26.8 ± 4.3 pA ($n = 17$) for L858H coexpressed with Na$_V$1.8 (*, $P < 0.05$). (D) Action potential overshoot in SCG neurons with L858H channel (23.8 ± 4.7 mV, $n = 17$) was increased when Na$_V$1.8 was coexpressed with L858H (41.5 ± 4.6 mV, $n = 17$; *, $P < 0.05$).

neurons because these cells also express $Na_V1.8$ channels that are, because of depolarized inactivation voltage-dependence, still available for activation.

We observed a similar depolarization, of ≈ 5 mV, in SCG neurons after the expression of L858H, but in these neurons the mutation produced hypoexcitability, i.e., increased threshold, attenuated repetitive firing, and reduced action potential amplitude. $Na_V1.3$, $Na_V1.6$, and $Na_V1.7$, but not $Na_V1.8$, are present in SCG neurons (figure 4). Because of the relatively hyperpolarized steady-state inactivation of $Na_V1.3$, $Na_V1.6$, and $Na_V1.7$ in neurons [$V_{1/2}$ values between -65 and -78 mV (refs. 31, 32)], the L858H-induced depolarizing shift in the RMP would be expected to inactivate sodium channels within SCG neurons, with a resultant decrease in excitability and action potential amplitude. Consistently with this, when we held SCG neurons expressing the L858H mutation at potentials hyperpolarized compared with their RMP, excitability and action potential amplitude increased (figure 3E).

To test the hypothesis that the selective presence within DRG neurons of $Na_V1.8$, with its depolarized $V_{1/2}$ of activation and inactivation,[14,15,23,24] contributes to the opposing functional effects of L858H in DRG and SCG neurons, we expressed $Na_V1.8$ within SCG neurons, where it is not normally present. In agreement with this hypothesis, the coexpression of $Na_V1.8$ with L858H tended to restore action potential threshold and amplitude toward the values seen with WT $Na_V1.7$, protecting against the hypoexcitability conferred by L858H in the absence of $Na_V1.8$, even though L858H produced a depolarizing shift of ≈ 5 mV in the RMP. Although we cannot exclude an additional contribution of differential expression of other molecules, such as potassium channels, to the opposing changes in excitability in DRG and SCG neurons expressing L858H, our results show that $Na_V1.8$, which is selectively expressed within DRG neurons, is a major contributor to this effect.

Our results show that the same sodium channel mutation can produce hyperexcitability in one type of neuron in which the channel gene is normally expressed, while producing hypoexcitability in another type of neuron where the gene is also expressed. Thus, the effects of sodium channel mutations on neuronal function should not be considered as unidirectional or predictable on the basis of the changes in channel function per se: they also depend on the cell background in which the mutation is expressed. More generally, we suggest the possibility that mutations of other ion channels, e.g., other sodium channel isoforms or calcium or potassium channels, may have different functional effects in different types of cells.

Materials and Methods

SCG and DRG Cultures

As described in ref. 33, we isolated SCG from deeply anesthetized (ketamine/xylazine, 80:10 mg/kg, i.p.) 1- to 5-day-old Sprague–Dawley rats, washed them with cold Hanks' balanced salt solution (HBSS) (Ca^{2+}- and Mg^{2+}-free), incubated them for 40 min at 37°C in HBSS (Ca^{2+}- and Mg^{2+}-free) containing 0.2% trypsin (Worthington), washed them twice in warm Leibovitz's L-15 medium (Invitrogen), and triturated them with a fire-polished Pasteur pipette in Leibovitz's L-15 medium containing 0.75 mg/ml BSA/trypsin inhibitor. SCG cells were pelleted by low-speed centrifugation, resuspended in modified Leibovitz's L-15 medium supplemented with 1 µg/ml nerve growth factor (Alomone, Jerusalem), 5% rat serum, 38 mM glucose, 24 mM sodium bicarbonate, and penicillin/streptomycin (each 50 units/ml), plated on 12-mm circular coverslips precoated with poly(D-lysine)/laminin (BD Biosciences, Franklin Lakes, NJ) and incubated at 37°C in 5% CO^2. DRG neurons from age-matched animals were cultured as described in ref. 34.

Cell Culture Immunocytochemistry

We incubated cultured DRG and SCG neurons sequentially in complete saline solution, 4% paraformaldehyde in 0.14 M Sorensen's buffer (pH 7.4) for 10 min, PBS, blocking solution (PBS containing 5% normal goat serum, 2% BSA, and 0.1% Triton X-100) for 30 min, and primary Ab [rabbit anti-$Na_V1.7$, 6 μg/ml, and rabbit anti-$Na_V1.8$, 3.2 μg/ml (Alomone)] in blocking solution overnight at 4°C. The next day, we incubated the coverslips sequentially in PBS, goat anti-rabbit IgG–Cy3 secondary Ab (0.5 μg/ml, Amersham Pharmacia), and PBS. Coverslips were mounted on slides with Aqua-Poly/Mount and examined with a Nikon E800 microscope equipped with epifluorescent optics by using METAVUE software (Universal Imaging, Downingtown, PA).

Tissue Immunocytochemistry

Adult Sprague–Dawley rats were deeply anesthetized (80 mg/kg ketamine/10 mg/kg xylazine, i.p.) and perfused with PBS and then 4% paraformaldehyde in 0.14 M Sorensen's buffer. SCG and DRG were excised, rinsed with PBS, and cryoprotected in 30% sucrose in PBS overnight at 4°C (ref. 35). Cryosections (10 μm) of DRG and SCG were incubated sequentially in (*i*) PBS containing 5% normal goat serum, 2% BSA, and 0.1% Triton X-100 for 30 min; (*ii*) primary Ab [rabbit anti-$Na_V1.7$, 6 μg/ml (Alomone), and rabbit anti-$Na_V1.8$, 0.3 μg/ml (ref. 35)] overnight at 4°C; (*iii*) PBS, six times for 5 min each time; (*iv*) goat anti-rabbit IgG–biotin (1:250); (*v*) PBS, six times for 5 min each time; (*vi*) avidin–horseradish peroxidase (1:250); (*vii*) PBS, six times for 5 min each time; (*viii*) 0.4% diaminobenzidine and 0.003% hydrogen peroxide in PBS for 7 min; and (*ix*) PBS containing 0.02% sodium azide and coverslipped with Aqua-Poly/Mount.

Reverse Transcription–Multiplex PCR

We synthesized first-strand cDNA from total cellular RNA isolated from L4–L5 DRG and SCG dissected from adult Sprague–Dawley rats, using the RNeasy Mini Kit (Qiagen, Valencia, CA).[19] We amplified fragments of sodium channel templates in the cDNA pool by multiplex PCR using four forward and three reverse primers (F1–F4 and R1–R3) designed against highly conserved sequences in domain 1 of *a*-subunits.[19] We investigated the presence of specific sodium channel templates by digesting 1/20th of the volume of the multiplex amplicons in a 10-μl final volume with restriction enzymes that produce distinct restriction products, as described in ref. 19.

Transfection of DRG and SCG Neurons and Current-Clamp Recordings

We transfected DRG and SCG neurons as described in ref. 3, using Rat Neuron Nucleofector Solution (Amaxa, Gaithersburg, MD) and a channel/GFP ratio of 5:1, with WT tetrodotoxin-resistant $Na_V1.7$ (ref. 36) or L858H mutant derivative,[7] and, in a cotransfection assay, we combined the L858H mutant channel and WT $Na_V1.8$ channel to transfect SCG neurons. Transfected DRG and SCG neurons were incubated in DMEM (Ca^{2+}- and Mg^{2+}-free) plus 10% FCS (for 5 min at 37°C) to allow recovery, diluted in regular culture medium (for DRG, DMEM/FCS; for SCG, modified Leibovitz's L-15) supplemented with nerve growth factor and glial cell-derived neurotrophic factor (50 ng/ml), plated on precoated 12-mm circular coverslips, and incubated at 37°C in 5% CO^2.

Whole-cell current-clamp recordings were made from transfected small-diameter ($\leq$25 μm) DRG or SCG neurons with robust GFP fluorescence, within 24–60 h, at room temperature (21–25°C) by using an Axopatch 200B amplifier (Axon Instruments, Union City, CA). The pipette solution contained 140 mM KCl, 0.5 mM EGTA, 5 mM Hepes, and 3 mM Mg·ATP (pH 7.3), adjusted to 315 mosM/liter with glucose. External solution contained 140 mM NaCl, 3 mM KCl, 2 mM $MgCl^2$, 2 mM $CaCl^2$, and 10 mM Hepes (pH 7.3), adjusted to 310 mosM/liter with glucose. Pipette potential was set to zero before seal formation without correction for liquid junction potentials. We canceled capacity transients before switching to current-clamp mode and compensated for series resistance (3–6 MΩ) by $\approx$70%. Traces were acquired from cells with stable RMP, excluding cells where RMP changed by >10%, by using CLAMPEX 8.1 software (Axon Instruments), filtered at 5 kHz, at a sampling rate of 20 kHz. Input resistances, measured by recording voltage changes evoked by injection of hyperpolarizing current, were not significantly different between groups. We measured action potential threshold at the beginning of the sharp upward rise of the action potential and determined current threshold by a series of depolarizing currents from 0 to $\approx$200 pA in 5-pA increments. We assessed repetitive firing by recording responses to sustained (950 ms) injection of depolarizing current.

Statistical Analysis

Data are presented as mean $\pm$ SEM. Data were analyzed by using CLAMPFIT 8.2 (Axon Instruments) and ORIGIN 6.1

(Microcal Software, Northampton, MA) software. Statistical significance was determined by using Student's t test, where we assumed that the apparent Gaussian nature of the data sets would be extended to the population.

Acknowledgments

We thank Lynda Tyrrell, Rachael Blackman, and Bart Toftness for technical assistance. This work was supported by the Medical Research Service and Rehabilitation Research Service, Department of Veterans Affairs, and by grants from the National Multiple Sclerosis Society and the Erythromelalgia Association. T.R.C. was supported by National Institutes of Health Research Grant NS053422. The Center for Neuroscience and Regeneration Research is a collaboration of the Paralyzed Veterans of America and the United Spinal Association with Yale University.

Conflict of interest statement: No conflicts declared.

About the Authors

Anthony M. Rush, Department of Neurology and Center for Neuroscience and Regeneration Research, Yale University School of Medicine, New Haven, CT; Rehabilitation Research Center, Veterans Affairs Connecticut Healthcare Center, West Haven, CT

Sulayman D. Dib-Hajj, Department of Neurology and Center for Neuroscience and Regeneration Research, Yale University School of Medicine, New Haven, CT; Rehabilitation Research Center, Veterans Affairs Connecticut Healthcare Center, West Haven, CT

Shujun Liu, Department of Neurology and Center for Neuroscience and Regeneration Research, Yale University School of Medicine, New Haven, CT; Rehabilitation Research Center, Veterans Affairs Connecticut Healthcare Center, West Haven, CT

Theodore R. Cummins, Department of Pharmacology and Toxicology, Stark Neurosciences Research Institute, Indiana University School of Medicine, Indianapolis, IN

Joel A. Black, Department of Neurology and Center for Neuroscience and Regeneration Research, Yale University School of Medicine, New Haven, CT; Rehabilitation Research Center, Veterans Affairs Connecticut Healthcare Center, West Haven, CT

Stephen G. Waxman, Department of Neurology and Center for Neuroscience and Regeneration Research, Yale University School of Medicine, New Haven, CT; Rehabilitation Research Center, Veterans Affairs Connecticut Healthcare Center, West Haven, CT

Notes

1. Waxman SG, Dib-Hajj S. 2005. *Trends Mol Med* 11: 555–562.

2. Yang Y, Wang Y, Li S, Xu Z, Li H, Ma L, Fan J, et al. 2004. *J Med Genet* 41: 171–174.

3. Dib-Hajj SD, Rush AM, Cummins TR, Hisama FM, Novella S, Tyrrell L, Marshall L, Waxman SG. 2005. *Brain* 128: 1847–1854.

4. Drenth JP, Te Morsche RH, Guillet G, Taieb A, Kirby RL, Jansen JB. 2005. *J Invest Dermatol* 124: 1333–1338.

5. Michiels JJ, Te Morsche RH, Jansen JB, Drenth JP. 2005. *Arch Neurol (Chicago)* 62: 1587–1590.

6. Han C, Rush A, Dib-Hajj S, Li S, Xu Z, Wang Y, Tyrrell L, Wang X, Yang Y, Waxman S. 2006. *Ann Neurol* 59: 553–558.

7. Cummins TR, Dib-Hajj SD, Waxman SG. 2004. *J Neurosci* 24: 8232–8236.

8. Toledo-Aral JJ, Moss BL, He ZJ, Koszowski AG, Whisenand T, Levinson SR, Wolf JJ, Silossantiago I, Halegoua S, Mandel G. 1997. *Proc Natl Acad Sci USA* 94: 1527–1532.

9. Sangameswaran L, Fish LM, Koch BD, Rabert DK, Delgado SG, Ilnicka M, Jakeman LB, et al. 1997. *J Biol Chem* 272: 14805–14809.

10. Renganathan M, Cummins TR, Waxman SG. 2001. *J Neurophysiol* 86: 629–640.

11. Waddell PJ, Lawson SN. 1990. *Neuroscience* 36: 811–822.

12. Blair NT, Bean BP. 2003. *J Neurosci* 23: 10338–10350.

13. Zhang XF, Zhu CZ, Thimmapaya R, Choi WS, Honore P, Scott VE, Kroeger PE, Sullivan JP, Faltynek CR, Gopalakrishnan M, Shieh CC. 2004. *Brain Res* 1009: 147–158.

14. Akopian AN, Sivilotti L, Wood JN. 1996. *Nature* 379: 257–262.

15. Sangameswaran L, Delgado SG, Fish LM, Koch BD, Jakeman LB, Stewart GR, Sze P, Hunter JC, Eglen RM, Herman RC. 1996. *J Biol Chem* 271: 5953–5956.

16. Black JA, Dib-Hajj S, McNabola K, Jeste S, Rizzo MA, Kocsis JD, Waxman SG. 1996. *Brain Res Mol Brain Res* 43: 117–131.

17. Cummins TR, Howe JR, Waxman SG. 1998. *J Neurosci* 18: 9607–9619.

18. Blair NT, Bean BP. 2002. *J Neurosci* 22: 10277–10290.

19. Dib-Hajj SD, Tyrrell L, Black JA, Waxman SG. 1998. *Proc Natl Acad Sci USA* 95: 8963–8968.

20. Freschi JE. 1983. *J Neurophysiol* 50: 1460–1478.

21. Nerbonne JM, Gurney AM. 1989. *J Neurosci* 9: 3272–3286.

22. Schofield GG, Ikeda SR. 1988. *Pflugers Arch* 411: 481–490.

23. Cummins TR, Waxman SG. 1997. *J Neurosci* 17: 3503–3514.

24. Sleeper AA, Cummins TR, Dib-Hajj SD, Hormuzdiar W, Tyrrell L, Waxman SG, Black JA. 2000. *J Neurosci* 20: 7279–7289.

25. Felts PA, Yokoyama S, Dib-Hajj S, Black JA, Waxman SG. 1997. *Brain Res Mol Brain Res* 45: 71–82.

26. Davis MD, Sandroni P, Rooke TW, Low PA. 2003. *Arch Dermatol* 139: 1337–1343.

27. Mork C, Kalgaard OM, Kvernebo K. 2002. *J Invest Dermatol* 118: 699–703.

28. Lehmann-Horn F, Kuther G, Ricker K, Grafe P, Ballanyi K, Rudel R. 1987. *Muscle Nerve* 10: 363–374.

29. Cummins TR, Zhou J, Sigworth FJ, Ukomadu C, Stephan M, Ptacek LJ, Agnew WS. 1993. *Neuron* 10: 667–678.

30. Djouhri L, Fang X, Okuse K, Wood JN, Berry CM, Lawson S. 2003. *J Physiol* 550: 739–752.

31. Cummins TR, Aglieco F, Renganathan M, Herzog RI, Dib-Hajj SD, Waxman SG. 2001. *J Neurosci* 21: 5952–5961.

32. Herzog RI, Cummins TR, Ghassemi F, Dib-Hajj SD, Waxman SG. 2003. *J Physiol* 551: 741–750.

33. Higgins D, Lein P, Osterhout D, Johnson M. 1991. In *Culturing Nerve Cells*, eds. Banker G., Goslin, K. (MIT Press, Cambridge, MA), pp. 177–205.

34. Rizzo MA, Kocsis JD, Waxman SG. 1994. *J Neurophysiol* 72: 2796–2815.

35. Black JA, Dib-Hajj S, Baker D, Newcombe J, Cuzner ML, Waxman SG. 2000. *Proc Natl Acad Sci USA* 97: 11598–11602.

36. Herzog RI, Cummins TR, Ghassemi F, Dib-Hajj SD, Waxman SG. 2003. *J Physiol* 551: 741–750.

6 EAVESDROPPING

Imagine trying to eavesdrop on a room full of people by thrusting a microphone, attached to a ramrod the size of telephone pole, through the wall. Although this technique of listening might allow one to hear some noises, the message would not be representative of what normally goes on within that room. Our intrusive microphone would blatantly disrupt any conversation. That is the type of challenge that is faced by neurophysiologists who wish to study the details of the electrical activity within single nerve cells. These cells measure, on average, less than 30 or 40 microns across, and in many cases, have a diameter of less than 20 microns, one-fiftieth of a millimeter and a fraction of the breadth of a human hair. Compounding the challenge, the electrical signals are tiny, ranging from 1/10 of a volt at largest to less than 1/1,000 of a volt (1/10,000 of the voltage of an AAA battery) at smallest, depending on the type of electrical activity one wants to record.

The largest of these signals are the all-or-none action potentials, the nerve impulses produced by any given neuron. Each neuron communicates with other neurons by producing action potentials, which propagate along its axon, finally reaching synapses at the axon terminals where the message is passed on to other ("postsynaptic") neurons by a process called synaptic transmission. The message of each neuron is encoded by the rate and pattern of its action potentials. Early neurophysiologists developed the capability to record the action potentials produced by single neurons in the brain and spinal cord, using tiny microelectrodes fashioned from stainless steel or tungsten, tapered to a very fine tip and insulated to within a few thousandths of a millimeter at the tip. These electrodes were inserted into the brain or spinal cord but did not enter neurons, so the nerve impulses were recorded without actually puncturing or touching the target nerve cells. This configuration was like placing a microphone just next to, but outside, of a room full of people. Nerve impulses from different neurons or "units" could be distinguished using this methodology on the basis of their size, with the signals from the neurons closest to the electrode being largest. This type of "single unit recording" turned out to be quite informative for researchers interested in determining *what* a neuron is saying. The rate and pattern of its action potentials are its message.

But what if one wants to understand *how* the neuron produces its message. In generating a nerve impulse or action potential, a neuron uses a rich repertoire of ion channels—several types of sodium channels, several types of potassium channels, and in some neurons, one or more types of calcium channels—which turn on and off in a complex but well-regulated way. If one wants to understand the molecular basis for neuronal signaling, or if one wants to target the molecules that generate nerve impulse activity for therapeutic purposes, one needs to discern the activity of these various types of ion channels. Imagine trying to dissect the contribution of one particular ion channel within the chatter of the nerve cell. Since a single neuron may contain dozens of types of ion channels, this is like trying to discern, microscopically, the contribution of one musical instrument within the music produced by an orchestra. How can neuroscientists accomplish this?

The electrical activity of nerve cells is produced by ion channels in the cell membrane and is most accurately measured by assessing the voltage drop across the cell membrane or the current flowing across it. These measurements require comparison of electrical activity inside and outside the cell. But how does one record electrical events inside single nerve cells? The first recordings from inside of nerve fibers took advantage of the presence in the squid of "giant" axons, which earned their name because they have diameters of nearly 1 millimeter, fifty times larger than the diameters of human nerve fibers. In the late 1940s, Hodgkin and Huxley, working at Cambridge University, succeeded at inserting tiny wires into squid giant axons and were able to record the actual currents that flowed across the nerve cell membrane to produce action potentials. This allowed them to predict the presence of sodium channels within the nerve cell membrane and to describe their basic properties. Generations of "axonologists" followed up on this seminal work, and, even today, some researchers continue to use the squid giant axon as a model and the Hodgkin–Huxley equations, developed on the basis of recordings in the squid giant axon, continue to form a basis for modern neurophysiological theory.

The squid giant axon, and other invertebrate preparations, provided invaluable information about the processes by which nerve cells generate electrical signals. Nevertheless, neuroscientists wanted to understand these processes in the nerve cells of vertebrates including mammals. At the end of the 1940s, Ralph Gerard, a physician-researcher in the Department of Physiology of the University of Chicago, developed "sharp intracellular microelectrodes," pulled from tiny glass capillary tubes so that they tapered to only several microns at the tip. He used these, as small harpoons, to directly impale nerve cells and record their electrical activity. This methodology propelled a generation of important investigations which included pioneering studies such as those of Bernard Katz, who, in seminal work at University College London, discovered that tiny, discrete packets of neurotransmitters are released at synapses by one neuron and act as signals on an adjacent nerve cell; and the studies of John Eccles in Canberra which demonstrated the ways in which excitatory and inhibitory synapses can both impinge on the same receiving nerve cell, which integrates them like a tiny computer chip. The following generation of electrophysiologists used the intracellular microelectrode to record the electrical activity within a multitude of types of neurons, and these studies gave us much of the basis for neurophysiology. Even the finely honed intracellular microelectrode, however, invaded the neurons from which it recorded, usually doing some damage and possibly distorting the message.

Against this background, Erwin Neher, Bert Sakmann, and their colleagues in Germany developed the "patch-clamp" recording method for studying electrical activity of nerve cells in the early 1980s (Neher and Sakmann 1992). Their innovative new method involved using finely crafted glass micropipettes that, rather than impaling neurons, fuse with their outer cell membranes, where they form a nearly perfect high-resistance "gigaseal." This permits relatively noninvasive recording, with high fidelity, of electrical activity within these neurons. Their development of the patch-clamp method was honored with the Nobel Prize in 1991.

This brings us to the question of how one can study, in a precisely quantitative manner, the effect of a mutated ion channel on the behavior of a particular type of neuron. One approach (Dib-Hajj et al. 2009) is to grow the neuron of interest in culture and insert the gene for the mutated ion channel into the cell. Patch-clamp recording can then be used for a head-to-head comparison of neurons transfected with mutant channels and neurons transfected with normal channels (termed "wild-type" by geneticists), so that the properties of the cells containing mutant and wild-type channels can be compared. This method can be very informative in providing a qualitative or semi-quantitative assessment of the effect of the mutant channel on neuronal firing. However, in experiments of this type, the level of expression of the transfected channels (the number of functional ion channels produced in each cell) cannot be precisely controlled, and thus it is not possible to ensure that the number and density of mutant channels within the transfected cell are similar to those in a naturally occurring neuron. An alternative approach is to use genetic "knock-out" strategies to silence one particular gene so that cells containing the channel of interest can be compared with cells that do not contain it. This approach, however, also has a limitation: It is usually constrained to studying cells from mice where knock-out is most readily achieved, and it limits the assessment to an "all-or-none" comparison. Still another potential alternative, recording from actual neurons from humans carrying the mutation, presents several challenges: In one approach, the nerve cells would have to be removed from a living human subject, which is ethically unacceptable. Alternatively, cells could be obtained from humans carrying the mutation at postmortem, but, in order to maintain the fragile cells and the molecules within them in a healthy state, the postmortem would have to be carried out and the neurons transported to the research laboratory within several hours of death, which is a substantial challenge.

The Vasylyev et al. paper (Vasylyev et al. 2014) addresses this problem by using the powerful technique of "dynamic clamping." The dynamic clamp method combines the strengths of patch-clamp recording with powerful computer simulation methods (Prinz, Abbott, and Marder 2004). We used it to study the effect of a precisely calibrated number of human $Na_V1.7$ channels, either wild-type or mutant, by virtually placing the simulated channels within an actual healthy pain-signaling DRG nerve cell removed from a rat or mouse. In our iteration of this method, to study mutations of $Na_V1.7$ we first used a patch-clamp electrode and powerful amplifiers to record the electrical currents (including the currents produced by $Na_V1.7$ channels) from a native, unperturbed nerve cell. We then used computational algorithms to subtract the current produced by the normal $Na_V1.7$ sodium channels and electronically injected, into the cell, electrical current that simulates the activity of a precisely calibrated number of mutated ion channels which substitute for the deleted normal channels.

The L858H mutation had been found in one of the early patients reported with inherited erythromelalgia (Yang et al. 2004), and we previously had used traditional patch-clamp methods to study the effect of the mutation on the behavior of the channel (Cummins, Dib-Hajj, and Waxman 2004). Now, we wanted to move closer to understanding the clinical effect of the mutation, and to understand the details of how the mutant channel altered the behavior of pain-signaling DRG nerve cells. The computational power of the dynamic clamp allowed us to precisely titrate the number of wild-type, normal $Na_V1.7$ channels, or mutant $Na_V1.7$ channels, that we sequentially placed in a real pain-signaling neuron. Thus, we could ask this question: What happens if you remove the normal $Na_V1.7$ channels in a DRG neuron and replace them *in the same cell* with a precisely calibrated number of mutant channels?

Dynamic clamp analysis required modeling of the $Na_V1.7$ channel. This, in turn, required development of a computer program that precisely simulated the dynamic behavior of the channel, so that we had to go back to the laboratory to assess, in detail, the properties of the channel in multiple functional states:

- resting

- nearly activated

- activated

- fatigued after activation

Next, these measurements were used to build a computer program which simulated the characteristics of the channel. Dmytro Vasylyev, a biophysicist who had received advanced mathematical training at the Bogomoletz Institute in his native Kiev, spent weeks constructing the model and writing the code for the program, which required calculating the current produced at a particular time by the channel, then recalculating again and again at intervals of 10 μsec (ten millionths of a second). Altogether, his computer had to repeat the calculations in an iterative manner for each 1/100,000 of a second of real time in a neuron, which was a substantial computational challenge. But he persevered, and, when this was done, we were finally ready to begin the experiment.

As a first step, while recording from a real cell, we subtracted the current produced by the endogenous $Na_V1.7$ channels. We then asked how the presence of normal $Na_V1.7$ channels alters the excitability of DRG neurons. To answer this question, we used the computer, which had virtually removed all $Na_V1.7$ channels from the cell, to add precisely calibrated amounts of the $Na_V1.7$ channel back into cell so that we could assess the effect of the cell's having no $Na_V1.7$ channels, or 20%, 40%, 60%, 80%, or 100% of its actual complement of $Na_V1.7$. These experiments taught us that $Na_V1.7$ channels act in a remarkably linear manner to increase the excitability of the cell. The more $Na_V1.7$ channels, the more excitable the cell became, with the relationship between amount of $Na_V1.7$ and threshold of the neuron falling on a straight line. The linear relationship showed us that the regulation of the number of $Na_V1.7$ channels in a cell can precisely control the cell's responsiveness. This is a beautiful example of elegance in the molecular architecture of the neuron. The strong effect of the number of $Na_V1.7$ channels within DRG neurons on the degree of excitability of these cells may also be relevant to disease because sensory neurons produce extra $Na_V1.7$ channels in response to inflammation and injury.

We next used the dynamic clamp to ask questions about mutant $Na_V1.7$ channels. We wanted to understand, for example, "Will a small number of mutant channels have an effect on the behavior of the cell?" and "How large an effect does the mutant channel—virtually inserted into a real cell at a density that mimics the situation in humans with inherited erythromelalgia—have on the behavior of the cell?" We learned, in terms of the first question, that "gain-of-function" changes, which increase the activity of $Na_V1.7$ mutant channels, are so powerful that even a small number of mutant $Na_V1.7$ channels will markedly increase the excitability of a pain-signaling DRG neuron. And we learned, in terms of the second question, that deployment of mutant channels at levels expected in humans has an even larger effect on the cells, making them even more overactive. These experiments showed very clearly that mutant $Na_V1.7$ channels, expressed at a physiologically relevant level, produce persistent sodium currents that, while tiny, are sufficient to depolarize neurons and reduce the threshold for nerve impulse generation, thus teaching us how, in a very fundamental sense, the mutant channels produce hyperexcitability of DRG neurons that underlies pain.

Shortly after completing our dynamic clamp study on $Na_V1.7$, Vasylyev returned to Kiev. The dynamic clamp method, however, was up and running. A few months thereafter, we used this methodology to study the human $Na_V1.8$ channel (Han et al. 2015) and the human $Na_V1.9$ channel (Huang et al. 2014), two cousins of $Na_V1.7$. Dynamic clamp gave us a quantitative, high-resolution picture of all three of the "peripheral" sodium channels and some of their mutants.

References

Cummins TR, Dib-Hajj SD, Waxman SG. 2004. Electrophysiological properties of mutant $Na_V1.7$ sodium channels in a painful inherited neuropathy. *J Neurosci* 24(38): 8232–8236.

Dib-Hajj SD, Choi JS, Macala LJ, Tyrrell L, Black JA, Cummins TR, Waxman SG. 2009. Transfection of rat or mouse neurons by biolistics or electroporation. *Nat Protoc* 4(8): 1118–1126.

Han C, Estacion M, Huang J, Vasylyev D, Zhao P, Dib-Hajj SD, Waxman SG. 2015. Human Nav1.8: Enhanced persistent and ramp currents contribute to distinct firing properties of human DRG neurons. *J Neurophysiol* 113(9): 3172–3185.

Huang J, Han C, Estacion M, Vasylyev D, Hoeijmakers JG, Gerrits MM, Tyrrell L, et al., and the Propane Study Group. 2014. Gain-of-function mutations in sodium channel Na(v)1.9 in painful neuropathy. *Brain* 137(Pt 6): 1627–1642.

Neher E, Sakmann B. 1992. The patch clamp technique. *Sci Am* 266(3): 44–51.

Prinz AA, Abbott LF, Marder E. 2004. The dynamic clamp comes of age. *Trends Neurosci* 27(4): 218–224.

Vasylyev DV, Han C, Zhao P, Dib-Hajj S, Waxman SG. 2014. Dynamic-clamp analysis of wild-type human Na$_V$1.7 and erythromelalgia mutant channel L858H. *J Neurophysiol* 111(7): 1429–1443.

Yang Y, Wang Y, Li S, Xu Z, Li H, Ma L, Fan J, et al. 2004. Mutations in SCN9A, encoding a sodium channel alpha subunit, in patients with primary erythermalgia. *J Med Genet* 41(3): 171–174.

DYNAMIC-CLAMP ANALYSIS OF WILD-TYPE HUMAN Na$_V$1.7 AND ERYTHROMELALGIA MUTANT CHANNEL L858H*

Dmytro V. Vasylyev, Chongyang Han, Peng Zhao, Sulayman Dib-Hajj, and Stephen G. Waxman

The link between sodium channel Na$_V$1.7 and pain has been strengthened by identification of gain-of-function mutations in patients with inherited erythromelalgia (IEM), a genetic model of neuropathic pain in humans. A firm mechanistic link to nociceptor dysfunction has been precluded because assessments of the effect of the mutations on nociceptor function have thus far depended on electrophysiological recordings from dorsal root ganglia (DRG) neurons transfected with wild-type (WT) or mutant Na$_V$1.7 channels, which do not permit accurate calibration of the level of Na$_V$1.7 channel expression. Here, we report an analysis of the function of WT Na$_V$1.7 and IEM L858H mutation within small DRG neurons using dynamic-clamp. We describe the functional relationship between current threshold for action potential generation and the level of WT Na$_V$1.7 conductance in primary nociceptive neurons and demonstrate the basis for hyperexcitability at physiologically relevant levels of L858H channel conductance. We demonstrate that the L858H mutation, when modeled using dynamic-clamp at physiological levels within DRG neurons, produces a dramatically enhanced persistent current, resulting in 27-fold amplification of net sodium influx during subthreshold depolarizations and even greater amplification during interspike intervals, which provide a mechanistic basis for reduced current threshold and enhanced action potential firing probability. These results show, for the first time, a linear correlation between the level of Na$_V$1.7 conductance and current threshold in DRG neurons. Our observations demonstrate changes in sodium influx that provide a mechanistic link between the altered biophysical properties of a mutant Na$_V$1.7 channel and nociceptor hyperexcitability underlying the pain phenotype in IEM.

The Na$_V$ voltage-gated sodium channel is preferentially expressed in primary nociceptors

* Previously published in *Journal of Neurophysiology* 111(7): 1429–1443, 2014. Copyright © 2014 Society for Neuroscience.

(Persson et al. 2010; Rush et al. 2007; Toledo-Aral et al. 1997) and activates at subthreshold membrane voltages so as to boost membrane responses to small depolarizing stimuli both in neuronal somata (Ahn et al. 2013; Cummins et al. 1998; Herzog et al. 2003; Rush et al. 2007) and at axon endings of small dorsal root ganglia (DRG) neurons (Vasylyev and Waxman 2012). Inherited erythromelalgia (IEM), the first human pain disorder linked to a sodium channel, is widely regarded as a genetic model of neuropathic pain. When studied in a mammalian heterologous expression system, the L858H mutation, one of the first Na$_V$1.7 mutations linked to IEM (Cummins et al. 2004; Rush et al. 2006; Yang et al. 2004), produces a hyperpolarizing shift in channel activation and increases the amplitude of the response of the channel to slow, small depolarizations. When small DRG neurons transfected with L858H and wild-type (WT) Na$_V$1.7 channels were studied by current-clamp, L858H was found to render DRG neurons hyperexcitable in a manner consistent with the severe pain characteristic of the erythromelalgia phenotype (Rush et al. 2006).

However, a mechanistic link between altered biophysical properties of mutant Na$_V$1.7 channels and hyperexcitability of primary nociceptor neurons carrying these mutant channels has not yet been established. In the present study, we used dynamic-clamp (Kemenes et al. 2011; Samu et al. 2012; Sharp et al. 1993) recordings to titrate levels of Na$_V$1.7 WT and L858H conductances so that we could study the effect of precisely calibrated, physiologically relevant levels of conductance on small DRG neuron excitability. This approach permitted us to vary the ratio of expression levels of WT and L858H within the physiological range within single neurons. This is important because, although the exact ratio of WT and L858H channels is not known, it is reasonable to suggest a 1:1 ratio of functional expressions of WT and L858H mutant allele in the affected individual (Yang et al. 2004). Using dynamic-clamp, we show that action potential (AP) current threshold of DRG neurons is regulated by $Na_V1.7$ conductance in a remarkably linear manner. We also show, in small DRG neurons in which we inserted the L858H mutant by dynamic-clamp, that the mutation substantially increases channel activity at membrane potentials below the AP threshold, producing a large persistent current that depolarizes the membrane potential. We also show that sodium influx via L858H mutant channels is increased not only during subthreshold membrane depolarizations, but also during interspike intervals. These observations on small DRG neurons within a physiologically relevant range of levels of conductance provide a quantitative mechanistic basis for understanding the role of WT $Na_V1.7$ in healthy DRG neurons and the enhanced excitability of primary nociceptors expressing L858H channels that underlies the pain phenotype in humans carrying this mutation.

Materials and Methods

Voltage-Clamp Recordings of $Na_V1.7$

Human $Na_V1.7$ channels were stably expressed in HEK-293 cell line (Cummins et al. 1998). Pipettes were pulled from glass capillaries (cat. no. PG10165-4; World Precision Instruments, Sarasota, FL) and had resistance 1.5–2 MD when filled with the intracellular solution in mM: 140 CsCl, 10 NaCl, 0.5 EGTA, 10 HEPES, 3 MgATP, 10 glucose, pH 7.3 with CsOH. The extracellular solution was HBSS (cat. no. 14025; Invitrogen) in mM: 1.3 $CaCl_2$, 0.5 $MgCl_2$, 0.4 $MgSO_4$, 5.3 KCl, 0.4 KH_2PO_4, 4.2 $NaHCO_3$, 138 NaCl, 0.3 Na_2HPO_4, 5.6 glucose, supplemented with 15 mM NaCl (320 mosM). The liquid junction potential (+3.7 mV) between pipette and bath solutions was measured according to Neher (1992) and was not compensated. Whole cell voltage-

clamp recordings were made using Axopatch 200B amplifier. Currents were low-pass filtered at 10 kHz and digitized/stored at 100 kHz by Digidata 1440A DAC using pCLAMP 10 software (Molecular Devices, Sunnyvale, CA). The series resistance was compensated by 80–85%. -P/4 protocol was used for current-voltage (I–V) and deactivation protocols to subtract uncompensated leak and capacitive currents. Recordings were made at room temperature (23–24°C). All data are presented as means ± SE. Data were analyzed using pCLAMP 10 and Origin 8.5 (OriginLab, Northampton, MA) software.

Assessment of $Na_V1.7$ Contribution to TTX-S Current in Small DRG Neurons

For assessment of the contribution of $Na_V1.7$ to the TTX-sensitive (TTX-S) current, DRG neurons were isolated from WT or $Na_V1.7$-knockout (KO) mice (11–16 wk old) and cultured as previously described (Dib-Hajj et al. 2009). Whole cell voltage-clamp recordings of small (20–25 μm) DRG neurons were obtained at room temperature (20–22°C) within 2–8 h in culture using an EPC 10 amplifier (HEKA Electronics) and fire-polished electrodes (1–2 MD) fabricated from 1.6-mm-outer-diameter borosilicate glass micropipettes (World Precision Instruments). The pipette potential was adjusted to zero before seal formation, and liquid junction potential was not corrected. Voltage errors were minimized with 80–90% series resistance compensation, and linear leak currents and capacitance artifacts were subtracted out using the P/6 method. Currents were acquired with PULSE software (HEKA Electronics) 5 min after establishing whole cell configuration, sampled at a rate of 50 kHz, and filtered at 2.9 kHz. The pipette solution contained in mM: 140 CsF, 10 NaCl, 1 EGTA, and 10 HEPES, pH 7.3 with CsOH (adjusted to 315 mosM with dextrose). The extracellular bath solution contained in mM: 70 NaCl, 70 choline chloride, 3 KCl, 1 $MgCl_2$, 1 $CaCl_2$, 20 TEACl, 5 CsCl, 1 4-AP, 0.1 $CdCl_2$, and 10 HEPES, pH 7.31 with NaOH (326 mosM). The amplitude of TTX-S sodium current was estimated by two protocols as previously described (Rush et al. 2005). Cells were first CsCl, 1 4-AP, 0.1 CdCl held at –80 mV, and a 500-ms depolarizing prepulse to –50 mV was applied to inactivate the TTX-S sodium channels while leaving $Na_V1.8$ current intact, followed by a series of step depolarizations from –70 to +20 mV (in 5-mV increments). Cells exhibiting $Na_V1.9$ currents were excluded from data analysis. For the second protocol, cells were held at −80 mV, a 500-ms hyperpolarizing prepulse to −120 mV was applied to rescue the TTX-S sodium channels from inactivation, and total sodium currents were evoked by a series of depolarizing steps from −70 to +20 mV (in 5-mV increments). The TTX-S sodium current was obtained by subtraction of the currents obtained from the two protocols.

Dynamic-Clamp Recording

DRG neurons (soma diameter 21–26 μm; 24.4 ± 0.3, *n* = 25) obtained from *postnatal day 0–5* Sprague-Dawley rats were grown in primary culture for 2–3 days (Ahn et al. 2013; Dib-Hajj et al. 2009). Small DRG neurons were dynamically clamped (Kemenes et al. 2011; Samu et al. 2012; Sharp et al. 1993) in whole cell configuration using patch pipettes pulled from glass capillaries (cat. no. PG10165-4; World Precision Instruments). Pipette resistance was 1.5–2 MD when filled with the intracellular solution in mM: 140 KCl, 3 MgATP, 0.5 EGTA, 5 HEPES, 10 glucose, pH 7.3 with KOH (adjusted to 325 mosM with sucrose). The extracellular solution was HBSS (cat. no. 14025; Invitrogen) in mM: 1.3 CaCl$_2$, 0.5 MgCl$_2$, 0.4 MgSO$_4$, 5.3 KCl, 0.4 KH$_2$PO$_4$, 4.2 NaHCO$_3$, 138 NaCl, 0.3 Na$_2$HPO$_4$, 5.6 glucose (adjusted to 325 mosM with sucrose). Liquid junction potential (+3.8 mV) between pipette and bath solutions was not compensated. Membrane voltages and currents were recorded in dynamic-clamp using Multi-Clamp 700B amplifier (Molecular Devices) interfaced with CED Power1401 mk II DAI and Signal software (Cambridge Electronic Design, Cambridge, United Kingdom), digitized by Digidata 1440A DAC, and stored on the hard disk using pCLAMP 10 software. Capacitance neutralization and bridge balance were rigorously employed to minimize the effect of electrode capacitance and series resistance on the dynamic-clamp recordings. *I–V* traces were filtered at 10 kHz and digitized at 50 kHz. Series resistance was compensated by 80–85%. Endogenous sodium current recorded in whole cell voltage-clamp was evoked from a holding potential of −50 mV by a test pulse to −10 mV with or without preceding 0.5-s prepulse to −100 mV to remove steady-state inactivation of TTX-S channels. TTX-S channels are mainly inactivated at −50 mV, whereas Na$_V$1.8 channels are still available for activation at this potential because steady-state inactivation of Na$_V$1.8 is shifted in a depolarized direction (Catterall et al. 2005).

Thus, as described by Cummins and Waxman (1997) and Rush et al. (2005), as a measure of total TTX-S current, we used a conditioning/subtraction protocol and assessed the peak current on the trace obtained by digital subtraction of the current trace evoked by the test voltage without preceding prepulse from that with the prepulse, respectively.

We estimated the contribution of Na$_V$1.7 to the total TTX-S current in our assay based on measurements of the total TTX-S current amplitude in WT and Na$_V$1.7-KO DRG neurons (see above). To evaluate the effect of defined levels of L858H functional expression on excitability of small DRG neuron using dynamic-clamp recording, we first estimated the endogenous Na$_V$1.7 conductance and then substituted graded amounts of endogenous conductance by equal amounts of L858H channel conductance, thus achieving a specified substitution ratio (SR) via a dynamic-clamp operation, SR × g_{max}(L858H − WT), where g_{max} is maximal Na$_V$1.7 endogenous conductance.

Recordings were made at room temperature (23–24°C). All data are presented as means ± SE. Data were analyzed using pCLAMP 10 and Origin 8.5 software. Unless specified otherwise, the hypothesis that population means are significantly different was checked using Mann-Whitney nonparametric test ($P < 0.05$, $P < 0.01$, and $P < 0.001$).

Kinetic Model of Na$_V$1.7 Channel

We developed our model of Na$_V$1.7 channel using Hodgkin–Huxley equations $dm/dt = \alpha_m(1 - m) - \beta_m m$; $dh/dt = \alpha_h(1 - h) - \beta_h h$, where *m* and *h* are channel activation and inactivation variable and α (β) are forward (backward) rate constants, respectively. Channel states were independent with a first-order reaction between states. Thus channel activation and deactivation were considered as transitions between closed and open states, whereas channel inactivation and repriming were assumed to be transitions between primed and inactivated states, respectively. Na$_V$1.7 channel steady-state parameters and kinetics obtained based on electrophysiological recordings were converted into appropriate rate constants at respective voltages using the equations $\alpha = m_\infty/\tau$, $\beta = (1 - m_\infty)/\tau$. These reaction rate constants were fitted with Boltzmann equations of the form $y = A2 + (A1 - A2)/\{1 + \exp[(V - V_{1/2})/k]\}$, where *V* is membrane voltage, $V_{1/2}$ is voltage when reaction rate is half-maximal, and *k* is slope coefficient. Fits were converted into steady-state inactivation (activation) variables and inactivation (activation) time constants according to $m_\infty = \alpha/(\alpha + \beta)$ and $\tau = 1/(\alpha + \beta)$. The latter curves were overplayed on the experimental data to provide feedback to the rate constants fitting step. This cycle was manually repeated until the best possible fit of the experimental data was achieved. We obtained the following rate constants for the WT $Na_V 1.7$ channel model:

$$\alpha_m = 10.22 - 10.22/\{1 + \exp[(V + 7.19)/15.43]\},$$
$$\beta_m = 23.76/\{1 + \exp[(V + 70.37)/14.53]\};$$

$$\alpha_h = 0.0744/\{1 + \exp[(V + 99.76)/11.07]\}, \beta_h = 2.54$$
$$- 2.54/\{1 + \exp[(V + 7.8)/10.68]\}.$$

We modeled the L858H IEM mutation because it has been well-studied at the voltage-clamp (Cummins et al. 2004) and current-clamp (Rush et al. 2006) levels. We focused on altered activation of the mutant channels because a hyperpolarizing shift in activation is common to all IEM mutant channels (Dib-Hajj et al. 2010). We did not model slow inactivation in the mutant channel because we limited stimulation to 1-s trains at 10 Hz where the development of slow inactivation is not appreciable. The L858H $Na_V 1.7$ channel model was described by the following equations:

$$\alpha_m = 9.1 - 9.1/\{1 + \exp[(V + 11.52)/22.49]\}, \beta_m = 23.76/$$
$$\{1 + \exp[(V + 87.6)/14.53]\};$$

$$\alpha_h = 0.0744/\{1 + \exp[(V + 99.76)/11.07]\}, \beta_h = 2.54$$
$$- 2.54/\{1 + \exp[(V + 7.8)/10.68]\}.$$

Sodium current was described by $I_{Na} = g_{max} \times m \times h \times (V_m - E_{Na})$, where V_m is membrane voltage potential and $E_{Na} = 65$ mV is sodium reversal potential. Currents evoked by different voltage protocols were calculated in 10-μs precision using a custom program written in Origin 8.5 LabTalk.

$Na_V 1.7$ current kinetics in response to square test pulses and the resulting I–V curve were identical either when calculated in LabTalk or obtained from dynamic-clamp recordings on a vendors-supplied physical cell model. All data are presented as means ± SE. Data were analyzed using pCLAMP 10 and Origin 8.5 software.

Results

Kinetic Model of WT $Na_V 1.7$ Based on Hodgkin–Huxley Equations

Channel kinetics were described based on a Hodgkin–Huxley model of sodium channel with several independent states and a first-order reaction between the states. Channel activation and deactivation were considered as transitions between closed and open states, whereas channel inactivation and repriming were assumed to be transitions between primed (open or closed) and inactivated states (Hille 1978; Hodgkin and Huxley 1952).

$Na_V 1.7$ currents were recorded in whole cell voltage-clamp to obtain channel steady-state and kinetics parameters. Steady-state inactivation (h_∞) was calculated as the ratio of peak current amplitude to the maximal peak current amplitude elicited by a 0-mV test voltage following a 1-s prepulse at different voltages ranging from −100 to −40 mV in 5-mV increments from a holding potential of −100 mV (figure 1A). Steady-state activation (m_∞) was defined as the ratio of $Na_V 1.7$ $g = I_{peak}/(V_m - E_{Na})$ determined at the respective membrane potentials to the $Na_V 1.7$ g_{max} (figure 1A). Steady-state relationships of recombinant $Na_V 1.7$ ($n = 8$ cells) were best fit using a Boltzmann equation with the following parameters: $V_{1/2} = -73.9$ mV, $k = 6.2$ mV and $V_{1/2} = -20.4$ mV, $k = 7.2$ mV for channel steady-state inactivation ($n = 8$) and steady-state activation ($n = 17$), respectively. Our model accurately described $Na_V 1.7$ channel steady-state properties as can be seen from the respective Boltzmann fits of the modeled steady-state curves, $V_{1/2} = -72.6$ mV, $k = 5.7$ mV and $V_{1/2} = -20.4$ mV, $k = 7.1$ mV (figure 1A).

$Na_V 1.7$ current activated in a sigmoidal manner with an apparent delay (figure 1, E and F), which suggests that the channel undergoes multiple closed-state transitions before activation. Channel activation kinetics were best described by a single exponential raised to the third power (figure 1E). Channel activation (figure 1B; $n = 8$) was determined from current traces elicited by test voltages ranging from –55 to 60 mV in 5- to 10-mV increments applied from –100-mV holding potential. Deactivation time constant (figure 1B; $n = 14$) was determined from a single-exponential fit of the respective portions of current traces ("tail currents") measured at different test voltages ranging from –100 to –20 mV following a 0.5-ms voltage step to –10 mV from a holding potential of –100 mV. The falling phase of the current (90 to 10% amplitude) was fitted with a single exponential to obtain the inactivation time constant (figure 1C; $n = 7$). The following protocol was used to evaluate channel repriming kinetics [for details, see Cummins et al. (1998)]. First, a 20-ms test voltage step to 0 mV was applied from a holding potential of –100 mV to inactivate the channel, and then repriming voltage steps of different durations (from 2 to 1,000 ms) were applied at a given voltage followed by the second 20-ms test voltage to 0 mV. The ratios of peak current amplitudes measured at the first and second test voltages were plotted as a function of the repriming step duration; this function was fitted with a single exponential to obtain a time constant of channel removal from inactivation (figure 1C; $n = 14$).

Our model effectively described channel kinetics as can be seen from the close match between the modeled and experimentally determined activation-deactivation (figure 1B) and inactivation-repriming (figure 1C) time constants at a wide range of physiological membrane voltages. The obtained Hodgkin–Huxley variables m^3 and h were both highly voltage-dependent with submillisecond activation kinetics resulting in a transient channel open probability in response to a series of voltage steps (figure 1D). Our model accurately followed the kinetics of Na$_V$1.7 current evoked by a series of depolarization steps (figure 1, F and G). The resulting I–V relationships also provided a match between modeled and experimentally determined data at a wide range of physiological membrane voltages (figure 1H). Thereafter, we utilized this model (WT) and its modification for the L858H mutant channel to study mechanisms of functional contribution of Na$_V$1.7 channel to neuronal excitability in normal and pathological conditions.

Na$_V$1.7 Conductance Regulates Current Threshold for AP Generation in a Linear Manner

We performed a quantitative analysis of the effect of graded additions or subtractions of sodium conductance resulting from Na$_V$1.7 channel function on small DRG neuron excitability using dynamic-clamp. Although we had the capability to transfect DRG neurons with Na$_V$1.7 channels to study the effect of the channel on neuronal excitability (Dib-Hajj et al. 2009; Rush et al. 2006), transfection does not permit accurate calibration of the level of Na$_V$1.7 channel that is being expressed. Thus we carried out dynamic-clamp recording in DRG neurons based on experimentally determined Na$_V$1.7 gating properties and an assumption that Na$_V$1.7 contributes on average 70% of the TTX-S current in small DRG neurons. We based our estimate of the Na$_V$1.7 contribution of 70% of the TTX-S current in small DRG neurons on our measurements of total TTX-S currents in mice that are deficient in Na$_V$1.7 (figure 2). Figure 2A shows representative family traces of TTX-S sodium currents recorded in DRG neurons from WT and Na$_V$1.7-KO mice, respectively. Peak current densities were 143 ± 17 pA/pF ($n = 16$) for TTX-S sodium channels recorded from WT DRG neurons. However, DRG neurons from Na$_V$1.7-KO mice produced significantly smaller TTX-S sodium currents with current densities ~32% (46 ± 9 pA/pF, $n = 16$) of that in WT DRG neurons (figure 2B).

Using dynamic-clamp with the Na$_V$1.7 channel model, we studied how increases in the level of Na$_V$1.7 conductance affect small DRG neuron

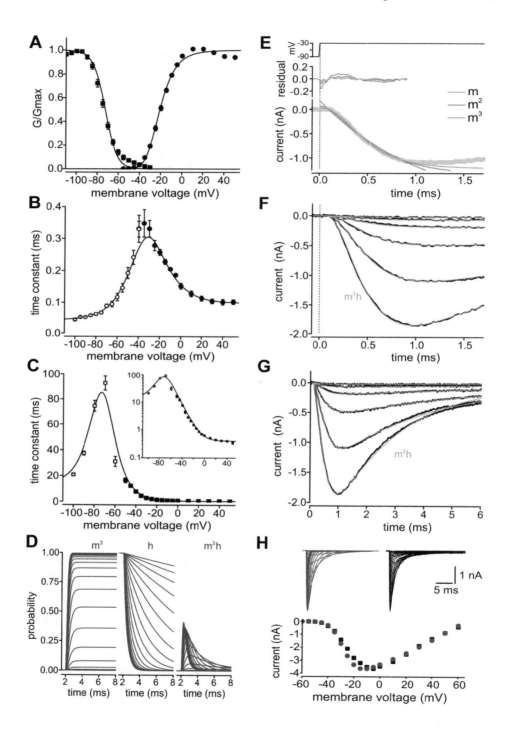

Figure 1
Kinetic model of Na$_V$1.7 voltage-gated sodium channel based on Hodgkin–Huxley equations. (A) Voltage dependence of conductance/maximal conductance (G/Gmax) at steady-state for inactivation (squares; $n = 8$) and activation (circles; $n = 17$) of Na$_V$1.7 channel. Solid lines are derived from the following equations: $h_\infty = \alpha_h/(\alpha_h + \beta_h)$; $(m_\infty)^3 = [\alpha_m/(\alpha_m + \beta_m)]^3$, where m and h are channel activation and inactivation variables and α and β are forward and backward rate constants (see Materials and Methods). (B) Voltage dependencies of activation (solid circles; $n = 8$) and deactivation (open circles; $n = 14$) time constants. Deactivation of the Na$_V$1.7 current was fitted with a single exponential, whereas channel activation was fitted with a single exponential raised to the 3rd power. (C) Inactivation (solid squares; $n = 13$) and removal of inactivation (open squares; $n = 7$) time constant obtained from a single-exponential fit of the respective data. *Inset* shows data replotted with time constants on a log scale. (D) Time sequences of m^3 and h variables along with the resulting open probability (m^3h) obtained in the model response to a series of voltage steps ranged from –60 to 40 mV in 5-mV increments from a holding potential of –110 mV. (E) Rising phase of the Na$_V$1.7 current (bottom) in response to a –30-mV test voltage (top) was fitted with a single exponential function of different powers. The best fit was obtained using 3rd-power exponential as determined based on the residual (middle); the residual of the 3rd-power exponential fit was not substantially different from the background noise, thus 4th-power exponential had not further improved the fit. (F and G) Na$_V$1.7 current evoked by test pulses ranged from –50 to –25 mV in 5-mV increments (black) and overlaid on the m^3h model (blue) at the respective voltages. Vertical dashed line denotes stimulus onset time. (H) Current traces (top) and the current-voltage (I–V) curve (bottom) of Na$_V$1.7 current (black) and the m^3h model (blue) at the respective test voltages.

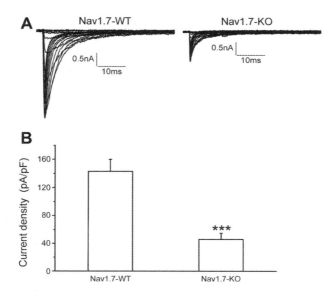

Figure 2
Measurement of Na$_V$1.7 contribution to TTX-sensitive (TTX-S) current in small dorsal root ganglia (DRG) neurons. (A) Representative I–V curve family traces of TTX-S sodium currents recorded from wild-type (WT) and Na$_V$1.7-knockout (KO) DRG neurons, respectively. (B) TTX-S currents in Na$_V$1.7-KO DRG neurons are significantly smaller than in WT DRG neurons. ***$P < 0.001$.

excitability. Dynamic-clamp allowed us to add graded increments of $Na_V1.7$ current to the cell, matching the injected conductances to the predicted contribution of $Na_V1.7$ channels to the TTX-S current (70% of total TTX-S current in each cell is assumed to be produced by $Na_V1.7$; see above). We found that the current threshold (defined when the 2nd differential of AP changes its sign) inversely correlated in a linear fashion ($r^2 = 0.97$, current threshold; $r^2 = 0.98$, incremental threshold change) with the addition of $Na_V1.7$ conductance (figure 3, A and B). Current threshold decreased from its original value (426 ± 82 pA, $n = 9$) to a value of 310 ± 65 pA ($n = 9$) when $Na_V1.7$ was doubled by dynamic-clamp. Since current threshold variability was large (current threshold in 9 control cells was 350, 230, 470, 525, 340, 240, 90, 840, and 750 pA) in small DRG neurons, we normalized the effect of the $Na_V1.7$ channel addition on current threshold and expressed it in the form $100\% \times \Delta CT/CT_0$, where ΔCT is current threshold change at the respective level of $Na_V1.7$ addition and CT_0 is native current threshold. The normalized current threshold change significantly decreased (Mann-Whitney, $P < 0.001$) from −5.6 ± 0.8% (addition of 12.5% $Na_V1.7$) to −28.1 ± 3.5% (addition of 100% $Na_V1.7$). Importantly, stimulation with a current equivalent to the current threshold when $Na_V1.7$ conductance was doubled did not elicit an AP in a DRG neuron with native levels of $Na_V1.7$ (figure 3, A and B). Electronic addition of $Na_V1.7$ conductance also resulted in an enhancement of AP firing probability (figure 3C). A 10-Hz train of 10 current pulses 10-ms duration each applied at the threshold level evoked 1.7 ± 0.3 APs in control cells vs. 4.3 ± 0.5 ($n = 8$; $P < 0.01$), 6.1 ± 0.7 ($n = 8$; $P < 0.01$), 8.4 ± 0.7 ($n = 8$; $P < 0.001$), and 9.4 ± 0.5 ($n = 8$; $P < 0.001$) after electronic addition of 12.5, 25, 50, and 100% $Na_V1.7$ conductance, respectively (figure 3D).

It is reasonable to suggest that electronic subtraction of $Na_V1.7$ conductance will reduce neuronal excitability. Indeed, incremental addition of graded levels of negative $Na_V1.7$ conductance resulted in an increase of current threshold in a linear fashion ($r^2 = 0.99$) and in incremental ($r^2 = 0.98$) reduction of AP firing probability (figure 4, A and B). A 10-Hz train of 10 current pulses applied at 1.5× threshold level evoked 9.9 ± 0.1 APs ($n = 15$) in control cells vs. 9.4 ± 0.4 ($n = 15$), 7.8 ± 0.6 ($n = 15$; $P < 0.001$), 5.3 ± 1.7 ($n = 15$; $P < 0.001$), and 2.0 ± 1.0 ($n = 15$; $P < 0.001$) after dynamic-clamp subtraction of 12.5, 25, 50, and 100% $Na_V1.7$ conductance, respectively (figure 4, A and B). In the same cells, current threshold increment significantly increased from 3.9 ± 0.7 to 9.4 ± 1.6% ($n = 13$; $P < 0.01$), 17.1 ± 2.3% ($n = 13$; $P < 0.001$), and 32.8 ± 3.4% ($n = 13$; $P < 0.001$) in response to 12.5, 25, 50, and 100% reduction of $Na_V1.7$ conductance. Since the $Na_V1.7$ channel begins to activate at −55 to −50 mV (figure 1A), it is possible that subtraction of $Na_V1.7$ conductance results in a reduced sodium current at subthreshold voltages, lowering the net current influx so that, to achieve AP threshold, the stimulus intensity would need to be increased to compensate for the lower sodium charge. Our measurements of $Na_V1.7$ channel activity in a dynamic-clamped DRG neuron support this hypothesis. $Na_V1.7$ began to activate at about −53 mV, reached 62% of its peak value at −32-mV threshold voltage, and reached peak amplitude at −19 mV (figure 4C). In the example shown, $Na_V1.7$ sodium influx at subthreshold voltages comprises ∼21% of the total sodium charge due to $Na_V1.7$ channel activity occurring in the time interval between stimulus onset and AP undershoot (figure 4C). Subsequently, the channel inactivates quickly, and the resulting current is not present during the interspike interval provided membrane potential is not ramping back to the threshold level (figure 4D, but see figure 5C). The relatively slow channel repriming kinetics at membrane voltages close to resting membrane potential (RMP; figure 1C) still allow the channel to recover from inactivation during 10-Hz stimulation cycle without significant accumulation

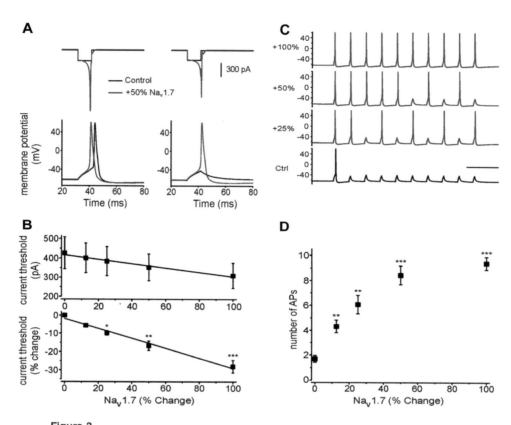

Figure 3

Additional Na$_V$1.7 conductance lowers current threshold for action potential (AP) generation and increases AP firing probability. (A) 10-ms-long test pulses (top) applied at the original threshold without additional conductance (left) and at the threshold after electronic addition of 50% Na$_V$1.7 conductance (right) elicited APs (bottom). Control stimulus and AP traces are shown in black, and those after addition of 50% Na$_V$1.7 conductance are shown in blue. (B) Averages of current threshold (top) and current threshold change (bottom) plotted as a function of additional Na$_V$1.7 conductance ($n = 9$). The solid line is a linear regression fit ($r^2 = 0.97$, top; $r^2 = 0.97$, bottom) of the data. Statistical analysis on the bottom was performed between threshold increments obtained at 12.5% and at the respective percentage of conductance increment. $*P < 0.05$, $**P < 0.01$, and $***P < 0.001$. (C) APs evoked by a 1-s-long, 10-Hz train of current pulses (10-ms pulse width) applied at the original threshold level (100% native Na$_V$1.7 conductance). Electronic addition of Na$_V$1.7 conductance (expressed as the incremental increase over the endogenous Na$_V$1.7 conductance) is noted on the y-axis. Scale bar, 200 ms. (D) Averages of the number of APs evoked by the protocol described in C plotted as a function of dynamically introduced Na$_V$1.7 conductance ($n = 8$).

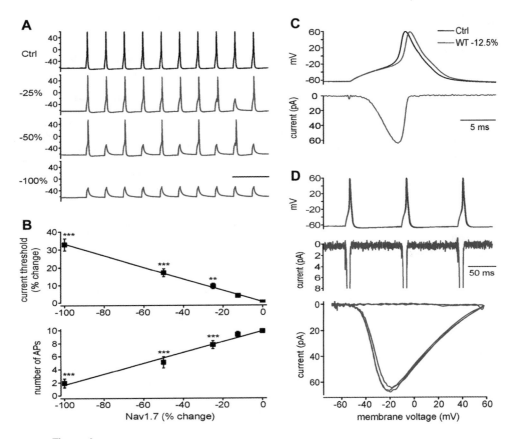

Figure 4

Removal of $Na_V1.7$ conductance raises current threshold for AP generation and reduces AP firing probability. (A) APs were evoked by 10-ms-long current pulses applied at 1.5× threshold amplitude in control (Ctrl; black) and after electronic subtraction of the incremental values of $Na_V1.7$ conductance. Dynamic-clamp subtraction of $Na_V1.7$ conductance (expressed as the incremental decrease over the endogenous $Na_V1.7$ conductance) is noted on the y-axis. Scale bar: 200 ms. (B, top) Averages ($n = 13$) of current threshold change in response to the subtraction of respective proportion of endogenous $Na_V1.7$ conductance. The solid line is a linear regression fit ($r^2 = 0.99$) of the data. Statistical analysis on the top was performed between threshold increments obtained at 12.5% and at the respective percentage of conductance increment. (B, bottom) Averages ($n = 15$) of the number of APs evoked by the protocol described in A and plotted as a function of dynamically subtracted $Na_V1.7$ conductance; the solid line is a linear regression fit ($r^2 = 0.98$) of the data. **$P < 0.01$ and ***$P < 0.001$. (C) AP (top) evoked by a 10-ms-long current stimulus of 1.5× threshold intensity in control (black) and after dynamic-clamp subtraction of 12.5% of $Na_V1.7$ conductance (blue) and the respective $Na_V1.7$ model current (bottom). (D) APs (top) evoked by the protocol described above in control (black) and after dynamic-clamp subtraction (middle) of 12.5% of endogenous $Na_V1.7$ conductance. The I–V phase plot of the model $Na_V1.7$ conductance dynamically subtracted during neuronal repetitive firing is shown on the bottom. Note that the positive-going (outward) dynamic-clamp current shown in C and D is flipped over 0 line to facilitate comparison of $Na_V1.7$ current across the manuscript.

of inactivation (figure 4D, bottom). These data suggest that Na$_V$1.7 channel activity at subthreshold membrane voltages drives the set point of current threshold for AP generation, thus regulating AP firing probability.

Model of Na$_V$1.7 L858H Mutant Predicts an Enhanced Level of Channel Activity during Repetitive Firing of DRG Neuron

The L858H mutation in human Na$_V$1.7 has been shown to be associated with a neuropathic pain syndrome, IEM (Yang et al. 2004). The mutation produces a hyperpolarizing shift in channel activation, slows channel deactivation, and causes an increase in amplitude of the Na$_V$1.7 current in response to slow, small depolarizations (Cummins et al. 2004). When expressed in the native cell environment, transfection with mutant channels renders small DRG neurons hyperexcitable and is associated with depolarized RMP and reduced current threshold (Rush et al. 2006). To study the mechanism of Na$_V$1.7 L858H-induced neuronal hyperexcitability in more detail, we performed quantitative evaluations of the effect of graded dynamic-clamp substitutions of L858H mutant conductance for WT Na$_V$1.7 conductance on the electrical excitability of small DRG neurons. In the absence of empirical data, we assumed that the level of functional WT and L858H channels in the DRG neuron plasma membrane was the same.

First, we constructed a Hodgkin–Huxley (Hodgkin and Huxley 1952) model of the L858H channel based on the previously reported data (Cummins et al. 2004) by appropriately modifying our kinetic model of WT Na$_V$1.7 channel. We adjusted activation rate constants to account for the -14-mV shift of L858H channel steady-state activation and for the altered mutant deactivation (figure 5B). The resulting kinetic model of L858H channel had a significantly enhanced window current (window current is defined as $m^3 \times h$ at steady-state; figure 5B) and an apparent leftward shift of I–V curve in a manner consistent with

data reported by Cummins et al. (2004) (figure 5, A and B). Maximal steady-state channel open probability increased 17-fold from 9.5×10^{-5} at -32.3 mV to 1.6×10^{-3} at -51.5 mV (figure 5B); when measured at -63-mV RMP, it increased 255-fold from 3.8×10^{-6} to 9.7×10^{-3} (figure 5B). Here and thereafter, both WT and L858H models were calculated in a 28-pF equipotential sphere of 1 μF/cm^2 capacitance; conductance density was set to 0.029 S/cm^2. We further studied differences of WT and L858H channel behavior in response to a voltage command shaped in the form of membrane potential previously recorded from spontaneously active small DRG neuron (figure 5C, top). Both WT and L858H channels were active at subthreshold levels during ramplike membrane depolarizations between APs (figure 5C, left) as well as during APs (figure 5C, right). L858H model channel was already activated at a -62-mV initiation point producing -115-pA inward current, whereas WT channel produced only -0.5-pA current at this voltage. During the second cycle of AP firing, L858H channel began to activate at -70-mV undershoot (-2 pA) and reached -209 pA at -54 mV, whereas WT channel just began to activate (-2 pA) at -54 mV. At the -33.5-mV AP voltage threshold, WT current was -115 pA, whereas L858H current was -657 pA. L858H current peaked (-659 pA) at -32.7 mV, and WT current peaked (-320 pA) at -2.9 mV. Within the postpeak 0.5 ms (WT) and 1 ms (L858H), current declined sharply to about -20 pA at the 56.8-mV AP overshoot. This pattern of L858H channel activity resulted in a substantial enhancement of the sodium influx at subthreshold membrane voltages (WT, 4.1×10^{-13} C and L858H, 1.1×10^{-11} C) as well as during AP (WT, 2.8×10^{-13} C and L858H, 7.7×10^{-13} C). The differences in the pattern of WT and L858H channel activity remain unchanged throughout the repetitive cycle of AP firing (figure 5, C and D). Steady-state inactivation and inactivation kinetics were not affected by L858H mutation. Hence, both WT and L858H channels

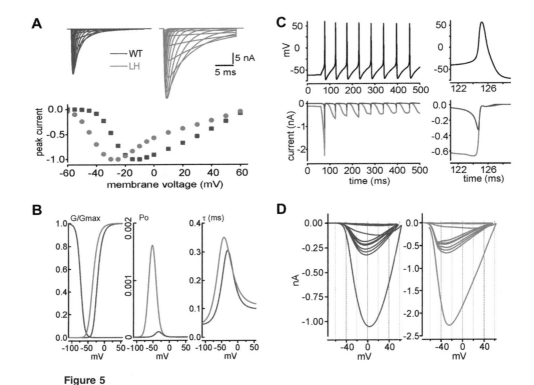

Figure 5

Kinetic model of L858H Na$_V$1.7 channel predicts a substantial enhancement of the persistent sodium current (I_{Na}) during repetitive firing of DRG neuron. (A) Normalized *I–V* relationships obtained from WT (blue) and L858H (LH; red) Na$_V$1.7 channel models. Respective traces of the $I_{Na} = g_{max}m^3h(V_m - E_{Na})$ model, where V_m is membrane voltage potential and $E_{Na} = 65$ mV is sodium reversal potential, used to obtain the *I–V* plot are presented on top. (B) Comparison of steady-state inactivation and steady-state activation (left), steady-state channel open probability (Po; middle), and activation time constant (τ; right) of the kinetic model of WT (blue) and L858H (red) Na$_V$1.7 channel. (C, top) The trace shows repetitive firing of a spontaneously active small DRG neuron. The neuron spontaneously fired APs under i=o current-clamp conditions, i.e., with no additional injected current. A small –50-pA constant current was injected to stop AP firing. The trace presented in C, top, was recorded in response to the removal of the stabilizing –50-pA current. (C, bottom) Modeled WT (blue) and L858H (red) Na$_V$1.7 currents obtained in response to the voltage command shaped in the form of the AP shown in C, top. Current-clamp recordings shown in C, *top*, were obtained from small DRG neuron in primary culture transfected by electroporation with WT Na$_V$1.7 (Dib-Hajj et al. 2009). *D*: *I–V* phase plots of WT (blue) and L858H (red) Na$_V$1.7 currents presented in C, bottom. Both models were calculated in a 28-pF equipotential sphere of 1 μF/cm^2 capacitance; conductance density was set to 0.029 S/cm^2.

showed a similar level of use-dependent inactivation (figure 5, C and D).

The model predicts a substantial enhancement of Na$_V$1.7 L858H mutant activity over a wide range of physiological membrane voltages during interspike intervals, at subthreshold levels of depolarization, and in the course of AP, thus increasing the sodium charge inflow.

Our kinetic model of the L858H mutant channel, consistent with the data published previously (Rush et al. 2006), predicted that expression of L858H mutant should enhance neuronal excitability. To test this hypothesis, we evaluated the effect of defined levels of L858H functional expression on electrical excitability of small DRG neurons using dynamic-clamp recording. A single-allele mutation of *SCN9A*, assuming equal efficiency of expression of WT and mutant channels, most probably results in 1:1 ratio of WT and L858H expressions in sensory neurons of the affected individual; however, the exact stoichiometry of WT-to-L858H expression is not known. We therefore used dynamic-clamp to assess the effect of substitutions of graded amounts of L858H current for WT current. In designing our experiments on rat DRG neurons, we first estimated the endogenous Na$_V$1.7 conductance (see above for details) and then dynamically substituted graded amounts of endogenous conductance by equal amounts of L858H channel conductance. Essentially, we performed dynamic-clamp operation SR × g_{max}(L858H – WT).

We first tested the effect of WT-to-L858H substitution on current threshold. An AP was first evoked in a control DRG neuron without any current substitution by a 10-ms current pulse of threshold intensity (figure 6A). WT-to-L858H substitution was then implemented and resulted in a substantial inward current that developed at subthreshold voltages during stimulation and an apparent shortening of the delay for AP generation. The amplitude of the AP was not affected and was (from overshoot to undershoot) 113.9 mV in control vs. 114.8 (112.6) mV at a 25%

(50%) SR [i.e., at 25% (50%) L858H]. At the same time, the maximal rate of AP rise became progressively smaller, being 114.2, 109.5, and 96.1 mV/ms in control and 25 and 50% SR, respectively (figure 6, A and B). We suggest that this deceleration of AP rate of rise could be the result of the additional inactivation of endogenous channels due to the depolarization of RMP described below; however, we cannot exclude the possibility that the reduction of net (L858H – WT) current seen at the respective voltage of AP maximal rise rate (20 mV; 527 pA at 25% SR and 385 pA at 50% SR) is a causative factor (figure 6B, right). Substitution of WT-to-L858H conductance in incremental amounts resulted in the reduction of AP current threshold in a linear manner (r^2 = 0.96, figure 6C, top; r^2 = 0.97, figure 6C, bottom). Current threshold was 668 ± 142 pA (control, n = 5) and was reduced to 598 ± 188, 457 ± 92, 328 ± 53, and 133 ± 20 pA (n = 5; P < 0.05) after 12.5, 25, 50, and 100% WT-to-L858H substitution, respectively (figure 6C). The reduction of current threshold was accompanied by enhancement of AP firing probability (figure 6D). A 10-Hz train of 10 current pulses applied at the threshold level evoked on average 1.3 ± 0.2 APs in control and 8.9 ± 0.5, 9.3 ± 0.6, 8.9 ± 1.0, and 8.4 ± 1.0 APs (n = 5; P < 0.01) after 12.5, 25, 50, and 100% WT-to-L858H substitution, respectively (figure 6E).

The present findings confirm earlier results (Rush et al. 2006) showing that the reduction of current threshold and the enhancement of AP firing probability are accompanied by RMP depolarization (figure 7C). At a mechanistic level, the present results add to the previous findings by showing that RMP depolarization is driven by the persistent window activity of L858H channel at membrane voltages close to RMP (figure 5B, middle). The effect of WT conductance subtraction in (L858H – WT) model on DRG neuron RMP was negligible since addition or subtraction of up to 100% of WT Na$_V$1.7 conductance, performed in a set of additional experiments, did

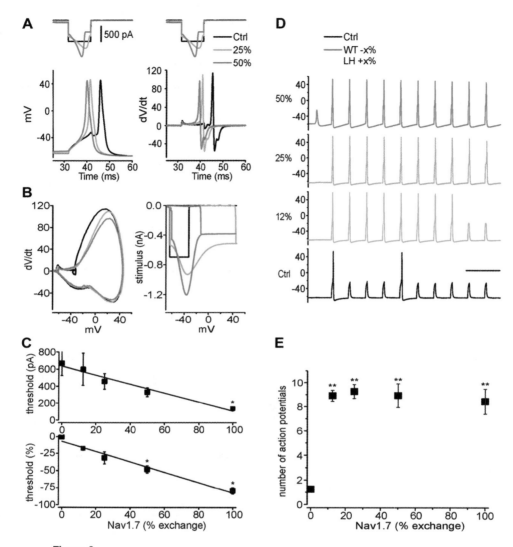

Figure 6

L858H mutant lowers current threshold and enhances AP firing probability of DRG neuron. (A) AP (bottom, left) evoked by 10-ms-long stimulus (on top) of threshold intensity in control (black) and after implementation of 25% (green) and 50% (red) WT-to-L858H substitution ratio (SR); traces of the respective AP rate of change are shown in bottom, right. (B) Trajectory plots of AP rate of change (left) and the respective trajectory of stimulus (right) recorded at incremental levels of WT-to-L858H substitution; data are obtained from APs shown in *A*. (C) Current threshold (top) and current threshold change (bottom) obtained at different levels of WT-to-L858H conductance substitution in dynamically clamped DRG neuron. Solid line represents linear regression fit of the data ($n = 5$; top, $r^2 = 0.96$; bottom, $r^2 = 0.97$). Statistical analysis on the bottom was performed between threshold increments obtained at 12.5% and at the respective percentage of conductance increment. *$P < 0.05$. (D) APs evoked by a 10-Hz train of 10-ms-long current pulses of threshold intensity in control (black) and after incremental levels (the value is depicted on the left to the *y*-axis) of WT-to-L858H conductance substitution. Scale bar, 200 ms. (E) Averages ($n = 5$) of the number of APs evoked by the protocol presented in *D* at different levels of WT-to-L858H conductance substitution. **$P < 0.01$.

not significantly affect RMP of DRG neurons in the −65- to −62-mV range of recorded RMP (figure 7, A and B). The average RMP of DRG neurons was (mean ± SE, $n = 6$; $P > 0.05$): −64 ± 0.6 mV in control and −63.5 ± 0.8, −63.8 ± 0.7, −64.0 ± 0.5, −63.6 ± 0.6, −63.6 ± 0.6, −63.7 ± 0.7, −63.9 ± 0.8, and −64.0 ± 1.0 mV after addition of −100, −50, −25, −12.5, +12.5, +25, +50, and +100% WT conductance, respectively

(figure 7, A and B). In contrast, WT-to-L858H substitution significantly depolarized RMP from −63.4 ± 0.6 mV in control to −62.3 ± 0.5 mV ($n = 6$; $P > 0.05$), −60.7 ± 0.8 mV ($n = 6$; $P < 0.05$), −58.4 ± 0.9 mV ($n = 6$; $P < 0.01$), and −56.6 ± 1.3 mV ($n = 6$; $P < 0.01$) after 12.5, 25, 50, and 100% WT-to-L858H conductance exchange, respectively (figure 7D).

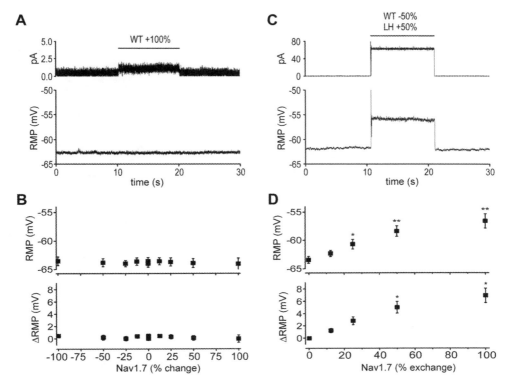

Figure 7
L858H mutant drives depolarization of resting membrane potential (RMP) of DRG neuron. (A) Dynamic-clamp recordings of RMP (bottom) and WT current (top) of DRG neuron in control and after addition of 100% WT Na$_V$1.7 conductance. (B) Averages ($n = 6$) of the RMP (top) and the RMP changes (bottom) as a function of addition or subtraction of the incremental values of WT Na$_V$1.7 conductance. (C and D) Data description is similar to A and B, but the RMP data were obtained as a response of WT-to-L858H substitution (WT conductance was dynamically subtracted while the equivalent amount of L858H conductance was added) at incremental levels ranging from 12.5 to 100% ($n = 6$). Statistical analysis on the bottom was performed between RMP changes obtained at 12.5% SR and at the respective percentage of conductance SRs. *$P < 0.05$ and **$P < 0.01$.

L858H Mutant Enhances DRG Neuron Excitability by Increasing Sodium Influx during Subthreshold Membrane Depolarizations and Interspike Intervals

Our model of the L858H mutant predicts an enhanced level of channel activity at subthreshold and suprathreshold voltages during repetitive firing of DRG neuron (see figure 5 and text above). The additional sodium charge inflow predicted by our results would be expected to be proexcitatory and should lead to enhanced neuronal excitability. We tested this hypothesis in dynamically clamped DRG neurons by assessing the response to a 10-Hz train of 10-ms depolarizing stimuli of two models: WT and (L858H – WT). We wanted to compare numerically the effect of these two models of channel activity on neuronal excitability side by side and first present data at 12.5% WT channel conductance addition and the respective 12.5% WT-to-L858H conductance exchange, since 12.5% SR is the minimal substitution studied for which AP firing is affected.

We found that L858H channels were already active at –63.4-mV RMP, producing current responsible for ~1-mV depolarizing shift of the RMP (–63.4 ± 0.6 mV in control and –62.3 ± 0.5 mV after 12.5% SR, $n = 6$, $P > 0.05$, but with a clear depolarizing trend of RMP), whereas

WT current was not detectable above the noise, thus having no effect on RMP (–64 ± 0.6 mV in control and –63.6 ± 0.6 mV after addition of 12.5% WT conductance; figure 8, A–D). WT current began to activate (–3 pA) at –50.9 mV and reached its –216-pA maximum amplitude at 12.4 mV, a value of membrane voltages well above –40-mV AP threshold. In contrast, (L858H – WT) net current was already active (–21 pA) at –63-mV RMP and reached its maximum (–452 pA) at –30.6 mV. During interspike intervals, the net current resulting from (L858H – WT) substitution gradually increased from –1 pA at –69.5 mV to –20 pA at –64 mV, contributing to the development of slow, ramplike depolarization of the membrane potential (figure 8, D and E), whereas current produced by WT model was not detectable above the noise (figure 8, B and E). Significantly more net charge was carried by the (L858H – WT) compared with WT (in pA*ms/nA, we normalized current charge to the amplitude of native $Na_V1.7$ current to account for cell-to-cell variability in the level of endogenous $Na_V1.7$ current): 6.6 ± 1.2 (WT, $n = 8$) vs. 48 ± 10 (L858H, $n = 5$; $P < 0.01$) during subthreshold depolarization; and –0.2 ± 0.32 (WT, $n = 8$) compared with 58.2 ± 10.4 (L858H, $n = 5$; $P < 0.01$) during interspike intervals; whereas the charge during AP actually was smaller for

Figure 8

L858H mutant augments DRG neuron excitability by enhancing sodium influx at subthreshold (subthresh) membrane voltages. (A) AP evoked by a 10-ms-long current pulse of threshold intensity in control (black) and after dynamically introduced +12.5% WT conductance (blue). APs are shown on the top (stimulation protocol is shown on top of APs), and the respective $Na_V1.7$ current is presented in the bottom. (B) AP repetitive firing (top) evoked by a 10-Hz train of 10-ms-long current pulses at threshold intensity in control (black) and after 12.5% WT addition (blue); dynamic-clamp recording of the 12.5% WT current addition is shown on the bottom. (C and D) Same protocols as shown in A and B, but the comparison is made between data obtained in control (black) and after dynamic-clamp substitution of 12.5% WT to 12.5% L858H conductance. (E) I–V phase plots of dynamic-clamp recordings of repetitive AP firing in DRG neuron presented in B and D at +12.5% WT (blue) and at 12.5% WT to 12.5% L858H substitution (red). (F) Modeled sodium currents were recorded in dynamic-clamp mode and subsequently integrated over 3 different time intervals: (1) from stimulus onset to AP threshold (threshold is defined when 2nd differential of AP changes its sign); this interval extends from arrow 1 to 2 in A and C; (2) from threshold to undershoot; this interval extends between arrows 2 and 3 in A and C; and (3) from undershoot to the next stimulus onset. Sodium charge (pA*ms) was normalized to the peak value of the native $Na_V1.7$ sodium current measured in each DRG neuron in voltage-clamp (see Materials and Methods). The data represent the model channel activity at +12.5% WT addition ($n = 8$, blue) and 12.5% WT-to-L858H substitution ($n = 5$, red). **$P < 0.01$.

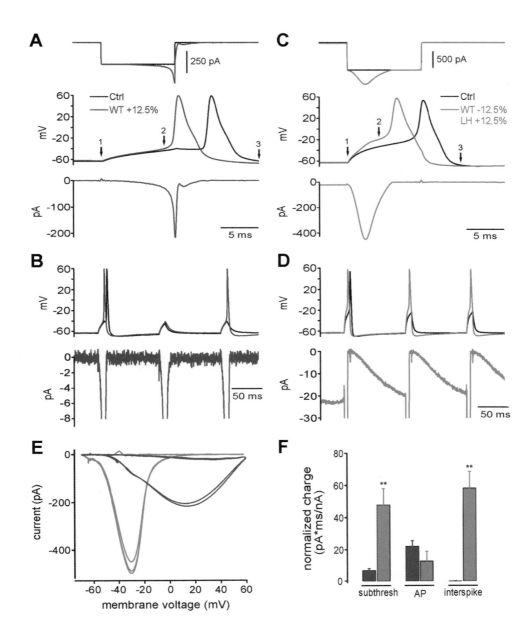

mutant cells, 12.6 ± 6.3 (L858H, *n* = 5), compared with WT, 22 ± 3.5 (*n* = 8). These data indicate that the substantial increase of L858H channel activity at subthreshold membrane voltages results in a significant amplification of net sodium influx, subsequent depolarization of the membrane potential, reduction of current threshold, and ensuing enhancement of AP firing probability. These observations reveal enhancement of small DRG neuron excitability by substitution of as little as 12.5% of the $Na_V1.7$ channels of the cell with L858H channel (i.e., with expression of the mutant channel at a density much lower than expected for a cell with 1 mutant allele) and demonstrate the powerful effect of the mutant channels on nociceptor excitability.

Finally, as a model of nociceptors in patients carrying the L858H mutation, where single-allele mutation of *SCN9A* probably results in a ratio close to 1:1 of WT and L858H, we assessed the effect of a 50% SR of L858H channels. The model produced −37 ± 2 pA (*n* = 6) persistent current at rest (figure 9, A and B), which depolarized RMP on average by 5 mV from −63.4 ± 0.6 mV in control to −58.4 ± 0.9 mV (*n* = 6; *P* < 0.01) after 50% WT-to-L858H conductance exchange (figure 7D and figure 9, A and B). This current activated further at subthreshold membrane potentials in response to depolarizing current injection, reached −432 ± 112 (*n* = 6) peak at 2.7 ± 0.4 ms poststimulus before AP threshold, and then promptly declined to essentially zero level within the next 3.6 ± 0.7 ms (figure 9A). The net charge inflow due to the (L858H − WT) model activity during subthreshold depolarization and during AP was 0.8 ± 0.3 pC and 0.3 ± 0.2 pC (*n* = 6), respectively (figure 9C). During first interspike intervals, the net current resulting from 50% (L858H − WT) SR produced 2.9 ± 0.5 pC charge inflow, contributing to the development of slow, ramp-like depolarization of the membrane potential (figure 9, B and C). These observations of increased sodium influx underlying enhancement of small DRG

Figure 9
A single-allele *SCN9A* mutation: L858H functional evaluation in small DRG neuron. (A) AP evoked by a current pulse of threshold intensity in control (black) and after dynamic-clamp 50% exchange of WT-to-L858H conductance (red). APs are shown on the top (stimulation protocol is shown on top of APs), and the respective $Na_V1.7$ current differential is presented in the bottom. (B) AP repetitive firing (top) evoked by a 10-Hz train of current pulses (same as in A) at threshold intensity in control (black) and after 50% WT-to-L858H SR (blue); dynamic-clamp recording of the 50% (L858H − WT) current is shown on the bottom. (C) Dynamic-clamp (L858H − WT) model currents at 50% SR of endogenous $Na_V1.7$ conductance were integrated over 3 different time intervals: (1) from stimulus onset to AP threshold (arrow 1 to *2* in A); (2) from threshold to undershoot (arrows 2 and 3 in A); and (3) from undershoot to the next stimulus onset. Sodium charge (pA*ms) was normalized to the peak value of the native $Na_V1.7$ sodium current (*n* = 6). Kruskal-Wallis ANOVA nonparametric test for 3 populations was used to determine whether the samples come from different populations (*P* < 0.01).

neuron excitability following L858H substitution provide a mechanistic link between altered function of mutant channels and nociceptor hyperexcitability underlying the pain phenotype in patients carrying the $Na_V1.7$ L858H mutation.

Discussion

Our dynamic-clamp recording in native rat DRG neurons shows that increasing the $Na_V1.7$ conductance density lowers threshold for a single AP and increases the number of APs fired in response to a train of depolarizing stimuli. Our data show a linear inverse relationship between functional $Na_V1.7$ conductance and current threshold (the minimal stimulus capable of eliciting an AP). Consistent with the latter, we found a direct correlation between $Na_V1.7$ conductance and AP firing probability. The relationship between $Na_V1.7$ conductance and AP firing probability was also linear in the 0–25% range of additional $Na_V1.7$ conductances. Saturation at 50–100% level was at least in part due to reach-

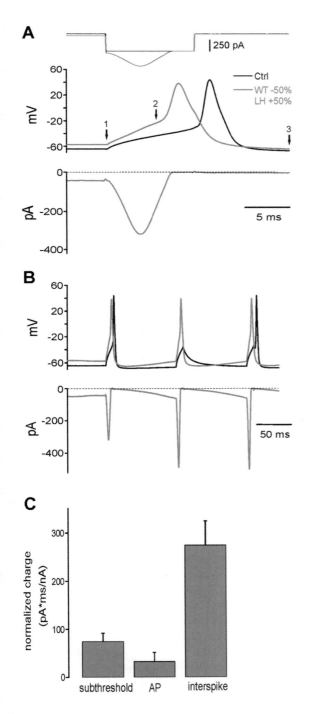

ing maximal possible number of APs that could be evoked by our stimulation protocol.

It is generally accepted that TTX-S channels, including Na$_V$1.7 channel, can function as a subthreshold sodium channel that amplifies membrane response to small depolarizing stimuli at subthreshold membrane voltages both in DRG neuron soma (Blair and Bean 2002; Choi and Waxman 2011; Kovalsky et al. 2009; Rush et al. 2007) and at the axon endings of primary sensory neurons (De Col et al. 2008; Pinto et al. 2008; Vasylyev and Waxman 2012). The functional impact of Na$_V$1.7 channel activity on neuronal excitability and pain signal processing has been generally studied using an "all-or-none" paradigm using genetic knockout (Nassar et al. 2004) of Na$_V$1.7 channel function. Functional contributions of Na$_V$1.7 to DRG neuron excitability, including current and voltage thresholds for AP generation and AP repetitive firing, have also been studied using computer simulations of DRG neurons (Choi and Waxman 2011; Herzog et al. 2001; Kouranova et al. 2008; Kovalsky et al. 2009; Sheets et al. 2007). However, dynamic-clamp recording is superior to computer simulation for quantitative study of Na$_V$1.7 channel function because it records the response of native neurons without making assumptions regarding which conductances to include in the computer model (Kemenes et al. 2011; Samu et al. 2012; Sharp et al. 1993). Our immediate and quite unexpected observation was that Na$_V$1.7, when studied in the native DRG neuron environment, regulated the set point for AP current threshold in a remarkably linear manner: increasing or reducing Na$_V$1.7 conductance by as little as 12.5% or as much as 100% produced a graded effect with a high degree of linearity over a 200% range of Na$_V$1.7 conductances. We found that substitution of as little as 12.5% of channels with L858H produces hyperexcitability in DRG neurons. This observation predicts that expression of L858H produces hyperexcitability of DRG neurons even if the 50% reduction of current density seen after expression of L858H in HEK-293 cells (Cummins et al. 2004) applies to nociceptors.

Within the domain permitted by our stimulation protocol, $Na_V1.7$ also regulated AP firing probability in a linear manner. This observation may be relevant to the pathophysiology of acquired pain since abnormal accumulations of $Na_V1.7$ have been demonstrated at nerve endings within painful neuromas in rats (Persson et al. 2011) and humans (Black et al. 2008), and $Na_V1.7$ levels and TTX-S current density have been shown to increase in DRG neurons in response to inflammation (Black et al. 2004) and in diabetic rats (Chattopadhyay et al. 2008, 2011). We would note, however, that although our previous patch-clamp analysis of small-diameter DRG neuron axons in vitro demonstrated a resting potential similar to that in DRG neuron somata, and sequential activation during AP clamp of TTX-S and TTX-resistant currents with characteristics attributed to $Na_V1.7$ and $Na_V1.8$ (Vasylyev and Waxman 2012) similar to that seen in DRG neuron somata (Blair and Bean 2002), we cannot exclude the possibility that the properties and functional role of $Na_V1.7$ are not identical in DRG neuron somata vs. sensory axons and their terminals.

Dynamic-clamp requires an input of a kinetic model of the channel under study. Several kinetic models of TTX-S sodium channels, including $Na_V1.7$ channel, have been recently proposed (Gurkiewicz et al. 2011; Herzog et al. 2001; Kovalsky et al. 2009; Sheets et al. 2007). These models rely on experimental data for TTX-S channels steady-state and kinetic properties with some degree of variability since these were obtained in different studies. This variability may be attributed, at least in part, to differences in recording solutions and in voltage protocols. TTX-S channel recordings were often performed using fluoride-based intracellular solution, which shifts the voltage dependence of $Na_V1.7$ channel steady-state and kinetic parameters (Coste et al. 2004; Meadows et al. 2002; Saab et al. 2003;

Sheets et al. 2007). At the same time, current-clamp recordings of AP firing in DRG neurons are commonly performed in a physiologically relevant chloride-based intracellular solution (Dib-Hajj et al. 2009; Estacion et al. 2011; Rush et al. 2006). It is reasonable to develop the kinetic model of $Na_V1.7$ channel based on voltage-clamp data obtained under conditions similar to those where this model is utilized. Thus we developed a kinetic model of recombinant $Na_V1.7$ channel based on voltage-clamp recordings obtained using intracellular solution essentially similar to that used for dynamic-clamp; the single difference between voltage-clamp and dynamic-clamp pipette solutions was that potassium chloride was replaced by cesium chloride on 1:1 basis (see Materials and Methods). We also used the same HBSS bath solution for voltage-clamp and dynamic-clamp recordings. Additionally, we performed a detailed analysis of $Na_V1.7$ channel activation kinetics. Although an m^3 model is generally accepted for sodium channel gating in squid giant axon (Hodgkin and Huxley 1952), mammalian skeletal muscles (Chanda and Bezanilla 2002), and mammalian sensory neurons (Herzog et al. 2001; Kostyuk et al. 1981; Ogata and Tatebayashi 1993; Sheets et al. 2007), an m^2 model of TTX-S sodium channel activation has been suggested in mammalian central neurons (Baranauskas and Martina 2006). Consistent with previous studies of TTX-S sodium current (Herzog et al. 2001; Kostyuk et al. 1981; McCormick et al. 2007; Ogata and Tatebayashi 1993; Sheets et al. 2007), we found that recombinant $Na_V1.7$ channel activated with an apparent delay, suggesting multiple transitions between closed states, in a sigmoidal manner with activation kinetics best described by m^3 model.

The $Na_V1.7$ L858H mutation was identified in a patient with hereditary primary erythromelalgia (Yang et al. 2004). Subsequent studies showed that the L858H mutation produces a -13.5-mV hyperpolarizing shift of $Na_V1.7$ channel activation, slows channel deactivation, and enhances

Na$_V$1.7 current amplitude in response to slow, small depolarizations in a manner consistent with its erythromelalgia phenotype (Cummins et al. 2004). We modeled kinetics of the L858H mutant by appropriately adjusting WT channel activation rate constants to obtain the respective alterations in kinetics and in *I–V* relationships similar to those reported for recombinant WT and L858H channels (Cummins et al. 2004). Our L858H model predicted enhancement of Na$_V$1.7 channel activity at subthreshold membrane voltages. In response to a voltage command shaped in the form of membrane voltage of spontaneously firing DRG neuron, substitution of only 12.5% of the channels of the cell with the L858H model, compared with WT, resulted in a 27-fold increase of sodium influx at subthreshold membrane voltages and in a 3-fold sodium influx increase during the AP. When we evoked APs in dynamic-clamp using a 10-ms depolarizing stimulus, persistent L858H channel activity at subthreshold voltages produced >600% additional sodium influx during small depolarizations and resulted in the appearance of a significant sodium influx during interspike intervals (−0.2 ± 0.32, WT; compared with 58.2 ± 10.4, L858H). Such a substantial increase of the sodium influx is proexcitatory, and we were not surprised to observe a hyperexcitable neuronal phenotype due to L858H introduced by dynamic-clamp. Substitution of 50% WT-to-L858H conductance in our dynamic-clamp experiments produced persistent current that depolarized RMP on average by 5 mV and resulted in a reduction of current threshold on average by 51% without changing AP overshoot. This persistent current activated further at subthreshold membrane potentials in response to depolarizing current injection, reached its peak before AP threshold, and then promptly declined to essentially zero level within the next few milliseconds. The net charge inflow due to (L858H − WT) model was larger during subthreshold depolarization than during the AP and produced a significant charge inflow during

interspike intervals driving a slow, ramplike depolarization of the membrane potential. On the basis of the present results, we attribute the L858H-induced RMP depolarization described by Rush et al. (2006) and seen in this study to the persistent current due to window channel activity. Steady-state open channel probability at −63-mV RMP increased 255-fold from 3.8 × 10^{-6} (WT) to 9.7 × 10^{-3} (L858H). Maximal conductance of endogenous Na$_V$1.7 current (see Materials and Methods and Results) was 317 ± 68 nS (*n* = 6, WT experiments) and 354 ± 64 nS (*n* = 6, L858H experiments). Addition of 50% of the respective conductance resulted, assuming the calculated steady-state open probability, in 0.08-pA (WT) and 22-pA (L858H) persistent current at −63-mV RMP for dynamic-clamped neuron.

Our results obtained via dynamic-clamp at physiological levels of WT and mutant Na$_V$1.7 conductance show, for the first time, that current threshold of small DRG neurons is regulated by Na$_V$1.7 in a linear manner. Our observations also demonstrate that persistent activity of the L858H mutant channel in small DRG neurons amplifies sodium influx at subthreshold membrane voltages, so as to depolarize RMP and reduce current threshold for AP generation, thus producing hyperexcitability in nociceptive DRG neurons. Taken together, these findings establish a quantitative mechanistic link between the altered biophysical properties of a mutant Na$_V$1.7 channel and nociceptor hyperexcitability underlying the pain phenotype in IEM.

Grants

This work was supported in part by grant from the Rehabilitation Research & Development Service and Medical Research Service, Department of Veterans Affairs to S. G. Waxman. The Center for Neuroscience and Regeneration Research is a collaboration of the Paralyzed Veterans of America with Yale University.

About the Authors

Dmytro V. Vasylyev, Department of Neurology and Center for Neuroscience and Regeneration Research, Yale University School of Medicine, New Haven, CT; and Rehabilitation Research Center, Veterans Affairs Connecticut Healthcare System, West Haven, CT

Chongyang Han, Department of Neurology and Center for Neuroscience and Regeneration Research, Yale University School of Medicine, New Haven, CT; and Rehabilitation Research Center, Veterans Affairs Connecticut Healthcare System, West Haven, CT

Peng Zhao, Department of Neurology and Center for Neuroscience and Regeneration Research, Yale University School of Medicine, New Haven, CT; and Rehabilitation Research Center, Veterans Affairs Connecticut Healthcare System, West Haven, CT

Sulayman Dib-Hajj, Department of Neurology and Center for Neuroscience and Regeneration Research, Yale University School of Medicine, New Haven, CT; and Rehabilitation Research Center, Veterans Affairs Connecticut Healthcare System, West Haven, CT

Stephen G. Waxman, Department of Neurology and Center for Neuroscience and Regeneration Research, Yale University School of Medicine, New Haven, CT; and Rehabilitation Research Center, Veterans Affairs Connecticut Healthcare System, West Haven, CT

Disclosures

No conflicts of interest, financial or otherwise, are declared by the author(s).

Author Contributions

D.V.V., S.D.-H., and S.G.W. conception and design of research; D.V.V., C.H., and P.Z. performed experiments; D.V.V. and C.H. analyzed data; D.V.V., C.H., S.D.-H., and S.G.W. interpreted results of experiments; D.V.V. and C.H. prepared figures; D.V.V. drafted manuscript; D.V.V., S.D.-H., and S.G.W. edited and revised manuscript; D.V.V., C.H., P.Z., S.D.-H., and S.G.W. approved final version of manuscript.

References

Ahn HS, Vasylyev DV, Estacion M, Macala LJ, Shah P, Faber CG, Merkies IS, Dib-Hajj SD, Waxman SG. 2013. Differential effect of D623N variant and wild-type Na(v)1.7 sodium channels on resting potential and interspike membrane potential of dorsal root ganglion neurons. *Brain Res* 1529: 165–177.

Baranauskas G, Martina M. 2006. Sodium currents activate without a Hodgkin- and-Huxley-type delay in central mammalian neurons. *J Neurosci* 26: 671–684.

Black JA, Liu S, Tanaka M, Cummins TR, Waxman SG. 2004. Changes in the expression of tetrodotoxin-sensitive sodium channels within dorsal root ganglia neurons in inflammatory pain. *Pain* 108: 237–247.

Black JA, Nikolajsen L, Kroner K, Jensen TS, Waxman SG. 2008. Multiple sodium channel isoforms and mitogen-activated protein kinases are present in painful human neuromas. *Ann Neurol* 64: 644–653.

Blair NT, Bean BP. 2002. Roles of tetrodotoxin (TTX)-sensitive Na$^+$ current, TTX-resistant Na$^+$ current, and Ca^{2+} current in the action potentials of nociceptive sensory neurons. *J Neurosci* 22: 10277–10290.

Catterall WA, Goldin AL, Waxman SG. 2005. International Union of Pharmacology. XLVII. Nomenclature and structure-function relationships of voltage-gated sodium channels. *Pharmacol Rev* 57: 397–409.

Chanda B, Bezanilla F. 2002. Tracking voltage-dependent conformational changes in skeletal muscle sodium channel during activation. *J Gen Physiol* 120: 629–645.

Chattopadhyay M, Mata M, Fink DJ. 2008. Continuous delta-opioid receptor activation reduces neuronal voltage-gated sodium channel (NaV1.7) levels through activation of protein kinase C in painful diabetic neuropathy. *J Neurosci* 28: 6652–6658.

Chattopadhyay M, Mata M, Fink DJ. 2011. Vector-mediated release of GABA attenuates pain-related behaviors and reduces Na(V)1.7 in DRG neurons. *Eur J Pain* 15: 913–920.

Choi JS, Waxman SG. 2011. Physiological interactions between Na$_V$1.7 and Na$_V$1.8 sodium channels: A computer simulation study. *J Neurophysiol* 106: 3173–3184.

Coste B, Osorio N, Padilla F, Crest M, Delmas P. 2004. Gating and modulation of presumptive Na$_V$1.9 channels in enteric and spinal sensory neurons. *Mol Cell Neurosci* 26: 123–134.

Cummins TR, Dib-Hajj SD, Waxman SG. 2004. Electrophysiological properties of mutant Na$_V$1.7 sodium channels in a painful inherited neuropathy. *J Neurosci* 24: 8232–8236.

Cummins TR, Howe JR, Waxman SG. 1998. Slow closed-state inactivation: A novel mechanism underlying ramp currents in cells expressing the hNE/PN1 sodium channel. *J Neurosci* 18: 9607–9619.

Cummins TR, Waxman SG. 1997. Downregulation of tetrodotoxin-resistant sodium currents and upregulation of a rapidly repriming tetrodotoxin-sensitive sodium current in small spinal sensory neurons after nerve injury. *J Neurosci* 17: 3503–3514.

De Col R, Messlinger K, Carr RW. 2008. Conduction velocity is regulated by sodium channel inactivation in unmyelinated axons innervating the rat cranial meninges. *J Physiol* 586: 1089–1103.

Dib-Hajj SD, Choi JS, Macala LJ, Tyrrell L, Black JA, Cummins TR, Waxman SG. 2009. Transfection of rat or mouse neurons by biolistics or electroporation. *Nat Protoc* 4: 1118–1126.

Dib-Hajj SD, Cummins TR, Black JA, Waxman SG. 2010. Sodium channels in normal and pathological pain. *Annu Rev Neurosci* 33: 325–347.

Estacion M, Han C, Choi JS, Hoeijmakers JG, Lauria G, Drenth JP, Gerrits MM, Dib-Hajj SD, Faber CG, Merkies IS, Waxman SG. 2011. Intra- and interfamily phenotypic diversity in pain syndromes associated with a gain-of-function variant of Na$_V$1.7. *Mol Pain* 7: 92.

Gurkiewicz M, Korngreen A, Waxman SG, Lampert A. 2011. Kinetic modeling of Na$_V$1.7 provides insight into erythromelalgia-associated F1449V mutation. *J Neurophysiol* 105: 1546–1557.

Herzog RI, Cummins TR, Ghassemi F, Dib-Hajj SD, Waxman SG. 2003. Distinct repriming and closed-state inactivation kinetics of Na$_V$1.6 and Na$_V$1.7 sodium channels in mouse spinal sensory neurons. *J Physiol* 551: 741–750.

Herzog RI, Cummins TR, Waxman SG. 2001. Persistent TTX-resistant Na$^+$ current affects resting potential and response to depolarization in simulated spinal sensory neurons. *J Neurophysiol* 86: 1351–1364.

Hille B. 1978. Ionic channels in excitable membranes: Current problems and biophysical approaches. *Biophys J* 22: 283–294.

Hodgkin AL, Huxley AF. 1952. A quantitative description of membrane current and its application to conduction and excitation in nerve. *J Physiol* 117: 500–544.

Kemenes I, Marra V, Crossley M, Samu D, Staras K, Kemenes G, Nowotny T. 2011. Dynamic clamp with StdpC software. *Nat Protoc* 6: 405–417.

Kostyuk PG, Veselovsky NS, Tsyndrenko AY. 1981. Ionic currents in the somatic membrane of rat dorsal root ganglion neurons-I. Sodium currents. *Neuroscience* 6: 2423–2430.

Kouranova EV, Strassle BW, Ring RH, Bowlby MR, Vasilyev DV. 2008. Hyperpolarization-activated cyclic nucleotide-gated channel mRNA and protein expression in large versus small diameter dorsal root ganglion neurons: Correlation with hyperpolarization-activated current gating. *Neuroscience* 153: 1008–1019.

Kovalsky Y, Amir R, Devor M. 2009. Simulation in sensory neurons reveals a key role for delayed Na$^+$ current in subthreshold oscillations and ectopic discharge: Implications for neuropathic pain. *J Neurophysiol* 102: 1430–1442.

McCormick DA, Shu Y, Yu Y. 2007. Neurophysiology: Hodgkin and Huxley model—still standing? *Nature* 445: E1–2; discussion E2–3.

Meadows LS, Chen YH, Powell AJ, Clare JJ, Ragsdale DS. 2002. Functional modulation of human brain Na$_V$1.3 sodium channels, expressed in mammalian cells, by auxiliary beta 1, beta 2 and beta 3 subunits. *Neuroscience* 114: 745–753.

Nassar MA, Stirling LC, Forlani G, Baker MD, Matthews EA, Dickenson AH, Wood JN. 2004. Nociceptor-specific gene deletion reveals a major role for Na$_V$1.7 (PN1) in acute and inflammatory pain. *Proc Natl Acad Sci USA* 101: 12706–12711.

Neher E. 1992. Correction for liquid junction potentials in patch clamp experiments. *Methods Enzymol* 207: 123–131.

Ogata N, Tatebayashi H. 1993. Kinetic analysis of two types of Na$^+$ channels in rat dorsal root ganglia. *J Physiol* 466: 9–37.

Persson AK, Black JA, Gasser A, Cheng X, Fischer TZ, Waxman SG. 2010. Sodium-calcium exchanger and multiple sodium channel isoforms in intraepidermal nerve terminals. *Mol Pain* 6: 84.

Persson AK, Gasser A, Black JA, Waxman SG. 2011. Nav1.7 accumulates and co-localizes with phosphorylated ERK1/2 within transected axons in early experimental neuromas. *Exp Neurol* 230: 273–279.

Pinto V, Derkach VA, Safronov BV. 2008. Role of TTX-sensitive and TTX-resistant sodium channels in Aδ- and C-fiber conduction and synaptic transmission. *J Neurophysiol* 99: 617–628.

Rush AM, Craner MJ, Kageyama T, Dib-Hajj SD, Waxman SG, Ransch B. 2005. Contactin regulates the current density and axonal expression of tetro-dotoxin-resistant but not tetrodotoxin-sensitive sodium channels in DRG neurons. *Eur J Neurosci* 22: 39–49.

Rush AM, Cummins TR, Waxman SG. 2007. Multiple sodium channels and their roles in electrogenesis within dorsal root ganglion neurons. *J Physiol* 579: 1–14.

Rush AM, Dib-Hajj SD, Liu S, Cummins TR, Black JA, Waxman SG. 2006. A single sodium channel mutation produces hyper- or hypoexcitability in different types of neurons. *Proc Natl Acad Sci USA* 103: 8245–8250.

Saab CY, Cummins TR, Waxman SG. 2003. GTP gamma S increases Nav1.8 current in small-diameter dorsal root ganglia neurons. *Exp Brain Res* 152: 415–419.

Samu D, Marra V, Kemenes I, Crossley M, Kemenes G, Staras K, Nowotny T. 2012. Single electrode dynamic clamp with StdpC. *J Neurosci Methods* 211: 11–21.

Sharp AA, O'Neil MB, Abbott LF, Marder E. 1993. Dynamic clamp: Computer-generated conductances in real neurons. *J Neurophysiol* 69: 992–995.

Sheets PL, Jackson JO 2nd, Waxman SG, Dib-Hajj SD, Cummins TR. 2007. A Na$_V$1.7 channel mutation associated with hereditary erythromelalgia contributes to neuronal hyperexcitability and displays reduced lidocaine sensitivity. *J Physiol* 581: 1019–1031.

Toledo-Aral JJ, Moss BL, He ZJ, Koszowski AG, Whisenand T, Levinson SR, Wolf JJ, Silos-Santiago I, Halegoua S, Mandel G. 1997. Identification of PN1, a predominant voltage-dependent sodium channel expressed principally in peripheral neurons. *Proc Natl Acad Sci USA* 94: 1527–1532.

Vasylyev DV, Waxman SG. 2012. Membrane properties and electrogenesis in the distal axons of small dorsal root ganglion neurons in vitro. *J Neurophysiol* 108: 729–740.

Yang Y, Wang Y, Li S, Xu Z, Li H, Ma L, Fan J, et al. 2004. Mutations in SCN9A, encoding a sodium channel alpha subunit, in patients with primary erythermalgia. *J Med Genet* 41: 171–174.

BEYOND THE SEARCH: EXPANDING HORIZONS

TWISTED NERVE: A GANGLION GONE AWRY[1]

The man on fire syndrome is very rare. Neuropathic pain is not. It occurs commonly in disorders as diverse as traumatic limb amputations, nerve or nerve root compression, and peripheral neuropathy due to many causes. The central molecular player in inherited erythromelalgia, $Na_V1.7$, is pivotal in these disorders too.

The eminent nineteenth-century physician Silas Weir Mitchell—one of the founders of the American Neurological Association—holds a place of special interest to military historians because he tended to wounded soldiers on the Civil War battlefields. At that time, amputation of the injured limb was all that was available to treat bullet wounds, and the concept of the ambulance—initially just a wagon to carry a wounded soldier away from the theater of active conflict—was just emerging. Mitchell was preoccupied with pain and is credited with publishing the first description of erythromelalgia (still called, by some, Mitchell's disease), although the cases he described came from patients without a family history. Mitchell also had a deep interest in pain following trauma to nerves, which he described in detail in his book *Injuries of Nerves and Their Consequences* (Mitchell 1872). As a clinician who treated soldiers wounded on the battlefield, Mitchell was aware of the nerve injury that necessarily accompanies traumatic limb amputation and of the long-lasting pain that can ensue, not just in the retained limb stump but also in a phantom limb. The phantom limb is a construct of the nervous system that frequently replaces the lost appendage with the sensation of a retained hand or foot, not in reality there but nonetheless felt, as a part of the body that feels as if it were present, sometimes twisted, and often painful. Mitchell coined the term "phantom limb" and documented the pain that can come with it. He was also aware of the propensity of high velocity missiles—gunshot injuries—to produce chronic pain (Mitchell, Morehouse, and Kenn 1864).

Following nerve injury, the injured nerve fibers within peripheral nerves have a propensity to regenerate. If the proximal and distal parts of the injured nerve are lined up and reattached and there are no obstacles in the way, the regenerating nerve fibers may find their way to appropriate peripheral tissues and even reinnervate them, reestablishing sensation in the territory supplied by the injured nerve. If, however, there is scar tissue at the site of the injury or if the limb has been severely traumatized or amputated, regenerating nerve fibers may not be able to find their way to appropriate peripheral locations and can profusely sprout in a futile attempt at regeneration, forming a knot-like collection of blindly ending nerve fibers that do not reestablish connections with the periphery. These tangled masses of blindly ending axons, mixed with proliferating connective tissue, are called neuromas. The injured axons within experimental neuromas (in laboratory animals), and in human neuromas, are the sites of abnormal, ectopic impulse generation which contributes to neuropathic pain (Amir and Devor 1993; Burchiel 1988). It was known, even before the entire deck of human sodium channels was cloned and sequenced, that hyperexcitability within pain-signaling neuromas depends on the activity of sodium channels (Chabal, Russell, and Burchiel 1989; Devor, Wall, and Catalan 1992; Matzner and Devor 1994). And, once sodium channels were cloned and their functional attributes understood, there was evidence for a contribution of $Na_V1.7$ to many types of acquired neuropathic pain as well as inflammatory pain in animal models (Black et al. 2004; Cummins, Sheets, and Waxman 2007; Rush, Cummins, and Waxman 2007). But, what about *human* neuromas?

In 2007, I began a collaboration with Lone Nikolajsen and Troels Jensen, two pain researchers, and their surgeon colleague Karsten Kroner, who were working at the Danish Pain Research Center at the University of Aarhus. Well-preserved human neuromas, and in particular human neuromas collected from patients who had been carefully characterized in clinical terms, were not easy to come by. My collaboration with the Aarhus pain researchers provided my laboratory with a source of tissue from well-studied patients. In a joint study (Black et al. 2008), we examined the expression of sodium channels within painful human neuromas from their patients, in some of whom there had been traumatic limb amputations.

Each of the patients described in this paper had a well-characterized peripheral nerve injury. These patients had been referred to the Aarhus Research Center because they had failed to respond to treatment with medications and had consented to participate in a clinical study in which the neuromas were surgically removed in an attempt to alleviate pain. The severity and pattern of pain had been carefully assessed by the Aarhus researchers in each patient. Following removal by the surgeon in the operating room, each neuroma was rapidly and carefully placed in a freezer and stored at −80°C until shipping by air express, on dry ice, from Denmark to our laboratory at Yale where it was cut into sections for viewing under the microscope. We used antibodies which bind specifically to each type of channel and fluoresce under the microscope (a technique called "immunocytochemistry"), to assess the presence of various types of sodium channels within axons in these precious human neuromas. As shown in Black et al. (2008), this allowed us to demonstrate that higher-than-normal levels of $Na_V1.7$ and $Na_V1.8$ accumulate within human painful neuromas. The presence of high levels of these channels would be expected to produce hyperexcitability in injured axons. A few years later we showed, using computer simulations and dynamic clamp, that even small elevations in the level of expression of either of these channels can produce hyperexcitability (Choi and Waxman 2011; Vasylyev et al. 2014). Interestingly, we also observed increased levels of an enzyme called MAP kinase ERK1/2 within the injured axons within neuromas. This may magnify the functional consequences of the accumulation of $Na_V1.7$ within neuromas, since ERK1/2 is known to interact with $Na_V1.7$ and make it easier to activate (Stamboulian et al. 2010). Irrespective of whether MAP kinase amplifies the effect of $Na_V1.7$, our observations pointed to a molecular target—$Na_V1.7$—in painful human neuromas.

These observations may help to explain the phantom limb phenomenon. One theory attributes the phantom limb experience to functional reorganization of the cerebral cortex, with the cortical areas originally receiving input from the amputated body part now deprived of input from that body part, and responding to other inputs to produce a message that is interpreted as indicating the presence of the lost limb (Ramachandran and Blakeslee 1998). Other experiments challenge this concept and posit a peripheral source of the abnormal pain signaling. For example, Vaso et al. (2014) provided data supporting the hypothesis that phantom limb pain is a result of exaggerated input to the brain, generated ectopically in the injured nerve fibers that, prior to injury, innervated the limb. In a series of amputees, they applied the local anesthetic lidocaine—a sodium channel blocker—to the DRG neurons whose axons had been amputated, and rapidly and reversibly extinguished phantom limb pain as well as nonpainful phantom limb sensations. The most parsimonious explanation of these observations is that, following injury to the distal ends of peripheral nerve fibers that accompanies traumatic limb amputation, sodium channels within the injured nerve cells produce aberrant barrages of nerve impulses, thereby producing pain. The importance of these results (Vaso et al. 2014), and of our observations on abnormal accumulations of $Na_V1.7$ and $Na_V1.8$ within neuromas (Black et al. 2008), is that they identify sodium channels as molecular targets, whose silencing would be expected to alleviate pain after traumatic nerve injury. Gene therapy approaches which "knock down" the genes for sodium channels have, in fact, been shown to alleviate pain after experimental nerve injury in rats (Samad et al. 2013). Identification of abnormal accumulations of $Na_V1.7$ and $Na_V1.8$ within human neuromas encourages us to think that targeting of these channels may provide pain relief not only in animal models of pain, but also in people who have sustained nerve injuries.

When Mitchell tended to wounded soldiers on the Civil War battlefield, amputation of an injured limb was one of the few options available to the doctor. Surgical excision of neuromas continues to be used for some patients today in attempts to alleviate pain. Previous assessments of the effects of surgical removal of neuromas, however, provided a mixed picture. There were some suggestions that this operation might relieve pain (Ducic et al. 2008; Krishnan, Pinzer, and Schackert 2005), but the results differed substantially in different series of patients. The patients we studied had continued to suffer from intractable and severe pain from their neuromas despite attempts at treatment with multiple medications. So, as a corollary to our study on sodium channels within neuromas, our Danish colleagues in Denmark wanted to assess the clinical efficacy of surgical excision of neuromas (Nikolajsen et al. 2010). These patients were told that surgical removal of neuromas was an experimental procedure that might result in reduced pain, but that there was a risk of worsened pain. Following surgical removal of the neuromas by a specialist in nerve surgery, patients were followed for six months, during which their pain was periodically assessed. We attempted to identify clinical features or responses to medications that might pinpoint patients who were more likely to respond favorably to surgery, but we did not find any predictors of successful outcome. We found that surgery produced long-lasting relief of spontaneous pain in only two out of the six patients we studied. Interestingly, one patient with relief of pain after surgery had a prior poor response to neuroma removal. We interpreted our findings as suggesting that, as a therapeutic maneuver, surgical excision of neuromas should be reserved for patients with intractable pain who have failed to respond to other therapies. We also noted, however, that a prior poor response to surgical neuroma removal does not preclude relief of pain after a new excision (Nikolajsen et al. 2010).

Overall, the limited efficacy of surgical removal of neuromas underscored the conclusions of our immunocytochemical study, which showed that nerve injury and neuroma formation trigger a change in the pattern of gene expression in the injured nerve cells that leads to hyperexcitability. These observations suggest that molecular targeting may be more effective than surgery in relieving pain from nerve injury and neuromas. New compounds that selectively block $Na_V1.7$ are being assessed in clinical studies. Blockers of $Na_V1.8$, which works in tandem with $Na_V1.7$ to produce high-frequency firing, may come next. It would be ironic if a cure for pain, after penetrating trauma from missiles or other weapons, were to be provided not by a surgeon's knife, but by therapeutic targeting of tiny molecules within nerve cells. That would signal a transformation of medicine from scalpel to the submicroscopic. And that seems to be where we are heading.

Note

1. From *Slaves,* published in the 1924 collection *The Three Sphinxes and Other Poems,* by George Sylvester Viereck.

References

Amir R, Devor M. 1993. Ongoing activity in neuroma afferents bearing retrograde sprouts. *Brain Res* 630(1–2): 283–288.

Black JA, Liu S, Tanaka M, Cummins TR, Waxman SG. 2004. Changes in the expression of tetrodotoxin-sensitive sodium channels within dorsal root ganglia neurons in inflammatory pain. *Pain* 108(3): 237–247.

Black JA, Nikolajsen L, Kroner K, Jensen TS, Waxman SG. 2008. Multiple sodium channel isoforms and mitogen-activated protein kinases are present in painful human neuromas. *Ann Neurol* 64(6): 644–653.

Burchiel KJ. 1988. Carbamazepine inhibits spontenous activity in experimental neuromas. *Exp Neurol* 102(2): 249–253.

Chabal C, Russell LC, Burchiel KJ. 1989. The effect of intravenous lidocaine, tocainide, and mexiletine on spontaneously active fibers originating in rat sciatic neuromas. *Pain* 38(3): 333–338.

Choi JS, Waxman SG. 2011. Physiological interactions between Na(v)1.7 and Na(v)1.8 sodium channels: A computer simulation study. *J Neurophysiol* 106(6): 3173–3184.

Cummins TR, Sheets PL, Waxman SG. 2007. The roles of sodium channels in nociception: Implications for mechanisms of pain. *Pain* 131(3): 243–257.

Devor M, Wall PD, Catalan N. 1992. Systemic lidocaine silences ectopic neuroma and DRG discharge without blocking nerve conduction. *Pain* 48(2): 261–268.

Ducic I, Mesbahi AN, Attinger CE, Graw K. 2008. The role of peripheral nerve surgery in the treatment of chronic pain associated with amputation stumps. *Plast Reconstr Surg* 121(3): 908–914, discussion 915–917.

Krishnan KG, Pinzer T, Schackert G. 2005. Coverage of painful peripheral nerve neuromas with vascularized soft tissue: Method and results. *Neurosurgery* 56(2 Suppl): 369–378, discussion 369–378.

Matzner O, Devor M. 1994. Hyperexcitability at sites of nerve injury depends on voltage-sensitive Na+ channels. *J Neurophysiol* 72(1): 349–359.

Mitchell SW. 1872. *Injuries of nerves and their consequences.* Philadelphia: Lippincott.

Mitchell SW, Morehouse GR, Kenn WW. 1864. *Gunshot wounds and other injuries of nerves.* Philadelphia: Lippincott.

Nikolajsen L, Black JA, Kroner K, Jensen TS, Waxman SG. 2010. Neuroma removal for neuropathic pain: Efficacy and predictive value of lidocaine infusion. *Clin J Pain* 26(9): 788–793.

Ramachandran VS, Blakeslee S. 1998. *Phantoms in the brain: Probing the mysteries of the human mind.* New York: William Morrow.

Rush AM, Cummins TR, Waxman SG. 2007. Multiple sodium channels and their roles in electrogenesis within dorsal root ganglion neurons. *J Physiol* 579(Pt 1): 1–14.

Samad OA, Tan AM, Cheng X, Foster E, Dib-Hajj SD, Waxman SG. 2013. Virus-mediated shRNA knockdown of Na(v)1.3 in rat dorsal root ganglion attenuates nerve injury-induced neuropathic pain. *Mol Ther* 21(1): 49–56.

Stamboulian S, Choi JS, Ahn HS, Chang YW, Tyrrell L, Black JA, Waxman SG, Dib-Hajj SD. 2010. ERK1/2 mitogen-activated protein kinase phosphorylates sodium channel Na(v)1.7 and alters its gating properties. *J Neurosci* 30(5): 1637–1647.

Vaso A, Adahan HM, Gjika A, Zahaj S, Zhurda T, Vyshka G, Devor M. 2014. Peripheral nervous system origin of phantom limb pain. *Pain* 155(7): 1384–1391.

Vasylyev DV, Han C, Zhao P, Dib-Hajj S, Waxman SG. 2014. Dynamic-clamp analysis of wild-type human Nav1.7 and erythromelalgia mutant channel L858H. *J Neurophysiol* 111(7): 1429–1443.

MULTIPLE SODIUM CHANNEL ISOFORMS AND MITOGEN-ACTIVATED PROTEIN KINASES ARE PRESENT IN PAINFUL HUMAN NEUROMAS*

Joel A. Black, Lone Nikolajsen, Karsten Kroner, Troels S. Jensen, and Stephen G. Waxman

Objective: Although axons within neuromas have been shown to produce inappropriate spontaneous ectopic discharges, the molecular basis for pain in patients with neuromas is still not fully understood. Because sodium channels are known to play critical roles in neuronal electrogenesis and hyperexcitability, we examined the expression of all the neuronal voltage-gated sodium channels (Na$_V$1.1, Na$_V$1.2, Na$_V$1.3, Na$_V$1.6, Na$_V$1.7, Na$_V$1.8, and Na$_V$1.9) within human painful neuromas. We also examined the expression of two mitogen-activated protein (MAP) kinases, activated p38 and extracellular signal-regulated kinases 1 and 2 (ERK1/2), which are known to contribute to chronic pain, within these human neuromas.

Methods: We used immunocytochemical methods with specific antibodies to sodium channels Na$_V$1.1, Na$_V$1.2, Na$_V$1.3, Na$_V$1.6, Na$_V$1.7, Na$_V$1.8, and Na$_V$1.9, and to activated MAP kinases p38 and ERK1/2 to study by confocal microscopy control and painful neuroma tissue from five patients with well-documented pain.

Results: We demonstrate upregulation of sodium channel Na$_V$1.3, as well as Na$_V$1.7 and Na$_V$1.8, in blind-ending axons within human painful neuromas. We also demonstrate upregulation of activated p38 and ERK1/2 MAP kinases in axons within these neuromas.

Interpretation: These results demonstrate that multiple sodium channel isoforms (Na$_V$1.3, Na$_V$1.7, and Na$_V$1.8), as well as activated p38 and ERK1/2 MAP kinases, are expressed in painful human neuromas, indicating that these molecules merit study as possible therapeutic targets for the treatment of pain associated with traumatic neuromas.

Injury to peripheral nerves associated with trauma, amputation, compression, or surgery can lead to the formation of painful neuromas,

* Previously published in *Annals of Neurology* 64(6): 644–653, 2008. © 2008 American Neurological Association

tangled masses of blind-ending axons, and proliferating connective tissue.[1] In humans, these neuromas can be debilitating, causing chronic and severe pain, which is frequently refractory to medical treatment. Axons in both experimental and human neuromas have been shown to produce spontaneous ectopic discharges,[2–4] which have been implicated in neuropathic pain,[5] but the molecular mechanisms responsible for this pain-producing hyperexcitability in neuromas are not fully understood.

Considerable attention has been focused recently on understanding the contribution of voltage-gated sodium channels in the pathogenesis of neuropathic pain.[6,7] It is now clear that there are nine distinct isoforms of sodium channels, with different amino acid sequences and distinct physiological profiles.[8] Sodium channel isoforms Na$_V$1.3, Na$_V$1.7, Na$_V$1.8, and Na$_V$1.9 have been shown to exhibit physiological properties and patterns of expression within the nervous system that poise them to play important roles in chronic pain. Significantly, Na$_V$1.3 is present at very low levels, if at all, in adult rat dorsal root ganglia (DRG) neurons, but the expression of Na$_V$1.3 is upregulated at the transcriptional level after peripheral axotomy of DRG neurons[9,10] or inflammation in their peripheral projection fields.[11] Na$_V$1.3 produces persistent currents and depolarizing responses that amplify small stimuli close to resting potential, and recovers rapidly from inactivation, thereby increasing neuronal excitability when expressed at higher than normal levels.[12–14] Na$_V$1.7 produces a depolarizing response to small, slow stimuli such as generator potentials,[15] thus setting the gain on nociceptors.[16] Consistent with a prominent role for this channel in nociception, Na$_V$1.7

is expressed in 85% of functionally identified nociceptive neurons within DRG[17] and has been localized to sensory nerve endings.[18] Gain-of-function mutations in $Na_V1.7$ have been shown to produce severe chronic pain,[15,19] whereas loss-of-function mutations in this channel produce profound insensitivity to pain in humans.[20–22] $Na_V1.8$, which is present within approximately 90% of C- and Aδ-nociceptive DRG neurons,[23] produces a majority of the current underlying the upstroke of the action potential in these neurons and supports repetitive firing when these cells are depolarized.[24] To date, two studies have examined expression of $Na_V1.7$ and $Na_V1.8$ in human neuromas.[25,26] However, there have been no studies on the expression of $Na_V1.3$ and other sodium channel isoforms within human neuromas.

Mitogen-activated protein kinases (MAPKs) transduce extracellular stimuli into intracellular posttranslational and transcriptional responses in a variety of cell types.[27] Current evidence has implicated activation of MAPK signaling pathways as a major contributor to the development and persistence of pain.[28,29] It has recently been demonstrated that sodium channels can be direct targets of activated MAPK. The activities of $Na_V1.6$,[30] $Na_V1.7$,[31] and $Na_V1.8$[32,33] have been shown to be modulated by MAPK. However, at this time, it is not known whether activated MAPKs are present in human painful neuromas.

Although the effect of surgical excision of neuromas is controversial, several studies in amputees have reported good results.[34–36] One goal of such neuroma surgeries is moving the nerve stump to a deeper location so that if a new neuroma re-forms, as it often does, it will not be so superficially located and vulnerable to mechanical stimulation. In this study, we have examined the expression of all the neuronal sodium channels, $Na_V1.1$, $Na_V1.2$, $Na_V1.3$, $Na_V1.6$, $Na_V1.7$, $Na_V1.8$, and $Na_V1.9$, and activated MAPKs p38 and extracellular signal-regulated kinases 1 and 2 (ERK1/2) within painful neuromas that were surgically extirpated from five patients. We

demonstrate that $Na_V1.3$, which is not detectable in control nerve, is accumulated together with $Na_V1.7$ and $Na_V1.8$ in human painful neuromas. We also show that activated p38 and ERK1/2 are accumulated in the majority of human painful neuromas. These results identify $Na_V1.3$, as well as $Na_V1.7$ and $Na_V1.8$, and MAPKs p38 and ERK1/2 as potential therapeutic targets in painful human neuromas.

Patients and Methods

Patients

Patients with verified peripheral nerve injury and palpable neuromas, referred by other physicians because of intractable pain to the neuropathic pain clinic at Aarhus University Hospital, were eligible to enter the study. The patients had tried a range of medications, including tricyclic antidepressants and anticonvulsants, but most of them wanted to stop these medications either because of side effects or because of lack of effect of treatment. The decision to operate and remove neuromas was made after discussion with a specialist in hand surgery, before patients consented to participate in the research study, and was based on the clinical status of patients, including elicitation of severe pain after palpation/percussion of the neuroma. Patients were told that removal of such neuromas and the subsequent burying of the excised nerve stump in surrounding muscle might result in reduced evoked pain, but that there was also a risk for worsened pain. Six patients were enrolled in the study (table 1). Patients were informed about the study, and written informed consent was obtained. The protocol was approved by the regional ethics committee (No. 2006–0044; Aarhus, Denmark).

Assessment of Pain

During the study period, the intensity of pain was recorded during the evening for a 1-week period commencing at 7 days before the operation and at 1, 3, and 6 months after the operation. A numerical rating scale with 0 as "no pain" and 10 as "worst possible pain" was used. Amputees recorded both stump and phantom pain; stump pain was defined as pain localized to the region of the stump, and phantom pain was defined as pain experienced in the

Table 1
Patient Baseline Characteristics

Patient No.	Sex/ Age (yr)	Cause of Pain/ Location	Injured Nerve	Previous Neuroma Removal	Pain Duration (mo)	Spontaneous Pain (NRS, 0–10): Stump/ Phantom[a]	Analgesic Treatment
1	M/37	Amputation (transmetacarpal)/5th finger, right hand	Ulnar	2003, 2004	71	9.4/6.7	None
2	M/58	Amputation/4th finger, left hand	Ulnar and median	—	24	6.1/5.2	None
3	M/61	Amputation/2nd finger, right hand	Median (common and proper palmar digital branches)	—	19	4.3/3.9	Pregabalin
4	F/26	Fracture and subsequent surgery/ right volar wrist	Radial	2004	28	1	None
5	M/38	Fracture and subsequent surgery/ left volar wrist	Median	—	82	5.3	Oxycodone, ibuprofen (Ibumetin)
6	F/57	Amputation/2nd finger, right hand	Median	1994, 1996	192	7.7/6.1	Tramadol, paracetamol

[a]NRS = numeric rating scale (0 = no pain; 10 = worst possible pain). Intensity of pain was calculated as a mean of the previous seven daily pain scores.

missing part of the limb. Mean intensity of pain was calculated from the previous seven daily pain scores (table 2).

Surgery and Handling of Neuromas

Patients underwent general anesthesia or axillary brachial plexus blockade, and the same hand surgeon performed all operations. The surgical approach was as follows: (1) any previous skin scar was reopened and excised; (2) the nerve lesion was shown, and soft tissue scars were carefully excised; the nerve was mobilized from the scar tissue and the nerve-end neuroma excised; and (4) the mobilized nerves were wrapped in a sheet of Divide® (Johnson, Johnson, Birkerod, Denmark), an adhesion barrier used to prevent scar adherences in areas close to joints, if considered appropriate by the surgeon. The neuromas were not locally anesthetized with lidocaine or similar agents. A small area of normal-appearing nerve trunk located approximately 2cm proximal to the neuroma was excised in most cases, providing nerve tissue outside of the neuroma from the same patient, to serve as control tissue.

Control and neuroma tissue were immediately snap-frozen in dry ice. Within 20 minutes after removal, the tissue was transferred to a freezer and stored at −80°C until shipping from Denmark to Connecticut. During shipping, the tissue was kept frozen in dry ice.

Immunocytochemistry

Ten-micrometer cryosections were processed for immunocytochemistry from six control nerves, and nine painful neuromas were removed from six patients as described previously.[37] Control and neuroma tissue were processed in parallel. Sections of control and neuroma tissue were mounted on the same slides, and were immersed for 5 minutes in 4% paraformaldehyde in 0.14M Sorensen's phosphate buffer, pH 7.4, rinsed several times in phosphate-buffered saline (PBS), and incubated in blocking solution (PBS with 5% normal goat serum, 1% bovine serum albumin, 0.1% Triton X-100 [Sigma, St. Louis, MO], 0.02% sodium azide) for 30 minutes at room temperature. Sections were then incubated individually or in combination with primary antibodies [rabbit anti-Na$_V$1.1 (1:100; Alomone, Jerusalem, Israel), rabbit anti-Na$_V$1.2

Table 2
Intensity of Pain (NRS: 0–10) before Surgery and after 1, 3, and 6 Months

Patient No.	Before	After 1 Month	After 3 Months	After 6 Months	Effect of Surgery on Pain
1	9.4/6.7	9.6/7.3	9.7/6.6	9/6.7	↔
2	6.1/5.2	4.9/3.3	7.9/5.3	7/5.6	↓ →
3	4.3/3.9	1.7/2.7	2.1/2	2.1/3.1	↓
4	1	1.6	2.6	5.4	↑
5	5.3	4.4	4.1	ND	→
6	7.7/6.1	3.6/3	1.6/1.4	2.4/3	↓

Intensity of pain (stump/phantom in patients with amputation) was calculated as a mean of the previous 7 daily pain scores.
NRS = numeric rating scale (0 = no pain; 10 = worst possible pain); ND = not determined.

(1:100, Alomone), rabbit anti-$Na_V 1.3$ (#16153; 1:500),[38] rabbit anti-$Na_V 1.6$ (PN4; 1:100; Sigma), rabbit anti-$Na_V 1.7$ (Y083, 1:250; generated from rat a.a. sequence 514–532), rabbit anti-$Na_V 1.8$ (1:200; Alomone), rabbit anti$Na_V 1.9$ (#6464; 1:500),[39] mouse anti-phosphorylated and anti-nonphosphorylated neurofilament (each 1:10,000; SMI 31 and SMI 32; Covance, Princeton, NJ), and guinea pig anti-Caspr (1:2,000)[40]] for 24 to 48 hours at 4°C. Sections were subsequently washed with PBS, incubated in appropriate secondary antibodies [goat anti–mouse IgG Alexa Fluor 488 or 633; 1:1,000; (Molecular Probes, Eugene, OR), goat anti–guinea pig IgG Alexa Fluor 488 (Molecular Probes), and goat anti–rabbit IgG Cy3 (1:2,000, Amersham, Piscataway, NJ)] for 12 to 24 hours at 4°C, washed with PBS, and coverslipped with Aqua Poly mount (Polysciences, Warrington, PA).

Tissue Analysis

To validate sodium channel antigenicity within control and neuroma samples, we initially reacted sections from all samples with antibodies to $Na_V 1.6$ and Caspr. $Na_V 1.6$ is the predominant sodium channel at nodes of Ranvier where it is expressed at a high density[41] and Caspr demarcates paranodal regions.[42] Samples that did not exhibit $Na_V 1.6$ labeling at nodes, as identified by paranodal Caspr staining, were not further examined for this study. Using this criterion, we included in our analyses five of six control samples from four patients and seven of nine neuroma samples from five patients (patients 1, 2, 3, 5, 6). For analyses of control and neuroma sections, multiple images were accrued with a Nikon C1 confocal microscope (Nikon USA, Melville, NY). Imaging settings

were selected with control tissue, and images of neuroma immunolabeling were acquired with the same settings. Control and neuroma images were composed and processed in parallel with enhanced contrast using Adobe Photoshop (Adobe Systems, Mountain View, CA).

Results

Six patients with neuropathic pain after peripheral nerve injury, not adequately controlled by medications, and palpable neuromas participated in the study (see table 1). Nine nerve-end neuromas and six control samples were obtained from these six patients. All neuromas were painful. Movement exacerbated pain in all patients, but Tinel's sign could not be elicited at locations proximal to the neuroma. Three patients had previously undergone neuroma removal, but the pain-attenuating effect of that surgery was transient. Medical treatment had limited or no effect on the painful neuromas analyzed in this study.

Voltage-Gated Sodium Channels

In this study, we analyzed seven painful human nerve-end neuromas from five patients who met our criterion for preserved sodium channel antigenicity. As exemplified in figure 1, neurofilament-positive axons, which run in parallel within the nerve trunk, course in a disorganized pattern throughout neuroma, which often becomes club shaped. Some of the axons within the neuroma are grouped into mini-fascicles, which consist of both myelinated and unmyelinated fibers.

Na$_V$1.3 Is Upregulated in Human Painful Neuromas Previous work with rat experimental neuromas demonstrated an accumulation of Na$_V$1.3 within the distal axon stumps.[10] Because Na$_V$1.3 produces persistent and ramp currents, and recovers rapidly from inactivation,[13,14] the expression of Na$_V$1.3 in injured neurons and their extensions has been suggested to contribute to their hyperresponsiveness.[7,12] In this study, we asked whether Na$_V$1.3 was accumulated within painful human neuromas. Na$_V$1.3 was not detectable in control nerves but was clearly present within axons in four of seven (approximately 60%) of the neuromas. In double-label immunofluorescence studies, Na$_V$1.3 immunolabeling was colocalized with neurofilament labeling, consistent with the accumulation of Na$_V$1.3 within axons in neuromas (figure 2). Na$_V$1.3 was present within the blindly ending tips of axons within these neuromas but did not appear to be confined to the tips of axons and was generally also present more proximally within the neuroma (see figure 2).

Na$_V$1.7 and Na$_V$1.8 Are Upregulated in Human Painful Neuromas In agreement with previous observations,[25] we detected substantially increased Na$_V$1.7 and Na$_V$1.8 immunofluorescence within axons in painful neuromas compared with that exhibited in control samples (figure 3). Increased Na$_V$1.7 immunoreactivity was always detected in the neuromas examined (7/7), whereas increased Na$_V$1.8 immunolabeling was observed in 3 of 7 (43%) of the neuromas.

Similar to the observation of Na$_V$1.8 localization at nodes of Ranvier in normal human tooth pulp,[43] we observed Na$_V$1.8 immunoreactivity at nodes in our control human tissue (see figure 3, inset); approximately 50% (16/31) of the nodes exhibited Na$_V$1.8 immunolabeling. Na$_V$1.8 was also observed at nodes within painful neuromas, where 60% (21/35) of the nodes displayed Na$_V$1.8 immunoreactivity.

Na$_V$1.1, Na$_V$1.2, Na$_V$1.6, and Na$_V$1.9 Are Not Upregulated in Human Painful Neuromas Na$_V$1.1 was present at low levels in both control nerves and neuromas, with no qualitative

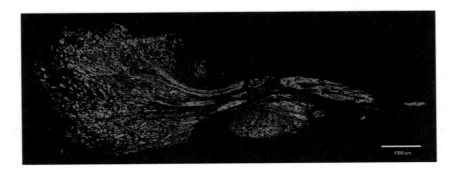

Figure 1
Human painful neuroma. A montage of low-magnification images of a neurofilament-labeled section from a human painful neuroma. Neurofilament-positive axons within the nerve trunk (right side of montage) are parallel in orientation, whereas within the club-shaped nerve-end neuroma, the axons are tangled and disorganized.

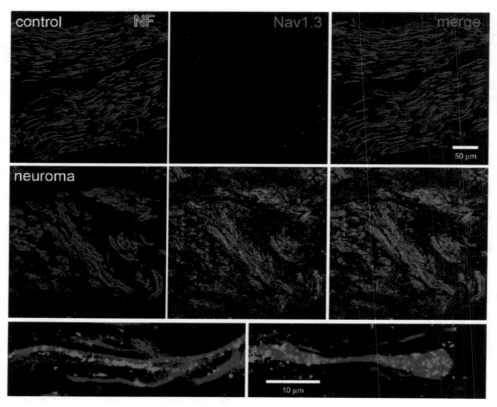

Figure 2
Sodium channel $Na_V1.3$ accumulates in human painful neuromas. Control human tissue exhibits low levels of $Na_V1.3$ immunolabeling. Painful neuromas display substantially increased $Na_V1.3$ immunoreactivity (red) compared with control tissue. Colocalization (magenta) of neurofilament (blue) and $Na_V1.3$ (red) demonstrates that $Na_V1.3$ is present within axons. At increased magnification (bottom two panels), axons (blue) within neuromas display $Na_V1.3$ immunolabeling. $Na_V1.3$ immunolabeling is exhibited by an apparently blind-ending axon (bottom right panel).

differences in the level of expression (figure 4). Only background levels of $Na_V1.2$ immunolabeling were observed in control nerves and neuromas (see figure 4). $Na_V1.9$ immunoreactivity was detected in neuromas at low levels, where its level of expression was similar to that in control nerves (see figure 4). Nodes of Ranvier in both control nerve and neuromas displayed strong $Na_V1.6$ immunoreactivity (e.g., figure 5), with no apparent difference in the degree of immunoreactivity. Faint immunolabeling

for $Na_V1.6$ along nonmyelinated axons was present in both control nerve and neuromas, but there were no apparent differences in the level of labeling.

Activated P38 and Extracellular Signal-Regulated Kinases 1 and 2 Are Upregulated in Painful Human Neuromas MAPK pathways have been implicated as contributing to the development of pain syndromes,[28,44] and modulation of sodium channels by p38

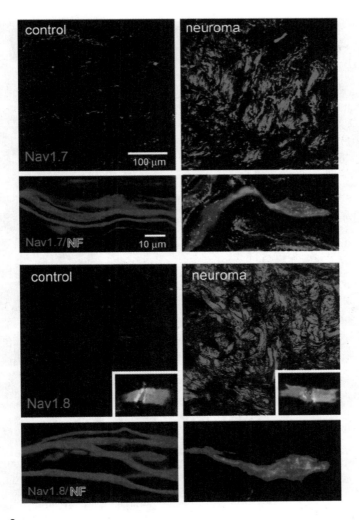

Figure 3

$Na_V1.7$ and $Na_V1.8$ accumulate in human painful neuromas. Control human tissue exhibits low levels of both $Na_V1.7$ and $Na_V1.8$ immunoreactivity. Human painful neuromas display increased $Na_V1.7$ and $Na_V1.8$ immunolabeling (red) compared with control tissue. At increased magnification, both $Na_V1.7$ and $Na_V1.8$ immunolabeling (red) is displayed in apparently blind-ending axons (blue) within neuromas (bottom right panels for $Na_V1.7$ and $Na_V1.8$); colocalization is indicated by magenta color. (insets) $Na_V1.8$ (red) immunolabeling is displayed at nodes of Ranvier (bounded by Casprpositive (green) paranodes) in both control nerve and neuromas.

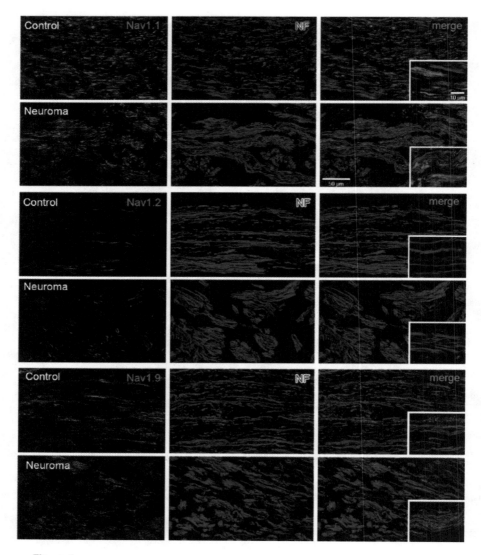

Figure 4

Na$_V$1.1, Na$_V$1.2 and Na$_V$1.9 are not accumulated in neuromas. Control and neuroma tissue sections were reacted with isoform-specific antibodies to Na$_V$1.1, Na$_V$1.2 and Na$_V$1.9. Low levels of Na$_V$1.1 immunolabeling are exhibited in both control nerves and neuromas, whereas only background levels of Na$_V$1.2 labeling are present in control tissue and neuromas. Low levels of Na$_V$1.9 immunolabeling are present in control nerves and neuromas. NF = neurofilament.

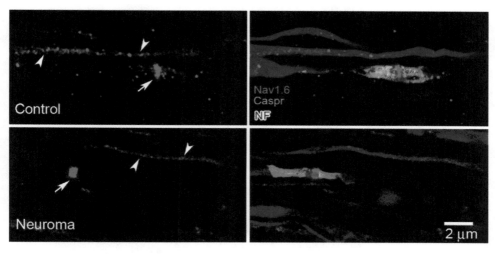

Figure 5
$Na_V1.6$ is expressed at nodes of Ranvier in control nerves and neuromas. Sections of control nerves and neuromas were triple immunolabeled for $Na_V1.6$, neurofilament (NF), and Caspr. Left column shows $Na_V1.6$ (red) signal only, whereas the right column shows merged image of $Na_V1.6$ (red), NF (blue), and Caspr (green) images. Nodes (arrows) in both control nerves and neuromas exhibit $Na_V1.6$ immunolabeling. Nonmyelinated axons (arrowheads) in control nerves and neuromas display a low level of $Na_V1.6$ immunoreactivity. There is no apparent accumulation of $Na_V1.6$ in neuromas compared with control nerves.

MAPK[30,32,33] and ERK1/2[31] has been reported. We therefore asked whether the expression of activated p38 and ERK1/2 was increased in painful human neuromas. We could not detect activated p38 or ERK1/2 in control nerve. In contrast, immunofluorescence for both activated p38 and ERK1/2 were clearly present in neuromas (figure 6). Double-label immunofluorescence studies with antibodies to activated p38 or ERK1/2 and neurofilament demonstrated that these activated MAPKs were expressed within axons. In favorable sections, activated p38 and ERK1/2 were detected in apparently blind-ending axons (see figure 6, inset). Accumulations of activated p38 and ERK1/2 were observed in 4 of 7 neuromas for each MAPK, and there was a tendency (3/7) for both p38 and ERK1/2 to be expressed in the same neuroma.

Discussion

The mechanisms underlying pain associated with nerve injury, including that seen after limb amputation, are not fully understood; the available evidence suggests, however, that both peripheral and central mechanisms may contribute.[45] Although it is clear that ectopic impulse activity in neuromas can contribute to chronic pain, the molecular basis for this hyperexcitability is not fully understood. In this study, we examined the expression of neuronal voltage-gated sodium channels $Na_V1.1$, $Na_V1.2$, $Na_V1.3$, $Na_V1.6$, $Na_V1.7$, $Na_V1.8$, and $Na_V1.9$, and the activated MAPK p38 and ERK1/2 in painful human neuromas. Consistent with previous reports,[25,26] we detected enhanced expression of $Na_V1.7$ and $Na_V1.8$ in human neuromas compared with control tissue obtained more proximally from the same nerves. In addition, we report novel observations of accumula-

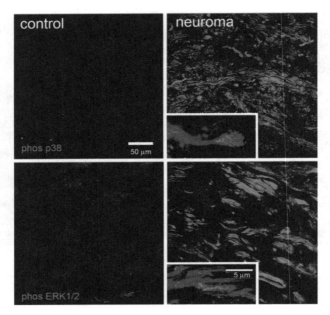

Figure 6
Mitogen-activated protein (MAP) kinases accumulate in human painful neuromas. Control human tissue displays low levels of activated (phosphorylated) p38 and extracellular signal-regulated kinases 1 and 2 (ERK1/2). In contrast, painful neuromas exhibit substantially increased immunolabeling for p38 and ERK1/2 compared with control tissue. (Insets) At increased magnification, activated p38 and ERK1/2 are localized within neurofilament-positive (blue) axons. In favorable section, activated p38 is accumulated at an apparent axon end-bulb.

tion of $Na_V1.3$ and activated MAPK in painful neuromas.

Current evidence strongly supports a major role for sodium channels[6,7,46,47] and MAPK pathways[28,29] in the cause of neuropathic pain. The presence of sodium channels $Na_V1.3$, $Na_V1.7$, and $Na_V1.8$, and activated p38 and ERK1/2 within these neuromas, at greater levels than within control tissue more proximally from these nerves, suggests that these proteins participate in the pathogenesis of pain associated with human neuromas.

Each of the neuromas examined in this study was associated with pain. Consistent with the neuroma per se being the site of ectopic impulse activity, the level of pain was reduced by one point or more on the numerical rating scale at

the first postoperative assessment (1 month) in three of the six patients studied (Patients 2, 3, and 6); in one of these three patients (Patient 2), pain subsequently returned, consistent with development of a new neuroma or development of hyperexcitability at a more proximal site. In three of the six patients (Patients 1, 4, and 5), pain was not ameliorated after excision of the neuroma. We did not find an association between the presence or absence of any particular sodium channel isoform or MAPK and the degree of pain or response to neuroma excision.

Although it might be argued that our use of nerve tissue obtained more proximally from the nerve causing the neuroma introduces the possibility of retrograde changes in the control tissue, we would stress that our use of this tissue as a control permitted comparison of axons within the neuroma, and axons outside of the neuroma, that were obtained nearly simultaneously from the same patient and processed in an identical manner. Importantly, we found that expression of $Na_V1.3$, $Na_V1.7$, $Na_V1.8$, and activated p38 and ERK1/2 were *increased* within the neuroma compared with the tissue obtained more proximally, where these channels and kinases were undetectable using our methods. Thus, although we cannot exclude the possibility that other channels such as $Na_V1.1$ or $Na_V1.2$ may have been upregulated in both the neuroma and more proximal parts of the nerve, our results demonstrate an accumulation of $Na_V1.3$, $Na_V1.7$, $Na_V1.8$, and activated p38 and ERK1/2 within the neuroma.

Ectopic spontaneous action potential discharges have been reported in experimental[3,4,48] and human[2] neuromas, and in humans with peripheral neuropathies and paresthesias.[49,50] Evidence that sodium channels contribute to the spontaneous ectopic discharges is provided by studies in which sodium channel blockers, including tetrodotoxin, lidocaine, and carbamazepine, inhibit the spontaneous activity in experimental neuromas.[51–53]

Our study examined, for the first time, expression of $Na_V1.3$ within human neuromas and demonstrates a distinct upregulation of $Na_V1.3$ in more than half of the painful neuromas that we studied. These results extend observations in experimental rat neuromas, in which increased $Na_V1.3$ immunolabeling was detected in the distal stumps of transected rat sciatic nerves,[10] and a report of increased $Na_V1.3$ immunoreactivity in injured axons within peripheral nerve trunks.[54] Significantly, contactin, which has been shown to associate with $Na_V1.3$ and to increase the density of this channel at the cell surface, has also been observed in experimental neuromas.[55] $Na_V1.3$ exhibits several properties that can contribute to neuronal hyperexcitability, including rapid recovery from inactivation, which can support high-frequency firing,

and production of persistent current and ramp responses to small, slow depolarizations.[12–14] In conjunction with their unique physiological properties, the localization of $Na_V1.3$ channels within blind-ending axons of painful human neuromas suggests that these channels can participate in the generation of ectopic discharges associated with chronic pain. We detected $Na_V1.3$ in four of seven painful neuromas; whether $Na_V1.3$ was present within the other three neuromas, at levels too low for immunocytochemical detection but high enough to support electrogenesis,[56] is not known.

We also detected increased immunoreactivity for sodium channels $Na_V1.7$ and $Na_V1.8$ in painful human neuromas compared with control tissue, but not for $Na_V1.1$, $Na_V1.2$, $Na_V1.6$, or $Na_V1.9$. Our observations extend previous reports of accumulation of $Na_V1.7$ and $Na_V1.8$ in human neuromas.[25,26] Interestingly, Kretschmer and colleagues[25] reported that painful neuromas of peripheral nerves exhibited greater $Na_V1.7$ labeling than nonpainful neuromas, whereas no difference was detected between painful and nonpainful human lingual nerve neuromas.[26] In our study, all seven neuromas, which were always from the upper extremity and were all painful, displayed enhanced $Na_V1.7$ immunoreactivity.

The prevalence of $Na_V1.7$ within painful neuromas, coupled with its voltage dependence and kinetic properties, support a major contributory role for this channel in neuroma neuropathic pain. $Na_V1.7$ is highly expressed in DRG neurons, where 100% of C-nociceptive and 93% of Aδ-nociceptive neurons exhibit $Na_V1.7$ immunolabeling.[17] The slow closed-state inactivation and voltage dependence of $Na_V1.7$ channels permit them to produce relatively large responses to small, subthreshold depolarizations,[57,58] and thus poise these channels to set the gain on nociceptors.[16] Point mutations that hyperpolarize the activation voltage dependence and slow deactivation of $Na_V1.7$ have been linked to the human pain disorder erythromelalgia,[15,19] whereas impaired inactivation has been linked to paroxysmal extreme pain disorder.[59] Recently, loss-of-function mutations in $Na_V1.7$ have been shown to produce insensitivity to pain.[20-22] These observations provide strong evidence that $Na_V1.7$ is essential to nociception in humans and suggest that the aberrant accumulation of $Na_V1.7$ within neuromas plays a role in the onset and/or maintenance of pain associated with the neuromas.

Accumulation of $Na_V1.8$ is also expected to make axons within neuromas hyperexcitable. $Na_V1.8$ has been shown to produce the majority of the inward current responsible for the action potential upstroke in the DRG neurons in which it is expressed and produces high-frequency firing of the cells when they are depolarized.[24] Moreover, experimental expression of $Na_V1.8$, in cells that do not normally express it, markedly enhances the excitability of these cells.[60,61]

MAPKs are a family of serine/threonine protein kinases that transduce extracellular stimuli into cellular responses via transcriptional and post-translational modifications.[27,62] MAPKs have received considerable attention for their involvement in nociception and sensitization.[28,63,64] For instance, ERK1/2 plays an important role in inflammatory responses,[65,66] and p38 activation is induced by noxious stimuli.[67] Recently, it has been demonstrated that sodium channels are substrates for MAPKs, which can modulate their activities. Phosphorylation of $Na_V1.8$ by activated p38 significantly increases the current density of this channel in DRG neurons[32,33] and would be expected to enhance the excitability of these cells. It has also been demonstrated that phosphorylation by ERK1/2 hyperpolarizes the activation curve of $Na_V1.7$,[31] lowering the threshold for activation of this channel.

In summary, our observations of upregulation of $Na_V1.3$, as well as $Na_V1.7$ and $Na_V1.8$, in conjunction with the localization of activated p38 and ERK1/2 within painful neuromas, implicate MAPKs and at least three isoforms of sodium channels as contributors to the pain associated with neuromas. Our results add to the evidence supporting the development of subtype-specific sodium channel blockers as potential treatments for neuropathic pain and suggest that, together with sodium channels, MAPKs may be opportune therapeutic targets for chronic pain after traumatic nerve injury in humans.

Acknowledgments

This work was supported by the Medical Research and Rehabilitation Research Services, Department of Veterans Affairs (S.G.W.), Erythromelalgia Association (S.G.W.), and Lundbeck Foundation and the Danish Research Council (K.K., T.S.J.). The Center for Neuroscience and Regeneration Research is a collaboration of the Paralyzed Veterans of America and the United Spinal Association with Yale University.

We thank Drs S. Dib-Hajj and P. Zhao for their contributions in the design and characterization of the $Na_V1.7$ antibody.

Potential conflict of interest: Nothing to report

About the Authors

Joel A. Black, PhD, Department of Neurology and Center for Neuroscience and Regeneration Research, Yale School of Medicine, New Haven; Rehabilitation Research Center, Veterans Affairs Connecticut Healthcare System, West Haven, CT

Lone Nikolajsen, MD, PhD, Department of Anesthesiology, Aarhus University Hospital; Danish Pain Research Center, University of Aarhus

Karsten Kroner, MD, Department of Orthopedic Surgery, Aarhus University Hospital, Aarhus, Denmark

Troels S. Jensen, MD, DMSc, Danish Pain Research Center, University of Aarhus

Stephen G. Waxman, MD, PhD, Department of Neurology and Center for Neuroscience and Regeneration Research, Yale School of Medicine, New Haven; Rehabilitation Research Center, Veterans Affairs Connecticut Healthcare System, West Haven, CT

References

1. Cravioto H, Battista A. 1981. Clinical and ultrastructural study of painful neuromas. *Neurosurgery* 8: 181–190.

2. Nystrom B, Hagbarth K. 1981. Microelectrode recording from transected nerves in amputees with phantom limb pain. *Neurosci Lett* 27: 211–216.

3. Devor M, Govrin-Lippmann R. 1983. Axoplasmic transport block reduces ectopic impulse generation in injured peripheral nerves. *Pain* 16: 73–85.

4. Burchiel KJ. 1984. Effects of electrical and mechanical stimulation on two foci of spontaneous activity which develop in primary afferent neurons after peripheral axotomy. *Pain* 18: 249–265.

5. Devor M. 2001. Neuropathic pain: What do we do with all these theories? *Acta Anaesthesiol Scand* 45: 1121–1127.

6. Amir R, Argoff CE, Bennett GJ, et al. 2006. The role of sodium channels in chronic inflammatory and neuropathic pain. *J Pain* 7: S1–S29.

7. Cummins TR, Sheets PL, Waxman SG. 2007. The roles of sodium channels in nociception: Implications for mechanisms of pain. *Pain* 131: 243–257.

8. Catterall WA, Goldin AL, Waxman SG. 2005. International union of pharmacology. XLVII. Nomenclature and structure-function relationships of voltage-gated sodium channels. *Pharmacol Rev* 57: 397–409.

9. Waxman SG, Kocsis JD, Black JA. 1984. Type III sodium channel mRNA is expressed in embryonic but not adult spinal sensory neurons, and is reexpressed following axotomy. *J Neurophysiol* 72: 466–472.

10. Black JA, Cummins TR, Plumpton C, et al. 1999. Upregulation of a silent sodium channel after peripheral, but not central, nerve injury in DRG neurons. *J Neurophysiol* 82: 2776–2785.

11. Black JA, Liu S, Tanaka M, et al. 2007. Changes in the expression of tetrodotoxin-sensitive sodium channels within dorsal root ganglia neurons in inflammatory pain. *Pain* 108: 237–247.

12. Cummins TR, Waxman SG. 1997. Downregulation of tetrodotoxin-resistant sodium currents and upregulation of a rapidly repriming tetrodotoxin-sensitive sodium current in small spinal sensory neurons after nerve injury. *J Neurosci* 17: 3503–3514.

13. Cummins TR, Aglieco F, Renganathan M, et al. 2001. $Na_V1.3$ sodium channels: Rapid repriming and slow closed-state inactivation display quantitative differences after expression in a mammalian cell line and in spinal sensory neurons. *J Neurosci* 21: 5952–5961.

14. Lampert A, Hains BC, Waxman SG. 2006. Upregulation of persistent and ramp sodium current in dorsal horn neurons after spinal cord injury. *Exp Brain Res* 174: 660–666.

15. Dib-Hajj SD, Cummins TR, Black JA, Waxman SG. 2007. From genes to pain: Nav 1.7 and human pain disorders. *Trends Neurosci* 30: 555–563.

16. Waxman SG. 2006. Neurobiology: A channel sets the gain on pain. *Nature* 444: 831–832.

17. Djouhri L, Newton R, Levinson SR, et al. 2003. Sensory and electrophysiological properties of guinea-pig sensory neurones expressing $Na_V1.7$ (PN1) Na^+ channel alpha subunit protein. *J Physiol* 546: 565–576.

18. Toledo-Aral JJ, Moss BL, Koszowski AG, et al. 1997. Identification of PN1, a predominant voltage-dependent sodium channel expressed principally in peripheral neurons. *Proc Natl Acad Sci USA* 94: 1527–1532.

19. Waxman SG, Dib-Hajj S. 2005. Erythermalgia: Molecular basis for an inherited pain syndrome. *Trends Mol Med* 11: 555–562.

20. Cox JJ, Reimann F, Nicholas AK, et al. 2006. An SCN9A channelopathy causes congenital inability to experience pain. *Nature* 444: 894–898.

21. Ahmad S, Dahllund L, Eriksson AB, et al. 2007. A stop codon mutation in SCN9A causes lack of pain sensation. *Hum Mol Genet* 16: 2114–2121.

22. Goldberg YP, MacFarlane J, MacDonald ML, et al. 2007. Loss-of-function mutations in the $Na_V1.7$ gene underlie congenital indifference to pain in multiple human populations. *Clin Genet* 71: 311–319.

23. Djouhri L, Fang X, Okuse K, et al. 2003. The TTX-resistant sodium channel $Na_V1.8$ (SNS/PN3): Expression and correlation with membrane properties in rat nociceptive primary afferent neurons. *J Physiol* 550: 739–752.

24. Renganathan M, Cummins TR, Waxman SG. 2001. Contribution of $Na_V1.8$ sodium channels to action potential electrogenesis in DRG neurons. *J Neurophysiol* 86: 629–640.

25. Kretschmer T, Happel LT, England JD, et al. 2002. Accumulation of PN1 and PN3 sodium channels in painful human neuroma: Evidence from immunocytochemistry. *Acta Neurochir (Wien)* 144: 803–810.

26. Bird EV, Robinson PP, Boissonade FM. 2007. $Na_V1.7$ sodium channel expression in human lingual nerve neuromas. *Arch Oral Biol* 52: 494–502.

27. Seger R, Krebs EG. 1995. The MAPK signaling cascade. *FASEB J* 9: 726–735.

28. Obata K, Noguchi K. 2004. MAPK activation in nociceptive neurons and pain hypersensitivity. *Life Sci* 74: 2643–2653.

29. Cheng J-K, Ji R-R. 2008. Intracellular signaling in primary sensory neurons and persistent pain. *Neurochem Res* 33: 1970–1978.

30. Wittmack EK, Rush AM, Hudmon A, et al. 2005. Voltage-gated sodium channel Na$_V$1.6 is modulated by p38 mitogen-activated protein kinase. *J Neurosci* 25: 6621–6630.

31. Stamboulian S, Choi J-S, Tyrrell LC, et al. 2008. The sodium channel Na$_V$1.7 is a substrate and is modulated by the MAP kinase ERK. *Soc Neurosci Abstr* 466.20.

32. Jin X, Gereau RW. 2006. Acute p38-mediated modulation of tetrodotoxin-resistant sodium channels in mouse sensory neurons by tumor necrosis factor-α. *J Neurosci* 26: 246–255.

33. Hudmon A, Choi J-S, Tyrrell L, et al. 2008. Phosphorylation of sodium channel Na$_V$1.8 by p38 mitogen-activated protein kinase increases current density in dorsal root ganglion neurons. *J Neurosci* 28: 3190–3201.

34. Koch H, Haas F, Hubner M, et al. 2003. Treatment of painful neu roma by resection and nerve stump transplantation into a vein. *Ann Plast Surg* 51: 45–50.

35. Krishnan KG, Pinzer T, Schackert G. 2005. Coverage of painful peripheral nerve neuromas with vascularized soft tissue: Method and results. *Neurosurgery* 56: 369–378.

36. Ducic I, Mesbahi AN, Attinger CE, Graw K. 2008. The role of peripheral nerve surgery in the treatment of chronic pain associated with amputation stumps. *Plast Reconstr Surg* 121: 908–914.

37. Black JA, Newcombe J, Trapp BD, Waxman SG. 2007. Sodium channel expression within chronic multiple sclerosis plaques. *J Neuropathol Exp Neurol* 66: 828–837.

38. Hains BC, Black JA, Waxman SG. 2002. Primary motor neurons fail to up-regulate voltage-gated sodium channel Na(v)1.3/brain type III following axotomy resulting from spinal cord injury. *J Neurosci Res* 70: 546–552.

39. Fjell J, Hjelmström P, Hormuzdiar W, et al. 2000. Localization of the tetrodotoxin-resistant sodium channel NaN in nociceptors. *Neuroreport* 11: 199–202.

40. Rush AM, Wittmack EK, Tyrrell L, et al. 2006. Differential modulation of sodium channel Na(v)1.6 by two members of the fibroblast growth factor homologous factor 2 subfamily. *Eur J Neurosci* 23: 2551–2562.

41. Caldwell JH, Schaller KL, Lasher RS, et al. 2000. Sodium channel Na$_V$1.6 is localized at nodes of Ranvier, dendrites and synapses. *Proc Natl Acad Sci USA* 97: 5616–5620.

42. Peles E, Nativ M, Lustig M, et al. 1997. Identification of a novel contactin-associated transmembrane receptor with multiple domains implicated in protein-protein interactions. *EMBO J* 16: 978–988.

43. Henry MA, Sorensen HJ, Johnson LR, Levinson SR. 2005. Localization of the Na$_V$1.8 sodium channel isoform at nodes of Ranvier in normal human radicular tooth pulp. *Neurosci Lett* 380: 32–36.

44. Ji R-R, Suter MR. 2007. p38 MAPK, microglial signaling, and neuropathic pain. *Mol Pain* 3: 33–41.

45. Nikolajsen L, Jensen TS. Phantom limb. 2006. In: McMahon SB, Kolzenburg M, eds. *Wall and Melzack's textbook of pain.* 5th ed. London: Churchill-Livingstone, 561–571.

46. Rogers M, Tang L, Madge DJ, Stevens EB. 2006. The role of sodium channels in neuropathic pain. *Semin Cell Dev Biol* 17: 571–581.

47. Hains BC, Waxman SG. 2007. Sodium channel expression and the molecular pathophysiology of pain after SCI. *Prog Brain Res* 161: 195–203.

48. Wall PD, Gutnick M. 1974. Ongoing activity in peripheral nerves: The physiology and pharmacology of impulses originated from a neuroma. *Exp Neurol* 43: 580–593.

49. Ochoa JL, Torebjörk HE. 1980. Paraesthesiae from ectopic impulse generation in human sensory nerves. *Brain* 103: 835–853.

50. Norden M, Nystrom B, Wallin U, Hagbarth K-E. 1984. Ectopic sensory discharge and paresthesiae in patients with disorders of peripheral nerves, dorsal roots and dorsal columns. *Pain* 20: 231–245.

51. Burchiel KJ. 1988. Carbamazepine inhibits spontaneous activity in experimental neuromas. *Exp Neurol* 102: 249–253.

52. Devor M, Wall PD, Catalan N. 1992. Systemic lidocaine silences ectopic neuroma and DRG discharge without blocking nerve conduction. *Pain* 48: 261–268.

53. Matzner O, Devor M. 1994. Hyperexcitability at sites of nerve injury depends on voltage-sensitive Na$^+$ channels. *J Neurophysiol* 72: 349–359.

54. Coward K, Aitken A, Powell A, et al. 2001. Plasticity of TTX-sensitive sodium channels PN1 and Brain III in injured human nerves. *Neuroreport* 12: 495–500.

55. Shah BS, Rush AM, Liu S, et al. 2004. Contactin associates with sodium channel Na$_V$1.3 in native tissues and increases channel density at the cell surface. *J Neurosci* 24: 7387–7399.

56. Waxman SG, Black JA, Kocsis JD, Ritchie JM. 1989. Low density of sodium channels supports action potential conduction in axons of neonatal rat optic nerve. *Proc Natl Acad Sci USA* 86: 1406–1410.

57. Cummins TR, Howe JR, Waxman SG. 1998. Slow closed-state inactivation: A novel mechanism underlying ramp currents in cells expressing the hNE/PN1 sodium channel. *J Neurosci* 18: 9607–9619.

58. Herzog RI, Cummins TR, Ghassemi F, et al. 2003. Distinct repriming and closed-state inactivation kinetics of $Na_V1.6$ and $Na_V1.7$ sodium channels in mouse spinal sensory neurons. *J Physiol* 551: 741–750.

59. Fertleman CR, Baker MD, Parker KA, et al. 2006. SCN9A mutations in paroxysmal extreme pain disorder: Allelic variants underlie distinct channel defects and phenotypes. *Neuron* 52: 767–774.

60. Renganathan M, Gelderblom M, Black JA, Waxman SG. 2003. Expression of $Na_V1.8$ sodium channels perturbs the firing patterns of cerebellar Purkinje cells. *Brain Res* 959: 235–242.

61. Rush AM, Dib-Hajj SD, Liu S, et al. 2006a. A single sodium channel mutation produces hyper- or hypoexcitability in different types of neurons. *Proc Natl Acad Sci USA* 103: 8245–8250.

62. Chang L, Karin M. 2001. Mammalian MAP kinase signalling cascades. *Nature* 410: 37–40.

63. Ji R-R. 2004. Mitogen-activated protein kinases as potential targets for pain killers. *Curr Opin Investig Drugs* 5: 71–75.

64. Ji RR, Kawasaki Y, Zhuang ZY, et al. 2007. Protein kinases as potential targets for the treatment of pathological pain. *Handb Exp Pharmacol* 177: 359–389.

65. Dai Y, Iwata K, Fukuoka T, et al. 2002. Phosphorylation of extracellular signal-regulated kinase in primary afferent neurons by noxious stimuli and its involvement in peripheral sensitization. *J Neurosci* 22: 7737–7745.

66. Zhuang ZY, Xu H, Clapham DE, Ji RR. 2004. Phosphatidylinositol 3-kinase activates ERK in primary sensory neurons and mediates inflammatory heat hyperalgesia through TRPV1 sensitization. *J Neurosci* 24: 8300–8309.

67. Mizushima T, Obata K, Yamanaka H, et al. 2005. Activation of p38 MAPK in primary afferent neurons by noxious stimulation and its involvement in the development of thermal hyperalgesia. *Pain* 113: 51–56.

8 CROSSING BORDERS

Popular legend has it that when Willie Sutton was asked why he robbed banks, he said "Because that's where the money is." I have sometimes been asked why I have worked together with researchers in Europe and Asia. Why travel thousands of miles for a collaboration when there are experts next door? The short answer is "Because those are the collaborations that worked." But that raises the following questions: What is a fruitful collaboration? How can one make it happen?

Scientific collaborations are driven by need or opportunity. My interest in finding pain genes, and my need to find the right patients, arose from watching my father spend the last years of his life sedated by the opiate medications that were used—unsuccessfully—in an attempt to treat the neuropathic pain that he experienced as a result of nerve damage from diabetes. As in many individuals with neuropathic pain, the medications produced a dulling of my father's sensorium, with only minimal relief from his discomfort. As I tried to think of ways to alleviate my father's pain, I was struck again and again by the remarkable fact that some patients with neuropathy experience excruciating pain while others describe mild tingling or electric-like sensations that are not severe and do not require medication. At this time I was already working on sodium channels. By understanding the differences in the sodium channels in these patients, I hoped that I might be able to silence the molecular machinery that generates their pain.

To find out whether patients with painful peripheral neuropathy might have mutations in their sodium channel genes, I needed access to two groups of people: patients with peripheral neuropathy and minimal or no pain, and patients with neuropathy and severe pain. By comparing the two groups, I hoped we could find a culprit gene causing or predisposing certain individuals to pain, or a protective gene that holds pain back.

Diabetes is of course quite prevalent in our society, and, because nerve damage occurs commonly as a complication of diabetes, patients with diabetic neuropathy are not hard to find. I asked colleagues throughout the United States—in general medicine, in endocrinology, and in neurology—if they could identify patients in these two groups, so that I could determine, from their DNA, whether there were mutations in sodium channel genes that correlated with the degree of pain. My vision, of a joint, focused effort with all of the contributors included as full partners in the work, was met with mixed responses including some enthusiasm. But enthusiasm, when present, was not accompanied by action. A common response was, "I'd like to help, but I'm too busy." A well-regarded diabetes expert signed on to a joint project but did not respond to drafts of the research plan. Another potential collaborator, a neurologist, agreed to send DNA, but, despite reminders, it never arrived.

So, what makes a collaboration succeed? Common purpose, complementary strengths, focus, and a bit of luck. I saw the first three up close as a graduate student in 1967 and 1968 at the Marine Biological Laboratory in Woods Hole, Massachusetts. Although the genes for sodium channels had not been discovered and I did not work on pain at that time, Woods Hole glowed with the theme of teamwork, a theme that continued in our conference room—the place where we planned experiments and which we called the War Room—after I moved to Yale in 1986. Decades after my time in Woods Hole, the search for a pain gene began.

Woods Hole

Nestled within a small peninsula jutting out from the base of Cape Cod, the village of Woods Hole was the departure point for the ferry to Martha's Vineyard. But more importantly, as the home of the Woods Hole Oceanographic Institution and the Marine Biological Laboratory, it was an oasis for scientists. The Marine Biological Laboratory was a unique institution. In the 1960s and 1970s biological researchers from around the world flocked to MBL each summer, drawn by a uniquely collaborative ethos and the availability of a rich ensemble of sea-dwelling species—squid, sea slugs, and even lobsters—whose large nerve cells and relatively simple brain circuitry provided useful experimental models. Several hundred investigators converged each June from leading institutions on both sides of the Atlantic and crammed themselves into small laboratories in the four buildings that made up MBL, within view of the ocean. There were very few organizational snafus, no administrative meetings, and not much paperwork. An investigator merely signed up, arranged for his or her grant to pay the appropriate fees to secure laboratory space, loaded equipment onto a rental truck or an airplane, and moved in.

Informality was the rule at Woods Hole. Lunches were eaten on Stony Beach, a small stretch of sand less than half of the size of a football field. Here, a towel occupied by graduate students might overlap a blanket belonging to a Nobel Prize winner, and a soft drink or a beer might be shared in both directions. My wife and I spent our first summer as a married couple in Woods Hole, and our marriage was celebrated at a party that also honored another newlywed, Sir John Eccles. Seminars as well as formal lectures provided a geyser of information, and the "Tuesday Night Fights" offered a public forum for the exchange of views, often violently different, between the giants of neurophysiology. In this open arena, notable neuroscientists like Stephen Kuffler of Harvard, Harry Grundfest of Columbia, and Mike Bennett of Albert Einstein tore each other's ideas to shreds, before adjourning for a beer at the local bar, the Cap'n Kidd. Equally important were chance encounters in MBL's hallways or at its tennis court. Investigators working at the MBL knew that they had to return to their home institutions in late August or early September, and it was understood by all that, for a collaboration to succeed, it had to advance within a short time window. Years later physiologist Ann Stuart summed up the Wood Hole ethos as "let's just do it." And it worked.

The War Room

I moved from Stanford University to Yale in 1986. At Yale I established a research center as a tripartite partnership between Yale University, the Department of Veterans Affairs, and the Paralyzed Veterans of America. Our overall goal was to capitalize on the "molecular revolution" to deliver new therapies for disorders of the nervous system. By design, the research center was multidisciplinary, bringing together cell and molecular biologists, neurophysiologists, ion channel biophysicists, pharmacologists, optical imaging experts, pain researchers, and clinicians in a concerted, focused effort. A key to our progress was seamless collaboration.

Next to my office, within our research center, was a room that I designated as the War Room. In reality, the War Room was a small conference room with a whiteboard on both walls and half a dozen chairs surrounding an oblong table. It was here that my colleagues and I jointly developed research proposals, strategized about experiments, reviewed data, and discussed progress, problems, and prospects. Although our wit did not match that of the Tuesday Night Fights at Woods Hole, our passion and bluntness did: "That will never work!" "You need to think that through more carefully!" "We'll never complete this experiment unless you come up with a better method!" An outsider, listening from the hall adjacent to the War Room, might have thought that the voices from within it represented adversaries. But we were not opponents. Candid discussion, to-the-point criticism, and a joint effort to wrestle challenges to the ground propelled our research and ultimately provided a template for our international collaborations.

Beijing

Soon after we published our 2004 paper on erythromelalgia (Cummins, Dib-Hajj, and Waxman 2004) we began two collaborations, one with a clinical researcher in China, Yong Yang, the second with a researcher in the Netherlands, Joost Drenth. Mutations of $Na_V1.7$ in people with the man on fire syndrome would, we hoped, provide "experiments of nature" that would help us to understand how $Na_V1.7$ causes pain. To hone in on the channel and how it works, we wanted to study as many mutations as possible. Both of these highly skilled physicians were receiving referrals of patients with inherited erythromelalgia.

Because patients from throughout China were sent to dermatologist Yong Yang in Beijing for diagnosis and treatment, he saw very rare diseases. Among these were kindreds with familial disorders involving the skin, including painful disorders. In late 2004, shortly after we published our initial paper on the functional profiles of erythromelalgia mutations, Yong Yang sent us a clinical history of a fifteen-year-old boy admitted to the Peking University First Hospital and asked if we were interested in working together to understand that child's disease. The boy suffered from debilitating burning pain in the feet, and there was a family history that included a similar disorder in a brother. Several weeks later Yong sent the coordinates of the previously undescribed mutation in these two children. The mutation, L858F, substituted a phenylalanine for a leucine at position 858 within the $Na_V1.7$ channel. This mutation was of special interest to us because we suspected, from earlier experiments on another amino acid substitution, L858H, at the same site within the channel (Cummins, Dib-Hajj, and Waxman 2004), that the presence of a leucine at position 858 was crucial for proper functioning of the $Na_V1.7$ channel.

Yong had the patients. The patients carried the mutations. We had the expertise to find out how the mutations worked. We agreed to work together, with Yong sending the coordinates of new $Na_V1.7$ mutations so that we could do the functional profiling in my laboratory. As part of this collaboration Yong spent some months on a sabbatical working directly with us. During this visit his family joined him for a week, and I gave them a tour of New Haven. I bought ice cream cones at a shop next to the Yale Art Gallery and ended up with as much chocolate on my shirt as Yong's five-year-old son had on his.

There was more to this collaboration. Yong wanted Chongyang Han, an energetic graduate student who had worked with him in Beijing, to learn how to physiologically analyze mutant $Na_V1.7$ channels, and our laboratory was to be the training ground. Chongyang traveled to New Haven from Beijing and spent seven months working in my laboratory. His analysis of the L858F mutation showed us that the substitution of this amino acid enhanced channel activation. This work also showed that, in some patients, a *founder* mutation (in this case in the patient's father) can act to launch a new family with erythromelalgia. We published this work together with Yang in 2006 (Han et al. 2006), and Chongyang returned to China to complete his PhD at the Chinese Academy of Medical Sciences. But this was not the end of this story. Chongyang returned to our laboratory in 2008 as a postdoctoral fellow. His initial plan was to return to China after a few years working with me. But this was not how it turned out. Chongyang and his wife decided to remain in America. He was promoted to a higher rank at Yale, associate research scientist, in 2011. After several very productive years in my laboratory Chongyang applied for a green card establishing his permanent residence status, and it was easy for me to write a letter highlighting his unique expertise as an ion channel researcher. He grew into a facile channel biophysicist, and he continues to be an important part of our research team.

Nijmegen

Shortly after our 2004 paper (Cummins, Dib-Hajj, and Waxman 2004) appeared, a Dutch medical investigator, Joost Drenth, published two articles describing additional erythromelalgia mutations of Na$_V$1.7 (Drenth et al. 2005; Michiels et al. 2005). An internist with a razor-sharp intellect, Drenth had trained in genetics in France and was best known for important discoveries—including identification of the gene for polycystic liver disease—in which he was unraveling the genetic basis for disorders of the liver, kidneys, and pancreas. More relevant to our interests, he was an erythromelalgia expert. As a medical student, Drenth had published papers on the diagnostic classification of erythromelalgia and on the role of certain medications in triggering the onset of erythromelalgia (Drenth 1989; Drenth and Michiels 1990). His linkage analysis (Drenth et al. 2001) had pointed to the site, on a specific chromosome, that housed the gene for erythromelalgia. Even though he was head of the Department of Gastrointestinal and Liver Diseases, a far cry from disorders involving neurons, Drenth's clinic at the Radboud University Medical Center in the Netherlands attracted patients from throughout Europe with the man on fire syndrome.

Because of Drenth's experience with erythromelalgia, and his expertise in medical genetics, we wanted to partner with him. He shared our interest in working together, and soon after we established contact in 2006, he made his first trip to New Haven. Over the ensuing years, working in tandem on a shoestring budget, we discussed interesting cases from throughout Europe as they were referred to Drenth, and we performed the functional profiling of the mutations in New Haven. Our partnership yielded a series of informative studies (Ahn et al. 2010; Cheng et al. 2011; Choi et al. 2011; Choi et al. 2010; Estacion et al. 2008; Estacion et al. 2011; Han, Hoeijmakers, Ahn, et al. 2012; Han, Hoeijmakers, Liu, et al. 2012), each teaching us something about Na$_V$1.7 and the ways it can go awry. One joint study allowed us to tease out the contribution to erythromelalgia of a process called slow inactivation, whereby a long-term silencing due to previous activity builds up to slowly inhibit the function of Na$_V$1.7 sodium channels. A Na$_V$1.7 mutation from another of Drenth's patients provided clues about why the pain of inherited erythromelalgia usually begins in infancy or early childhood but waits until later in some families. Working together, we learned about the role of alternative splicing, or the use of alternative gene subparts, as the Na$_V$1.7 gene is transcribed during different stages of development. Each mutation taught us something about how Na$_V$1.7 works, and about how its abnormal activity leads to pain. And, in each instance, the mutations that Drenth sent were accompanied by sage comments. Nearly a decade after his first visit, Joost Drenth continues to be a valued collaborator and a friend.

Maastricht

In mid-2010, I received an email from two neurologists, Catharina (Karin) Faber and Ingemar Merkies from Maastricht University in the Netherlands. They had an impressive record of assembling cohorts of patients for clinical studies, and they were experts on peripheral nerve disease. They wrote as follows:

Dear Professor Waxman,

We are two neurologists from The Netherlands (Maastricht University Medical Centre) with particular interest in peripheral neuropathies.

We have read your papers that helped us in creating a genetic hypothesis. In the last 3 years we have succeeded in creating a comprehensive database with > 60 patients with neuropathy, containing data ranging from aspects like pain and autonomic symptoms, skin biopsy findings (intraepidermal nerve fibre density [IENFD]), temperature threshold testing, to disability and quality of life assessments.

Some of these patients are believed to have (new) mutations in the SCN9A gene. ... Based on these findings, we ask whether you would be interested in interchanging ideas and perhaps come to a scientific joined venture. ... We would be very honoured if we could meet and we are certainly willing to fly over to your institute to discuss things. Tentatively, these are some dates that we could come over: July 16th–July 20th, September 25th–Sept 29th, October 18th–October 20th, October 25th–October 28th.

We thank you beforehand for your time and hope that you would be interested in meeting us.

Sincerely yours,

Catharina Faber / Ingemar Merkies

Every scientist studying a rare disease hopes that it will hold lessons about more common disorders. Now Karin Faber and Ingemar Merkies were suggesting a springboard, from which to extrapolate from a rare genetic disorder, inherited erythromelalgia, to a common disease, painful neuropathy. It took me only a few minutes to reply:

Dear Drs. Faber and Merkies,

It was good to hear from you. We would like to collaborate with you. Working together, I think we can come up with a significant story, spanning from the clinical to the molecular and biophysical, on the relationship of $Na_V1.7$ mutations and neuropathies.

With respect to your questions:

Yes, we would be very interested in exchanging ideas and shaping a collaboration. Our research center possesses unique resources for the profiling and functional characterization of mutant $Na_V1.7$ channels. Each mutation's analysis is labor-intensive, so we prioritize the mutations in order of interest. Do you have any mutations in patients with i) a definitive and well-characterized small fiber neuropathy (e.g. in terms of IENFD) and ii) a strong family history, with the mutation segregating with disease (if we know that all affected patients within a family house the mutation, it provides strong evidence that the mutation is linked to disease). If you could send us the history etc. and the mutation from such families, we could move those mutations to the front of the line and get our physiologists and biophysicists to work on them now, in advance of your visit, so that we might have data waiting for you.

Finally, yes, we would love to have you visit. ... Yale University is located in New Haven ... a relatively European city (for the U.S.!) and a pleasant place to visit this time of year.

I look forward to hearing from you, and to meeting you,

Steve Waxman

It was clear to all of us, even prior to July 2010 when Faber and Merkies made their first visit to New Haven, that our two groups, working together, were poised to make exciting progress. Our research team, which at that time included Sulayman Dib-Hajj, Mark Estacion, Chongyang Han, Jin Choi, Xiaoyang Cheng, Hye-Sook Ahn, and Jianying Huang, was highly talented. In Maastricht, Faber and Merkies had established a peripheral neuropathy clinic that attracted patients from throughout Europe. Faber, Merkies, and I recognized that we had the makings of a fruitful collaboration. But my team worked in New Haven, while Faber and Merkies lived and worked in the Netherlands three thousand miles away. Would it work?

Faber, Merkies, and I spent the first part of their 2010 visit talking about logistics. We had the manpower to make things work. Rather than looking for additional funds, we decided to move ahead using existing resources. Patients would be studied clinically in Maastricht, and then their mutations would be functionally analyzed at Yale. It was perhaps fortuitous that all of us worked on a "let's do it now!" time clock. Remarkably, by late August 2010 we reached, together with our institutions in Maastricht and New Haven, a streamlined agreement which established the official basis for our collaboration.

In 2010, the term "translational research"—research that linked the laboratory bench and the clinic—was evoking excitement throughout the biomedical community. The Maastricht–Yale partnership, like our transoceanic collaborations with Drenth and Yong Yang, was translational and brought together multiple parts—on the European end, highly effective accrual of human subjects, quantitative clinical evaluation, assessment of peripheral nerve pathology, computerized sensory testing, human electrophysiology, and clinical genetics; in New Haven, molecular and cell biology, ion channel biophysics, cellular neurophysiology, computer modeling, and pharmacology. The results of this collaboration exceeded our expectations. Faber, Merkies, and their co-workers in Maastricht made a major contribution even at the outset of this work, providing a series of twenty-eight "gold standard" patients in whom a diagnosis of small-fiber neuropathy had been confirmed, both by demonstrating nerve damage by analysis of skin biopsies, and by computerized testing which could detect subtle deficits in sensation (Faber et al. 2012). Their clinical acumen echoed throughout the project.

As we moved forward, we stayed in close touch by email and phone, the only ground rule being that we would try to not wake each other in the middle of the night. On at least a few occasions, I violated this rule, with calls to a sleeping Netherlands announcing, for example, "We have it! The mutation in patient XX destabilizes the closed state of the $Na_V1.7$ channel!" Only a science addict could appreciate such a call. Candor, reminiscent of the Tuesday Night Fights at Woods Hole and echoing debates in our War Room at Yale, punctuated our progress. In commenting on each others' ideas, none of us was hesitant to drive a point home. Emails and telephone discussions incorporated friendly queries about families or intermittent quips about Ingemar Merkies's golf game ("It's just physics with a little ball," he would insist). But other than this, our conversations included few niceties. Summaries of progress and drafts of articles bounced from one side of the ocean to the other filled with comments such as "how do you know?," "that doesn't make sense," or "provide a strong rationale or TAKE THIS OUT." Sometimes a comment was accompanied by "NO!!" We made up for our lack of social graces when we met face-to-face, over good food, cappuccino, and fine wine.

Within three years, from this initial group of patients and additional patients that followed, we identified a string of mutations in $Na_V1.7$ linked to small fiber neuropathy, each instructive in its own way. A series of papers (Ahn et al. 2013; Estacion et al. 2011; Faber et al. 2012; Han, Hoeijmakers, Ahn, et al. 2012; Han, Hoeijmakers, Liu, et al. 2012; Persson et al. 2013; Lauria et al. 2012; Hoeijmakers et al. 2012; Estacion et al. 2015) emanated from these discussions. In this work, we made the leap from inherited erythromelalgia, a rare disease, to a common disorder and showed that mutations of $Na_V1.7$ play a major role in painful neuropathy.

Neither Yong Yang nor Drenth nor the Maastricht group nor my team would have made so much progress alone. We did it well, and quickly, and together. So, what makes a collaboration work? Did we have to cross borders? As I wrote this book I posed that question to my Dutch colleagues. Drenth cited our complementary strengths, "We all need each other." And he said that he appreciated "constantly being pushed." I don't think anybody else has ever thanked me for being a nag! Karin Faber answered with a Dutch saying: "Trust arrives by foot, but leaves on a horse." This means, she explained, that trust is precious but fragile: It can easily evaporate. And indeed, we steered clear of horses as we built these collaborations. Only a little money was involved, and we shared what there was. There were no committees. We said what we thought, rapidly reached consensus or agreed to disagree, and moved ahead quickly. I'm reminded of animated discussions on Woods Hole's Stony Beach where scientists from both sides of the globe could watch the sun set, plan an experiment, and return to the laboratory with a simple sense of "let's just do it."

References

Ahn HS, Dib-Hajj SD, Cox JJ, Tyrrell L, Elmslie FV, Clarke AA, Drenth JP, Woods CG, Waxman SG. 2010. A new Nav1.7 sodium channel mutation I234T in a child with severe pain. *Eur J Pain* 14(9): 944–950.

Ahn HS, Vasylyev DV, Estacion M, Macala LJ, Shah P, Faber CG, Merkies IS, Dib-Hajj SD, Waxman SG. 2013. Differential effect of D623N variant and wild-type Na(v)1.7 sodium channels on resting potential and interspike membrane potential of dorsal root ganglion neurons. *Brain Res* 1529: 165–177.

Cheng X, Dib-Hajj SD, Tyrrell L, Te Morsche RH, Drenth JP, Waxman SG. 2011. Deletion mutation of sodium channel Na(V)1.7 in inherited erythromelalgia: Enhanced slow inactivation modulates dorsal root ganglion neuron hyperexcitability. *Brain* 134(Pt 7): 1972–1986.

Choi JS, Boralevi F, Brissaud O, Sanchez-Martin J, Te Morsche RH, Dib-Hajj SD, Drenth JP, Waxman SG. 2011. Paroxysmal extreme pain disorder: A molecular lesion of peripheral neurons. *Nat Rev Neurol* 7(1): 51–55.

Choi JS, Cheng X, Foster E, Leffler A, Tyrrell L, Te Morsche RH, Eastman EM, et al. 2010. Alternative splicing may contribute to time-dependent manifestation of inherited erythromelalgia. *Brain* 133(Pt 6): 1823–1835.

Cummins TR, Dib-Hajj SD, Waxman SG. 2004. Electrophysiological properties of mutant Nav1.7 sodium channels in a painful inherited neuropathy. *J Neurosci* 24(38): 8232–8236.

Drenth JP. 1989. Erythromelalgia induced by nicardipine. *BMJ* 298(6687): 1582.

Drenth JP, Finley WH, Breedveld GJ, Testers L, Michiels JJ, Guillet G, Taieb A, Kirby RL, Heutink P. 2001. The primary erythermalgia-susceptibility gene is located on chromosome 2q31-32. *Am J Hum Genet* 68(5): 1277–1282.

Drenth JP, Michiels JJ. 1990. Three types of erythromelalgia. *BMJ* 301(6758): 985–986.

Drenth JP, te Morsche RH, Guillet G, Taieb A, Kirby RL, Jansen JB. 2005. SCN9A mutations define primary erythermalgia as a neuropathic disorder of voltage gated sodium channels. *J Invest Dermatol* 124(6): 1333–1338.

Estacion M, Dib-Hajj SD, Benke PJ, Te Morsche RH, Eastman EM, Macala LJ, Drenth JP, Waxman SG. 2008. NaV1.7 gain-of-function mutations as a continuum: A1632E displays physiological changes associated with erythromelalgia and paroxysmal extreme pain disorder mutations and produces symptoms of both disorders. *J Neurosci* 28(43): 11079–11088.

Estacion M, Han C, Choi JS, Hoeijmakers JG, Lauria G, Drenth JP, Gerrits MM, Dib-Hajj SD, Faber CG, Merkies IS, Waxman SG. 2011. Intra- and interfamily phenotypic diversity in pain syndromes associated with a gain-of-function variant of NaV1.7. *Mol Pain* 7: 92.

Estacion M, Vohra BP, Liu S, Hoeijmakers JG, Faber CG, Merkies IS, Lauria G, Black JA, Waxman SG. 2015. Ca2+ toxicity due to reverse Na+-Ca2+ exchange contributes to degeneration of neurites of DRG neurons induced by a neuropathy-associated Nav1.7 mutation. *J Neurophysiol* 114(3): 1554–1564.

Faber CG, Hoeijmakers JG, Ahn HS, Cheng X, Han C, Choi JS, Estacion M, et al. 2012. Gain of function $Na_V1.7$ mutations in idiopathic small fiber neuropathy. *Ann Neurol* 71(1): 26–39.

Han C, Hoeijmakers JG, Ahn HS, Zhao P, Shah P, Lauria G, Gerrits MM, et al. 2012. Nav1.7-related small fiber neuropathy: Impaired slow-inactivation and DRG neuron hyperexcitability. *Neurology* 78(21): 1635–1643.

Han C, Hoeijmakers JG, Liu S, Gerrits MM, te Morsche RH, Lauria G, Dib-Hajj SD, Drenth JP, Faber CG, Merkies IS, Waxman SG. 2012. Functional profiles of SCN9A variants in dorsal root ganglion neurons and superior cervical ganglion neurons correlate with autonomic symptoms in small fibre neuropathy. *Brain* 135(Pt 9): 2613–2628.

Han C, Rush AM, Dib-Hajj SD, Li S, Xu Z, Wang Y, Tyrrell L, Wang X, Yang Y, Waxman SG. 2006. Sporadic onset of erythermalgia: A gain-of-function mutation in Nav1.7. *Ann Neurol* 59(3): 553–558.

Hoeijmakers JG, Han C, Merkies IS, Macala LJ, Lauria G, Gerrits MM, Dib-Hajj SD, Faber CG, Waxman SG. 2012. Small nerve fibres, small hands and small feet: A new syndrome of pain, dysautonomia and acromesomelia in a kindred with a novel NaV1.7 mutation. *Brain* 135(Pt 2): 345–358.

Lauria G, Faber CG, Merkies IS, Waxman SG. 2012. Diagnosis of neuropathic pain: Challenges and possibilities. *Expert Opin Med Diagn* 6(2): 89–93.

Michiels JJ, te Morsche RH, Jansen JB, Drenth JP. 2005. Autosomal dominant erythermalgia associated with a novel mutation in the voltage-gated sodium channel alpha subunit Nav1.7. *Arch Neurol* 62(10): 1587–1590.

Persson AK, Liu S, Faber CG, Merkies IS, Black JA, Waxman SG. 2013. Neuropathy-associated Nav1.7 variant I228M impairs integrity of dorsal root ganglion neuron axons. *Ann Neurol* 73(1): 140–145.

9   FROM ZEBRAS TO HORSES

A common admonition at rounds on the wards of teaching hospitals is "when you hear hoofbeats, think of horses," to which the attending physician might add "and don't limit your thoughts to zebras." Zebras, in this setting, refer to rare diseases, while horses stand for common disorders. Our demonstration that gain-of-function changes in mutant $Na_V1.7$ channels cause inherited erythromelalgia (Cummins, Dib-Hajj, and Waxman 2004; Dib-Hajj et al. 2005) and, following that, discovery that other gain-of-function mutations of $Na_V1.7$ cause pain in paroxysmal extreme pain disorder (PEPD) (Fertleman et al. 2006), had shown that hyperactivity of $Na_V1.7$ channels can produce disorders characterized by intense pain. But these were very rare diseases, zebras. Might $Na_V1.7$ be a player in chronic pain within broader populations?

Peripheral neuropathy has increasingly been recognized as a source of pain in large numbers of patients. Diabetic neuropathy, for example, occurs in about one-half of people with diabetes and often causes pain that is not relieved by existing medications. Cancer chemotherapy can trigger the onset of painful neuropathy, and exquisite pain can occur in postherpetic neuralgia which follows shingles and with the neuropathies that occur as a complication of certain inflammatory disorders. Worldwide, millions of people suffer from pain that accompanies peripheral neuropathy.

Our peripheral nerves contain large-, medium-, and small-diameter axons, and neuropathy can affect any of these groups of nerve fibers. Peripheral axons carry information from our body surface and organs via nerves such as the sciatic nerve to the spinal cord, and they vary in size—axons that relay information about muscle tension, involved in deep tendon reflexes, are about 10 microns in diameter, while nerve fibers that convey information about pain are much smaller, usually with a diameter of less than one micron or 1/1,000th of a millimeter. Because of their diminutive size the small-diameter axons had been less well studied.

"Small fiber neuropathy" is a form of peripheral neuropathy that affects small-diameter, unmyelinated and thinly myelinated axons within peripheral nerve, including pain-signaling nerve fibers. We now know that the clinical picture of small fiber neuropathy is dominated by pain, often with a burning quality, which is usually first felt within the territories innervated by the longest nerves (Gorson and Ropper 1995; Hoeijmakers, Faber, et al. 2012; Holland et al. 1998; Lacomis 2002). Patients with small fiber neuropathy typically come to the doctor complaining of burning pain in the feet or the hands. This characteristic of peripheral neuropathy is widely taught to medical students as a "stocking-glove" pattern of clinical abnormality.

Although small fiber neuropathy is not rare—Faber, Merkies, and their colleagues estimated a prevalence of about 50 per 100,000, or 1 in 2,000 (Peters et al. 2013)—it was not widely recognized as a clinical entity until the 1990s. The reason was that, until then, it was difficult to diagnose. In its pure form small fiber neuropathy specifically affects small-diameter nerve fibers within peripheral nerves, sparing the large-diameter nerve fibers that support deep tendon reflexes and perception of vibration, which were assessed in the routine neurological examination. Because their large nerve fibers were not affected, patients with small fiber neuropathy presented to clinicians with *symptoms* such as pain but did not manifest objective *signs* such as loss of reflexes when tested with the neurologist's hammer or impaired vibration sensibility when tested with a tuning fork. Since their neurological examinations were often normal, the complaints of patients with small fiber neuropathy—which occurred without physical signs of disease of the nervous system that can be seen by the physician— were, in the past, often dismissed as being of little consequence, or as having a psychological origin.

A crucial step forward in recognition of small fiber neuropathy as a disease came with the development of techniques for assessing the number, and health, of small nerve fibers. A breakthrough, led by clinical investigations at Johns Hopkins, came with recognition that the tips of the tiny nerve fibers, most distant from the DRG neurons that give rise to them, terminate within the skin where they can be assessed by microscopic examination of biopsies (Kennedy and Wendelschafer-Crabb 1999; McCarthy et al. 1995). A relatively noninvasive method for skin biopsy uses a small punch to remove a core of skin 3 mm across, about the size of a large pencil lead. Following removal, the skin sample is preserved, cut into sections, stained, and examined in the microscope, where the number of small nerve fibers can be counted and compared with normal, healthy controls (usually age-matched and gender-matched) so that loss of nerve fibers can be assessed. Injured nerve fibers can also be identified since they form abnormal bulb-like swellings (figure 9.1).

As another measure of the status of small nerve fibers, sensitivity to warmth, coolness, heat-induced pain, and cold-induced pain could be quantitatively assessed in human subjects using computerized techniques, in a test called quantitative sensory testing, or QST. The development of methods for assessment of small nerve fibers within skin biopsies, and QST, made it possible for small fiber neuropathy to be diagnosed on the basis of objective, quantifiable criteria (Bakkers et al. 2009; Herrmann et al. 1999; McArthur et al. 1998; Walk et al. 2007).

Our characterization of $Na_V1.7$ mutations in patients with small fiber neuropathy began in mid-2010, when I started to work with Catharina Faber and Ingemar Merkies of Maastricht University. Working as a team, these peripheral neuropathy experts had assembled a cohort of patients with painful small fiber neuropathy. They now wanted to know whether there were disease-causing $Na_V1.7$ mutations in these patients. Here we had an obvious scaffold for collaboration.

My interest in sodium channels in peripheral neuropathy was partly based on some clinical similarities—burning pain in the feet and hands—to inherited erythromelalgia. It was also partly propelled by work carried out nearly two decades previously in my laboratory by Peter Stys, then a research fellow and now a distinguished professor of neuroscience at the University of Calgary. In studies on small axons within the optic nerve that connects the eye and the brain in the rat, Stys had demonstrated that sodium channels play an important role in axonal injury. His work showed that in various forms of axonal injury, the channels provide a route for a small but persistent flow of sodium ions into the axons. This tiny but sustained sodium influx, in turn, triggers the activity of a molecule called the sodium-calcium exchanger (Stys, Waxman, and Ransom 1992). The sodium-calcium exchanger is an antiporter or see-saw molecule that normally carries a small amount of sodium from the outside of cells where its concentration is high, to the inside of cells where its concentration is normally low. As implied by its name, the sodium-calcium exchanger, in a swap for the influx of sodium, normally moves calcium ions out of cells, thereby maintaining the intracellular concentration of calcium at low levels where it cannot activate injurious enzymes. Stys's experiments showed that, after various insults to axons in the optic nerve, a small but sustained influx of sodium ions increases the concentration of sodium within these fragile nerve fibers, forcing the sodium-calcium exchanger to work in a "reverse" mode where, instead of extruding calcium, it imports calcium into axons. The high levels of calcium

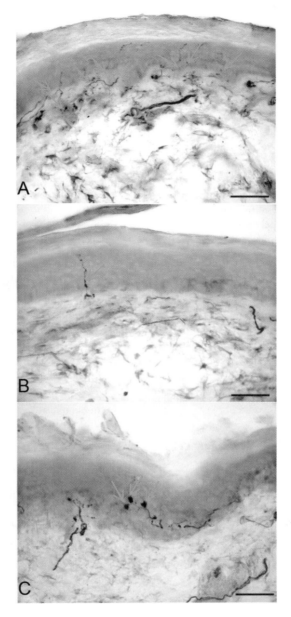

Figure 9.1

Small fiber neuropathy can be diagnosed using skin biopsy to demonstrate degeneration of the endings of nerve fibers within the skin. Panel A shows a skin biopsy from a normal individual in whom multiple nerve fibers within the skin (green arrows) can be seen. Panel B shows a skin biopsy from a patient with small fiber neuropathy, in whom there is a depletion of nerve fibers. Panel C shows swellings of nerve fibers (green arrows) in the skin, from another patient with small fiber neuropathy. These are predegenerative changes. Scale bars: 50 μm. From Hoeijmakers, Faber et al. (2012).

then activate deleterious enzymes that lead to axonal demise (figure 9.2). Importantly, experiments we had done with Stys in the 1990s showed that blockade of sodium channels could protect axons so that they did not degenerate after various insults (Stys, Ransom, and Waxman 1992; Stys, Waxman, and Ransom 1992). These earlier studies established sodium channels as key players in axonal injury within the optic nerve, which is an extension of the brain. Now, twenty years later, it was logical to ask whether sodium channels might also play a role in axonal injury within peripheral nerves.

Joel Black, working in my lab, had shown that small nerve fibers in our peripheral nerves and their terminals in the skin contain $Na_V1.7$ channels (figure 9.3A) (Black et al. 2012). I also knew, from the observations of Swedish pain researcher Anna-Karin Persson, who was working in my lab, that small nerve fibers in the skin contain the sodium-calcium exchanger, located in the same regions as $Na_V1.7$ (figure 9.3B). And as shown in figure 9.4, Dymtro Vasylyev was able to use tiny microelectrodes in my laboratory to accomplish the challenging task of directly recording the electrical activity from small nerve fibers. These recordings showed us that $Na_V1.7$ channels were not only present within these tiny axons, but were also inserted into the axon membrane in a normal manner so that they are functional (Vasylyev and Waxman 2012).

Another feature of small nerve fibers also drove my interest. Earlier studies in our laboratory and others (Donnelly 2008; Waxman et al. 1989) had shown us that small-diameter axons are especially sensitive to small changes in sodium channel activity. These studies had shown that small axons are poised to fire in response to very small stimuli, or to degenerate in response to small, subtle changes in the number or properties of the channels. Neuroscientists attribute this to a characteristic of small nerve fibers called "high input impedance." The effect of input impedance can be appreciated by considering, for example, the impact of a small whistle on rooms of various sizes. Within a large auditorium, the whistle sounds may be lost or drowned out. In contrast, within the confines of a small room, the whistle can be heard and may even echo and disrupt conversation. Similar to a small room

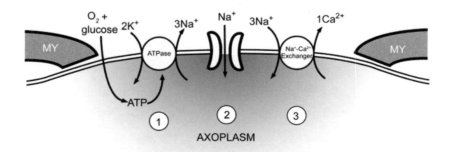

Figure 9.2
Diagram showing how, in injured axons (1) energy reserves (ATP) are depleted, leading to failure of the ATPase and collapse of ionic gradients; (2) Na^+ ions enter through sodium channels; (3) the resultant increase in Na^+ within the axon causes the Na^+-Ca^{2+} exchanger to operate in reverse mode, carrying damaging quantities of Ca^{2+} into the axon. MY, myelin. Modified from Stys, Ransom, and Waxman (1992).

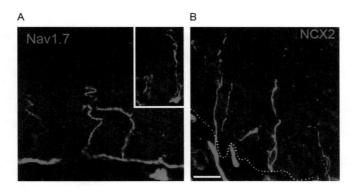

Figure 9.3
(A) A micrograph showing small-diameter nerve fibers within the skin, in which red staining indicates the presence of $Na_V1.7$. Scale bar: 20 μm (Black et al. 2012). (B) A micrograph showing small nerve fibers in the skin, in which red staining indicates the presence of the sodium-calcium exchanger. Scale bar: 20 μm. From Persson et al. (2010).

where the sound of a whistle can be impactful, we knew that small nerve fibers are highly sensitive to changes—even small changes—in the sodium channels within them. And based on this, it seemed logical to me that even minor degrees of hyperactivity of sodium channels might have a dramatic impact on small-diameter axons.

Now, working with Faber and Merkies, I wanted to find out whether $Na_V1.7$ mutations contributed to development of peripheral neuropathy. Faber and Merkies described themselves as "just clinicians." In my view this understated their contributions to our work together. They began with a series of 248 patients referred to them with a presumptive diagnosis of small fiber neuropathy. Pain was a common presenting symptom. In some of these patients, even the touch of a bedsheet was painful. To winnow this large group down to a smaller cohort of patients with small fiber neuropathy with a low likelihood of a nongenetic cause, they excluded cases in which there were underlying conditions such as diabetes, treatment with medications known to produce peripheral neuropathy as a side effect, inflammatory disorders, or other diseases that were known to be accompanied by neuropathy. This left 63 patients with small fiber neuropathy and no apparent underlying medical disease.

Forty-four of these patients agreed to participate in a research study; this was testimony to the close bond that Faber and Merkies established with their patients. But still another layer of filtering was needed before the ball moved to my court. Functional analysis, to determine whether any particular mutation was pathogenic, was going to require a substantial effort in my laboratory. Because of this, we decided to focus on patients in whom the diagnosis of small fiber neuropathy had been confirmed by the most stringent criteria. To accomplish this, after obtaining consent, Faber and Merkies studied all 44 patients by skin biopsy and by QST. These tests were both abnormal in 28 patients who, using these stringent criteria, gave us a "gold standard" cohort of subjects with well-documented, biopsy-confirmed small fiber neuropathy, pain, and no identifiable nongenetic cause. Remarkably, within this group of 28 patients, mutations of $Na_V1.7$ were present in eight, or nearly 30%.

Some mutations are pathogenic and alter the function of ion channels in a way that contributes to disease, while others are functionally silent and clinically inconsequential. The challenge was to determine whether these mutations were functionally significant. Eight mutations may not sound like

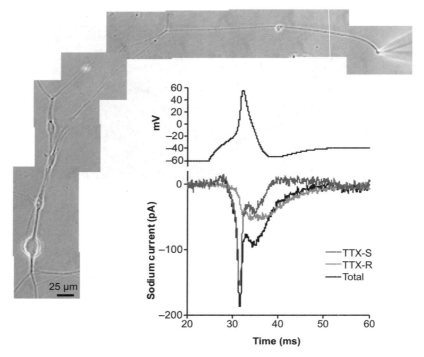

Figure 9.4
Patch-clamp recording from a small nerve fiber with a diameter of approximately 1 μm extending
from a dorsal root ganglion neuron in tissue culture. The micrograph shows (upper right) the tip
of the electrode where it contacts the nerve fiber. The top trace shows a nerve impulse (action
potential) from this nerve fiber. The bottom trace shows the sodium currents, produced by $Na_V1.7$
(blue trace) and then $Na_V1.8$ channels (red), which underlie the action potential. The black trace
indicates the summed $Na_V1.7$ and $Na_V1.8$ currents. From Vasylyev and Waxman (2012).

a large number, but functional assessment of eight sodium channel mutations represented an immense
task. Each mutation required production of the gene for $Na_V1.7$ containing the mutation and then, insertion of the DNA into cells in the laboratory. After the cells had grown in sterile tissue culture dishes
and made the mutant channels, we could do a voltage-clamp analysis using patch-clamp recording to
assess the effect of the mutation on the function of the ion channel. We also decided to assess each
mutation by current clamp so that we could examine the effect of the mutant channels on the behavior
of pain-signaling neurons. For each of the eight mutations, this analysis required extended study by
a team that included an experienced electrophysiologist supported by a molecular biology technician
to produce the mutant genes and a tissue culture technician who prepared tissue cultures containing
DRG neurons in which the mutant channels could be expressed. We knew, at the outset, that analysis
of each mutation could take up to three or four months if things went smoothly. Or even longer if they
did not.

   Faced with eight mutations, I decided to deploy our entire electrophysiology team, including five
highly skilled PhD electrophysiologists, each with substantial expertise in sodium channels, to work

in parallel with the necessary support staff. This was a heavily leveraged bet. It was going to divert precious manpower from other projects. Indeed, if the bet did not work out, we would have invested several years of work by more than half a dozen team members, with no reward.

The ensuing months were very busy, as members of our team marched forward day by day, completing the intricate measurements needed for analysis of each of the eight mutations. We met nearly every day in the War Room to review progress. From our knowledge of the molecular architecture of the channel, and from the coordinates of the substituted amino acids which were located outside of the membrane-spanning segments of the channel protein molecule, we expected that the mutations would cause relatively subtle changes in channel function. This turned out to be the case, and it meant that we had to make an especially large number of measurements to detect small but functionally important changes in how the mutant channels worked. Our sense of urgency was amplified by frequent inquiries from Maastricht—"Have you found anything yet?" "What about D623N?" I did not regard this as a bother. Our Dutch collaborators were cheering us on.

As the months rolled by, the work progressed. The data from one, then another, then a third mutation arrived in the War Room, and a striking picture began to emerge. Some mutations impaired a process called slow inactivation, which essentially immobilizes channels in an inoperable state after prolonged depolarization. Other mutations produced a small impairment of slow inactivation together with a small impairment of fast inactivation, a process that temporarily locks channels in an inoperable state after brief periods of depolarization. And still another mutation enhanced resurgent current, which is triggered by repolarization at the end of a sustained depolarization so as to produce additional firing. The common thread was that every one of the mutations produced pro-excitatory changes that enhanced the activity of the channel.

When we put the mutant $Na_V1.7$ channels into DRG neurons (the sensory neurons where they normally reside), each of the mutations produced hyperexcitability. The abnormal excitability was manifested by a decrease in current threshold (making it easier to excite the neuron) and a higher-than-normal frequency of firing in response to stimulation. These changes provided a basis for understanding the pain that could be evoked by even a light touch in our patients. Making the story even more complete, the mutations produced abnormal spontaneous firing in DRG neurons. This provided an explanation for the spontaneous pain, in the absence of stimulation, that brought most of our patients to the clinic. Here we had, in patients with a relatively common disorder, another example of the role of $Na_V1.7$ in pain.

Our studies in this initial gold-standard cohort of 28 patients with painful small neuropathy had demonstrated gain-of-function mutations in about 28% (Faber, Hoeijmakers, et al. 2012). In follow-up studies on a larger cohort of more than 100 patients, in whom biopsy confirmation was not available and diagnosis rested on clinical criteria, $Na_V1.7$ mutations were again found, although the percentage of patients carrying $Na_V1.7$ mutations was about 15%. As I discussed this with our Maastricht collaborators, we speculated that the discrepancy might have reflected inclusion of some patients without neuropathy, or with mild neuropathy, in the larger group of patients, in which confirmation of the diagnosis by biopsy was not required. Irrespective of the precise percentage, we had demonstrated gain-of-function mutations in $Na_V1.7$ in a substantial number of patients with painful neuropathy, a relatively common disorder. Subsequent to our 2012 report, we documented the gain-of-function changes in other $Na_V1.7$ mutations linked to painful neuropathy (Estacion et al. 2011; Han, Hoeijmakers, Ahn, et al. 2012; Han, Hoeijmakers, Liu, et al. 2012; Hoeijmakers, Han, et al. 2012).

What about the patients with neuropathy who did not carry mutations of $Na_V1.7$? To examine that question, we first searched in the DNA of these patients for mutations of $Na_V1.8$, another "peripheral" sodium channel. For this study (Faber, Lauria, et al. 2012) we assessed a series of 104 patients with painful neuropathy in which a $Na_V1.7$ mutation had not been found. Seven mutations in $Na_V1.8$ were identified in nine of these 104 patients. Computer algorithms that assessed the potential functional effects of these mutations, on the basis of their effects on channel structure, suggested that three of these mutations were likely to be pathogenic. We assessed these mutations by voltage-clamp and current-clamp. Two of these mutations were found to enhance the channel's response to depolarization and produced hyperexcitability in DRG neurons (Faber, Lauria, et al. 2012). We subsequently studied two additional $Na_V1.8$ mutations from patients with painful neuropathy and found that these, too, conferred gain-of-function changes on the channel and produced DRG neuron hyperexcitability (Han et al. 2014; Huang et al. 2013).

In other studies together with our European collaborators, we asked whether mutations of the third peripheral sodium channel, $Na_V1.9$, might be present in patients with painful peripheral neuropathy in whom $Na_V1.7$ or $Na_V1.8$ mutations were not present. For this study, we assessed a cohort of 344 patients with painful neuropathy without mutations in $Na_V1.7$ or $Na_V1.8$ and found four mutations of $Na_V1.9$ in conserved, membrane-spanning regions of the channel. The biophysical effects of these mutations were especially interesting. The normal $Na_V1.9$ channel is unusual in displaying a large overlap between activation and inactivation. As a result of this overlap, $Na_V1.9$ channels produce a "window current," which is a small, sustained inward sodium current that depolarizes neurons. Functional analysis of the $Na_V1.9$ mutations from patients with painful neuropathy is ongoing as this book is being written. We have thus far found three $Na_V1.9$ mutations from patients with painful neuropathy that shift channel gating so as to increase the window current, to a degree that depolarizes DRG neurons to a level that makes them hyperexcitable, providing an explanation for the pain that these patients' experience (Han et al. 2015; Huang et al. 2014). We have also studied a $Na_V1.9$ mutation from a patient with a loss of pain sensation. Interestingly, in this case a massive change in channel gating produces a larger increase in the window current that profoundly depolarizes DRG neurons, inactivating the sodium channels within these cells so that they lose the ability to generate nerve impulses, thus explaining the loss of pain sensibility (Huang et al., 2017). In the aggregate, these studies are showing us that, while less common than $Na_V1.7$ mutations, $Na_V1.8$ and $Na_V1.9$ mutations also contribute to disorders of pain signaling.

These findings may have therapeutic implications. New agents designed to selectively block each of the peripheral sodium channels—$Na_V1.7$, $Na_V1.8$, and $Na_V1.9$—are under development. The basic idea is that, because $Na_V1.7$, $Na_V1.8$, and $Na_V1.9$ do not play substantial roles within the brain, selective blockade of these peripheral sodium channels would not be expected to affect the brain; consequently, subtype-specific $Na_V1.7$, $Na_V1.8$, or $Na_V1.9$ blockers would be expected to provide pain relief without "central" side effects such as double vision, loss of balance, confusion, or sleepiness. And, because they do not act on the brain, these peripheral sodium channel blockers would be expected to be devoid of addictive potential. Development of $Na_V1.7$ blockers is the most advanced. Particularly promising, as described in chapter 11, are the results of early-phase clinical trials on $Na_V1.7$ blockers as a treatment for pain.

There is another dimension to these observations. These studies may help us to understand the events that lead to degeneration of nerve fibers in peripheral neuropathy. Identification of specific molecules that play key roles in axonal injury might provide a basis for therapies that would prevent, or slow, the degeneration of axons, thus halting or slowing the progression of peripheral neuropathy. In thinking about injury to axons in peripheral neuropathy, we built upon lessons learned in our earlier studies (Stys, Waxman, and Ransom 1992) on degeneration of axons within the optic nerve. Since small pain-signaling axons were known to express the sodium-calcium exchanger in proximity to $Na_V1.7$ (Persson et al. 2010), we hypothesized that increased sodium influx into axons expressing mutant $Na_V1.7$ channels might trigger calcium influx via reverse (calcium-importing) sodium-calcium exchange, as we had shown in 1992 in the optic nerve. To begin to assess this hypothesis, we developed a tissue culture model in which we could study the effect of mutant $Na_V1.7$ sodium channels on the axons of DRG neurons. These studies showed that the length of axons of DRG transfected with mutant $Na_V1.7$ channels was reduced compared to similar neurons transfected with normal, wild-type channels (Persson, Liu, et al. 2013). This suggested that the mutant $Na_V1.7$ channels might impair the integrity of these axons. To examine this hypothesis, we asked whether a sodium channel blocker would protect axons transfected with the $Na_V1.7$ mutant channels, preventing the decrease in length. For a variety of reasons we started with the sodium channel blocker carbamazepine, and we found that it does, in fact, have a protective effect. We also assessed the effect of a pharmacological blocker of reverse sodium-calcium exchange and found that it, too, was protective, preventing injury to the axons of DRG neurons expressing the mutant channels (Persson, Liu, et al. 2013).

Of course there is more to learn. Several aspects of peripheral neuropathy remain especially enigmatic. For example, we still have not solved the question "why does peripheral neuropathy become manifest in most patients relatively late in life?" Given that patients with $Na_V1.7$-associated neuropathy carry their mutations throughout their entire lives, it is possible that axonal injury in peripheral neuropathy may build up via a multihit process: The sodium channel mutations may drive axonal degeneration in concert with other factors—genetic, or epigenetic, or environmental—that accumulate over time. Our recent observations suggest, for example, that dysfunction of mitochondria—intracellular organelles which act as energy generators for the cell—occurs with aging and accumulates as ever-increasing numbers of mitochondria are injured, finally combining with the gain-of-function in $Na_V1.7$ channels to trigger axonal degeneration. As a postdoctoral fellow in 1976 I had demonstrated, using the computational methods available at that time, that multiple, cumulative insults to a nerve fiber, occurring at different times, could account for length-dependent injury (Waxman et al. 1976). We recently carried out experiments that show sodium channels contribute to degeneration of DRG axons induced by mitochondrial injury in tissue culture (Persson, Kim, et al. 2013), providing support for a multihit mechanism of axonal injury that involves mitochondrial dysfunction together with gain-of-function of $Na_V1.7$. This work is ongoing (Estacion et al. 2015; Rolyan et al. 2016). These observations raise the possibility that in the future, it may be possible to devise neuroprotective strategies that will slow or prevent axonal degeneration in peripheral neuropathy.

Men on fire are very rare. In the parlance of medical rounds, they are "zebras." But their genes pointed to $Na_V1.7$ as a major player in pain. And helped us to discover that $Na_V1.7$ is a participant in a more common disorder, peripheral neuropathy. People with peripheral neuropathy are "horses" and are seen every day in clinics around the world. The DNA of men on fire has helped to explain a disease in "the rest of us."

References

Bakkers M, Merkies IS, Lauria G, Devigili G, Penza P, Lombardi R, Hermans MC, van Nes SI, De Baets M, Faber CG. 2009. Intraepidermal nerve fiber density and its application in sarcoidosis. *Neurology* 73(14): 1142–1148.

Black JA, Frezel N, Dib-Hajj SD, Waxman SG. 2012. Expression of Nav1.7 in DRG neurons extends from peripheral terminals in the skin to central preterminal branches and terminals in the dorsal horn. *Mol Pain* 8: 82.

Cummins TR, Dib-Hajj SD, Waxman SG. 2004. Electrophysiological properties of mutant Nav1.7 sodium channels in a painful inherited neuropathy. *J Neurosci* 24(38): 8232–8236.

Dib-Hajj SD, Rush AM, Cummins TR, Hisama FM, Novella S, Tyrrell L, Marshall L, Waxman SG. 2005. Gain-of-function mutation in Nav1.7 in familial erythromelalgia induces bursting of sensory neurons. *Brain* 128(Pt 8): 1847–1854.

Donnelly DF. 2008. Spontaneous action potential generation due to persistent sodium channel currents in simulated carotid body afferent fibers. *J Appl Physiol* 104(5): 1394–1401.

Estacion M, Han C, Choi JS, Hoeijmakers JG, Lauria G, Drenth JP, Gerrits MM, Dib-Hajj SD, Faber CG, Merkies IS, Waxman SG. 2011. Intra- and interfamily phenotypic diversity in pain syndromes associated with a gain-of-function variant of NaV1.7. *Mol Pain* 7: 92.

Estacion M, Vohra BP, Liu S, Hoeijmakers JG, Faber CG, Merkies IS, Lauria G, Black JA, Waxman SG. 2015. Ca2+ toxicity due to reverse Na+-Ca2+ exchange contributes to degeneration of neurites of DRG neurons induced by a neuropathy-associated Nav1.7 mutation. *J Neurophysiol* 114(3): 1554–1564.

Faber CG, Hoeijmakers JG, Ahn HS, Cheng X, Han C, Choi JS, Estacion M, et al. 2012. Gain of function $Na_V1.7$ mutations in idiopathic small fiber neuropathy. *Ann Neurol* 71(1): 26–39.

Faber CG, Lauria G, Merkies IS, Cheng X, Han C, Ahn HS, Persson AK, et al. 2012. Gain-of-function Nav1.8 mutations in painful neuropathy. *Proc Natl Acad Sci USA* 109(47): 19444–19449.

Fertleman CR, Baker MD, Parker KA, Moffatt S, Elmslie FV, Abrahamsen B, Ostman J, Klugbauer N, Wood JN, Gardiner RM, Rees M. 2006. SCN9A mutations in paroxysmal extreme pain disorder: Allelic variants underlie distinct channel defects and phenotypes. *Neuron* 52(5): 767–774.

Gorson KC, Ropper AH. 1995. Idiopathic distal small fiber neuropathy. *Acta Neurol Scand* 92(5): 376–382.

Han C, Hoeijmakers JG, Ahn HS, Zhao P, Shah P, Lauria G, Gerrits MM, et al. 2012. Nav1.7-related small fiber neuropathy: Impaired slow-inactivation and DRG neuron hyperexcitability. *Neurology* 78(21): 1635–1643.

Han C, Hoeijmakers JG, Liu S, Gerrits MM, te Morsche RH, Lauria G, Dib-Hajj SD, Drenth JP, Faber CG, Merkies IS, Waxman SG. 2012. Functional profiles of SCN9A variants in dorsal root ganglion neurons and superior cervical ganglion neurons correlate with autonomic symptoms in small fibre neuropathy. *Brain* 135(Pt 9): 2613–2628.

Han C, Vasylyev D, Macala LJ, Gerrits MM, Hoeijmakers JG, Bekelaar KJ, Dib-Hajj SD, Faber CG, Merkies IS, Waxman SG. 2014. The G1662S NaV1.8 mutation in small fibre neuropathy: Impaired inactivation underlying DRG neuron hyperexcitability. *J Neurol Neurosurg Psychiatry* 85(5): 499–505.

Han C, Yang Y, de Greef BT, Hoeijmakers JG, Gerrits MM, Verhamme C, Qu J, et al. 2015. The Domain II S4-S5 linker in $Na_V1.9$: A missense mutation enhances activation, impairs fast inactivation, and produces human painful neuropathy. *Neuromolecular Med* 17(2): 158–169.

Herrmann DN, Griffin JW, Hauer P, Cornblath DR, McArthur JC. 1999. Epidermal nerve fiber density and sural nerve morphometry in peripheral neuropathies. *Neurology* 53(8): 1634–1640.

Hoeijmakers JG, Faber CG, Lauria G, Merkies IS, Waxman SG. 2012. Small-fibre neuropathies—advances in diagnosis, pathophysiology and management. *Nat Rev Neurol* 8(7): 369–379.

Hoeijmakers JG, Han C, Merkies IS, Macala LJ, Lauria G, Gerrits MM, Dib-Hajj SD, Faber CG, Waxman SG. 2012. Small nerve fibres, small hands and small feet: A new syndrome of pain, dysautonomia and acromesomelia in a kindred with a novel NaV1.7 mutation. *Brain* 135(Pt 2): 345–358.

Holland NR, Crawford TO, Hauer P, Cornblath DR, Griffin JW, McArthur JC. 1998. Small-fiber sensory neuropathies: Clinical course and neuropathology of idiopathic cases. *Ann Neurol* 44(1): 47–59.

Huang J, Han C, Estacion M, Vasylyev D, Hoeijmakers JG, Gerrits MM, Tyrrell L, et al, and the Propane Study Group. 2014. Gain-of-function mutations in sodium channel Na(v)1.9 in painful neuropathy. *Brain* 137(Pt 6): 1627–1642.

Huang J, Vanoye CG, Cutts A, Goldberg YP, Dib-Hajj SD, Cohen CJ, Waxman SG, George AL Jr. 2017. Sodium channel Na$_v$1.9 mutations associated with insensitivity to pain dampen neuronal excitability. *J Clin Invest* 127(7): 2805–2814.

Huang J, Yang Y, Zhao P, Gerrits MM, Hoeijmakers JG, Bekelaar K, Merkies IS, Faber CG, Dib-Hajj SD, Waxman SG. 2013. Small-fiber neuropathy Nav1.8 mutation shifts activation to hyperpolarized potentials and increases excitability of dorsal root ganglion neurons. *J Neurosci* 33(35): 14087–14097.

Kennedy WR, Wendelschafer-Crabb G. 1999. Utility of the skin biopsy method in studies of diabetic neuropathy. *Electroencephalogr Clin Neurophysiol* 50(Supplement): 553–559.

Lacomis D. 2002. Small-fiber neuropathy. *Muscle Nerve* 26(2): 173–188.

McArthur JC, Stocks EA, Hauer P, Cornblath DR, Griffin JW. 1998. Epidermal nerve fiber density: Normative reference range and diagnostic efficiency. *Arch Neurol* 55(12): 1513–1520.

McCarthy BG, Hsieh ST, Stocks A, Hauer P, Macko C, Cornblath DR, Griffin JW, McArthur JC. 1995. Cutaneous innervation in sensory neuropathies: Evaluation by skin biopsy. *Neurology* 45(10): 1848–1855.

Persson AK, Black JA, Gasser A, Cheng X, Fischer TZ, Waxman SG. 2010. Sodium-calcium exchanger and multiple sodium channel isoforms in intra-epidermal nerve terminals. *Mol Pain* 6: 84.

Persson AK, Kim I, Zhao P, Estacion M, Black JA, Waxman SG. 2013. Sodium channels contribute to degeneration of dorsal root ganglion neurites induced by mitochondrial dysfunction in an in vitro model of axonal injury. *J Neurosci* 33(49): 19250–19261.

Persson AK, Liu S, Faber CG, Merkies IS, Black JA, Waxman SG. 2013. Neuropathy-associated Nav1.7 variant I228M impairs integrity of dorsal root ganglion neuron axons. *Ann Neurol* 73(1): 140–145.

Peters MJ, Bakkers M, Merkies IS, Hoeijmakers JG, van Raak EP, Faber CG. 2013. Incidence and prevalence of small-fiber neuropathy: A survey in the Netherlands. *Neurology* 81(15): 1356–1360.

Rolyan H, Liu S, Hoeijmakers JG, Faber CG, Merkies IS, Lauria G, Black JA, Waxman SG. 2016. A painful neuropathy-associated Nav1.7 mutant leads to time-dependent degeneration of small-diameter axons associated with intracellular Ca2+ dysregulation and decrease in ATP levels. *Mol Pain* 12.

Stys PK, Ransom BR, Waxman SG. 1992. Tertiary and quaternary local anesthetics protect CNS white matter from anoxic injury at concentrations that do not block excitability. *J Neurophysiol* 67(1): 236–240.

Stys PK, Waxman SG, Ransom BR. 1992. Ionic mechanisms of anoxic injury in mammalian CNS white matter: Role of Na+ channels and Na(+)-Ca2+ exchanger. *J Neurosci* 12(2): 430–439.

Vasylyev DV, Waxman SG. 2012. Membrane properties and electrogenesis in the distal axons of small dorsal root ganglion neurons in vitro. *J Neurophysiol* 108(3): 729–740.

Walk D, Wendelschafer-Crabb G, Davey C, Kennedy WR. 2007. Concordance between epidermal nerve fiber density and sensory examination in patients with symptoms of idiopathic small fiber neuropathy. *J Neurol Sci* 255(1–2): 23–26.

Waxman SG, Black JA, Kocsis JD, Ritchie JM. 1989. Low density of sodium channels supports action potential conduction in axons of neonatal rat optic nerve. *Proc Natl Acad Sci USA* 86(4): 1406–1410.

Waxman SG, Brill MH, Geschwind N, Sabin TD, Lettvin JY. 1976. Probability of conduction deficit as related to fiber length in random-distribution models of peripheral neuropathies. *J Neurol Sci* 29(1): 39–53.

GAIN OF FUNCTION Na$_V$1.7 MUTATIONS IN IDIOPATHIC SMALL FIBER NEUROPATHY*

Catharina G. Faber, Janneke G. J. Hoeijmakers, Hye-Sook Ahn, Xiaoyang Cheng, Chongyang Han, Jin-Sung Choi, Mark Estacion, Giuseppe Lauria, Els K. Vanhoutte, Monique M. Gerrits, Sulayman Dib-Hajj, Joost P. H. Drenth, Stephen G. Waxman, and Ingemar S. J. Merkies

Objective: Small nerve fiber neuropathy (SFN) often occurs without apparent cause, but no systematic genetic studies have been performed in patients with idiopathic SFN (I-SFN). We sought to identify a genetic basis for I-SFN by screening patients with biopsy-confirmed idiopathic SFN for mutations in the *SCN9A* gene, encoding voltage-gated sodium channel Na$_V$1.7, which is preferentially expressed in small diameter peripheral axons.

Methods: Patients referred with possible I-SFN, who met the criteria of 2:2 SFN-related symptoms, normal strength, tendon reflexes, vibration sense, and nerve conduction studies, and reduced intraepidermal nerve fiber density (IENFD) plus abnormal quantitative sensory testing (QST) and no underlying etiology for SFN, were assessed clinically and by screening of *SCN9A* for mutations and functional analyses.

Results: Twenty-eight patients who met stringent criteria for I-SFN including abnormal IENFD and QST underwent *SCN9A* gene analyses. Of these 28 patients with biopsy-confirmed I-SFN, 8 were found to carry novel mutations in *SCN9A*. Functional analysis revealed multiple gain of function changes in the mutant channels; each of the mutations rendered dorsal root ganglion neurons hyperexcitable.

Interpretation: We show for the first time that gain of function mutations in sodium channel Na$_V$1.7, which render dorsal root ganglion neurons hyperexcitable, are present in a substantial proportion (28.6%; 8 of 28) of patients meeting strict criteria for I-SFN. These results point to a broader role of Na$_V$1.7 mutations in neurological disease than previously considered from studies on rare genetic syndromes, and suggest an etiological basis for

I-SFN, whereby expression of gain of function mutant sodium channels in small diameter peripheral axons may cause these fibers to degenerate.

* Previously published in *Annals of Neurology* 71(1): 26–39, 2012. Additional supporting information can be found in the online version of this article (doi: 10.1002/ana.22485). © 2011 American Neurological Association.

Small nerve fiber neuropathy (SFN) is a relatively common disorder of thinly myelinated and unmyelinated nerve fibers recently recognized as a distinct clinical syndrome.[1] The clinical picture is typically dominated by onset in adulthood of neuropathic pain, often with a burning quality, and autonomic symptoms.[2–6] The diagnosis of pure SFN, in which small diameter nerve fibers are affected but large diameter fibers are spared, is usually made on the basis of the clinical picture, preservation of large fiber functions (normal strength, tendon reflexes, and vibration sense), and normal nerve conduction studies (NCS), and is confirmed by demonstration of reduced intraepidermal nerve fiber density (IENFD) or abnormal quantitative sensory testing (QST).[7] Despite intensive search for underlying causes such as diabetes mellitus, impaired glucose tolerance, Fabry disease, celiac disease, sarcoidosis, human immunodeficiency virus (HIV), and other systemic illnesses that may be treatable,[5,8] the proportion of patients with idiopathic SFN (I-SFN), in which no cause can be identified, remains substantial, ranging in different series from 24% to 93%.[5,6,9] Observations of autosomal dominant inheritance suggest a genetic origin for the small fiber involvement that is seen in burning feet syndrome.[10] However, no specific gene has been linked to, or mutations identified in, patients with adult onset I-SFN.

Voltage-gated sodium channel Na$_V$1.7 is preferentially expressed in dorsal root ganglion

(DRG) and sympathetic ganglion neurons[11,12] and their axons,[13] and opens in response to small depolarizations close to resting potential.[14] Gain of function mutations in the *SCN9A* gene encoding $Na_V1.7$ have been found to cause the painful disorders inherited erythromelalgia (IEM)[15,16] and paroxysmal extreme pain disorder (PEPD),[17] which are characterized by increased excitability of DRG neurons, and loss of function mutations of $Na_V1.7$ have been linked to channelopathy-associated insensitivity to pain.[18] Sodium channel mutations have not, however, been linked to axonal degeneration. Reasoning that $Na_V1.7$ is present in small diameter peripheral axons,[13] in this study we asked whether mutations in the *SCN9A* gene could be found in a clinically well-defined cohort of patients with biopsy-confirmed I-SFN.

Our results demonstrate, for the first time, the presence of sodium channel mutations in a substantial proportion of patients with I-SFN, show that these missense mutations occur in an ion channel that is preferentially expressed in peripheral axons and share the common feature of rendering DRG neurons hyperexcitable, and point to a broader role of $Na_V1.7$ mutations in neurological diseases than previously considered from studies on rare genetic hyperexcitability syndromes.

Patients and Methods

Patients

Inclusion/Exclusion Criteria: Preselection

To accrue a cohort of patients with I-SFN, we initially assessed all patients aged ≥18 years seen at Maastricht University Medical Center neurological clinic with a clinical diagnosis of SFN between 2006 and 2009 and excluded those in whom, after full workup, a cause for SFN was identified. All patients with a clinical diagnosis of I-SFN were asked to participate in this study. Eligibility criteria were normal strength, tendon reflexes, and vibration sense; normal NCS; and presence of at least 2 of the following symptoms:

burning feet, allodynia, diminished pain and/or temperature sensation, dry eyes or mouth, orthostatic dizziness, bowel disturbances (constipation/diarrhea/gastroparesis), urinary disturbances, sweat changes (hyper-/hypohidrosis), accommodation problems and/or blurred vision, impotence, diminished ejaculation or lubrication, hot flashes, and palpitations. Exclusion criteria were symptoms or signs of large nerve fiber involvement (muscle weakness, loss of vibration sense, hypo-/areflexia), abnormal NCS, and history or detection after screening of illnesses known to cause SFN, including diabetes mellitus, impaired glucose tolerance, hyperlipidemia, liver, kidney, or thyroid dysfunction, monoclonal gammopathy, connective tissue disorders, sarcoidosis, Sjogren syndrome, amyloidosis, Fabry disease (alpha-galactosidase, in females combined with GLA gene sequencing), celiac disease, HIV, alcohol abuse, hemochromatosis, antiphospholipid syndrome, B6 intoxication, and neurotoxic drugs (e.g., chemotherapy). Patients were not screened for mutations associated with hereditary sensory and autonomic neuropathy, which usually has an early onset and clinical characteristics[19] that are different from those seen in our cohort of patients with I-SFN, or for antibodies to peripherin, which have recently been associated with small fiber neuropathy.[20]

Final Patient Selection, Biopsy, and QST Confirmation of SFN

Of 248 patients initially screened following referral with a suspected clinical diagnosis of SFN, 44 patients met inclusion/exclusion criteria and underwent skin biopsy and QST. From this group, 28 met strict criteria for I-SFN (i.e., reduced IENFD and abnormal QST compared to normative values). *SCN9A* gene analysis was carried out in all 28 patients with biopsy-confirmed I-SFN. The current study describes 8 patients, from this group of 28 patients with I-SFN, who were found to carry a mutation in the *SCN9A* gene (figure 1).

Clinical Characterization

Skin Biopsy Punch biopsy (10cm above lateral malleolus) specimens were fixed (2% paraformaldehyde-lysine-sodium periodate at 4°C), cryoprotected, and stored at −80°C in cryoprotective solution (20% glycerol) before sectioning (50μm).[21] The numbers of individual nerve fibers crossing the dermal–epidermal junctions

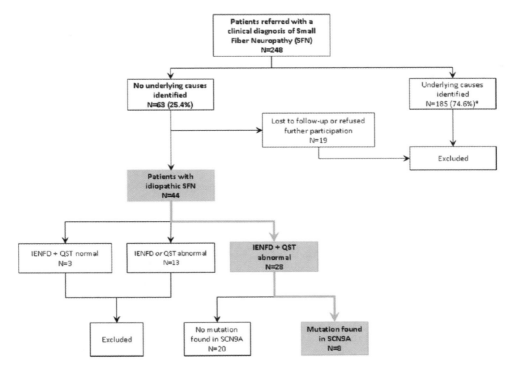

Figure 1
*Causes identified for SFN: sarcoidosis, n=150; medication, n=9; hemochromatosis, n=5; diabetes mellitus, n=4; thyroid dysfunction, n=4; alcohol abuse, n=4; gammopathy related, n=3; hypercholesterolemia, n=2; vitamin B6 intoxication, n=1; Lyme disease, n=1, Wegener granulomatosis, n=1; antiphospholipid syndrome, n=1. The Maastricht University Medical Hospital is a referral center for sarcoidosis in the Netherlands. IENFD, intraepidermal nerve fiber density; QST, quantitative sensory testing.

were analyzed in each of 3 sections, immunostained with polyclonal rabbit antiprotein gene product-9.5 antibody (Ultraclone; Wellow, Isle-of-Wight, UK), by bright field microscopy using a stereology workstation (Olympus [Tokyo, Japan] BX50, PlanApo oil-objective ×40/numerical aperture (NA)=1.0). Linear quantification of intraepidermal nerve fiber density was compared with available age- and gender-adjusted normative values.[22]

QST   QST, performed in accordance with previous guidelines,[23] using a TSA-2001 (Medoc, Ramat-Yishai, Israel) instrument, assessed thresholds at the dorsum of both feet and thenar eminences, using ascending/descending (warm/cool) thermal ramp stimuli delivered

through a thermode.[24] Heat pain modality was also examined. Results were compared with reported normative values.[25] Measurements were considered abnormal when Z values exceeded 2.5. A sensory modality was classified as abnormal if results of both method of limits and method of levels were abnormal.[26]

SFN Symptom Inventory Questionnaire   The validated SFN Symptom Inventory Questionnaire (SIQ) includes 13 questions (sweating abnormalities, sudden diarrhea, constipation, urination problems (e.g., incontinence), dry eyes and/or mouth, orthostatic dizziness, palpitations, hot flashes, skin sensitivity of legs, burning feet, sheet intolerance, and restless legs; each having 4 response options: 0=never, 1=sometimes,

$2 = \text{often}$, $3 = \text{always}$) derived from the SIQ[22] and a composite autonomic symptoms scale.[27]

Neuropathic Pain Scale/Visual Analogue Pain Scale

The Neuropathic Pain Scale (NPS) was used to assess neuropathic pain, each of 10 qualities being scored from 0 (no pain) to 10 (most intense pain imaginable).[28] The Visual Analogue Pain Scale (VAS) ranges from 0 (no pain) to 100 (most severe pain).[29]

SCN9A Mutation Analysis

Exon Screening   Genomic DNA was extracted from 300μL whole blood using the Puregene genomic DNA isolation kit (Gentra-Systems, Minneapolis, MN). All coding exons and flanking intronic sequences, and exons encoding 5′ and 3′-untranslated sequences within the complementary DNA, were amplified and sequenced as described previously.[30] Genomic sequences were compared with reference $Na_V1.7$ cDNA (NM_002977.3) to identify sequence variations,[31] using Alamut Mutation-Interpretation Software (Interactive-Biosoftware, Rouen, France). A control panel of DNA from 100 healthy Dutch (Caucasian) individuals (200 chromosomes) was screened for all new mutations.

Functional Analysis

Previous studies have demonstrated the importance of profiling the effects of $Na_V1.7$ mutations on channel function (voltage clamp), and on DRG neuron firing properties (current clamp).[15,32] This multimodal analysis of 7 mutations was carried out by 5 electrophysiologists using previously published voltage clamp and current clamp methods in HEK293 cells[16] and DRG neurons,[33,34] transfected with $Na_V1.7$ wild-type (WT) or mutant channels as described previously.[34] To minimize inherent culture to culture variation and to overcome the possibility of error introduced by pooling the results of experiments on DRG neurons harvested from multiple animals and cultured over many months, each mutant was compared with contemporaneous controls (WT $Na_V1.7$ expressed in cultures of cells prepared, transfected, and recorded under identical conditions by the same electrophysiologist).[15] Previous studies have demonstrated that some $Na_V1.7$ mutations do not produce biophysical changes after expression within heterologous systems such as HEK293 cells, but do produce functional changes after expression in DRG neurons, where voltage clamp is more difficult to achieve due to neurite outgrowth,

but the channels are expressed in a native cell background.[33,34] Voltage clamp analysis was therefore carried out after transfection into HEK293 cells together with β-1 and β-2 subunits[16] or, if biophysical changes were not detected in this cell background, within adult small (<30μm diameter) DRG neurons.[33,34] If changes were not found in activation, fast inactivation, slow inactivation, or ramp current, the proportion of cells producing resurgent current, which has been found to be enhanced by some $Na_V1.7$ mutations[35] and the amplitude of resurgent current, was assessed as previously described.[35] Current clamp analysis was carried out after transfection into DRG neurons.[33,34]

Study Design

The study was approved by medical ethical committees at Yale University and Maastricht University Medical Center. All aspects of the study were explained and written informed consent obtained prior to study. After examination, patients completed the SFN-SIQ, NPS, and VAS in random order. The study was performed between December 2008 and March 2011. Normative values of IENFD were obtained in an earlier study.[22]

Data Analysis

Clinical characteristics are descriptively presented. Electrophysiological data were analyzed using PulseFit 8.74 (HEKA Electronics, Lambrecht, Germany) or Clamp-Fit (Molecular Devices, Sunnyvale, CA) and Origin 8.1 (Microcal, Northampton, MA), and presented as means ± standard error. Statistical significance was determined by unpaired Student t tests (voltage clamp except resurgent currents; current clamp except firing frequency and spontaneous activity), Mann-Whitney test (firing frequency), or 2-proportion z test (comparison of proportion of cells producing resurgent currents or spontaneous activity).

Results

Patient Selection and *SCN9A* Analysis

Of 248 Dutch patients referred with a suspected clinical diagnosis of SFN and screened, underlying causes were identified in 185 patients. Nineteen patients were lost to follow-up or refused participation. Forty-four patients met inclusion/

exclusion criteria and underwent skin biopsy and QST. From this group, 28 Dutch Caucasian patients met strict criteria for I-SFN (i.e., reduced IENFD compared with age- and gender-adjusted normative values,[22] plus abnormal QST and no apparent cause) and underwent *SCN9A* gene analysis (see figure 1 and supplementary figure).

Eight (28.6%) of these 28 patients with biopsy-confirmed I-SFN had mutations in *SCN9A* (table 1, and figure 2). In each case, the mutation was missense (c.554G>A, p.R185H, in 2 unrelated patients; c.1867G>A, p.D623N; c.2215A>G, p.I739V; c.2159 T>A, p.I720K; c.4596G>A, p.M1532I; c.2794A>C, p.M932L + c.2971G>T, p.V991L; c.684C>G, p.I228M), and the patient was heterozygous for the mutation. None of these mutations was found in a control panel (DNA from 100 healthy Caucasian Dutch individuals; 200 chromosomes).

Clinical characteristics of the 8 patients with *SCN9A* mutations (table 2) were similar to those of the 20 patients without *SCN9A* mutations Here, we describe these 8 patients with I-SFN and *SCN9*A mutations.

General Characteristics

Mean age of these 8 patients with *SCN9A* mutations was 32.4 (standard deviation [SD], 20.7; median, 23.5; range, 14–68 years; 4 females/4 males). Mean duration of symptoms was 14.5 (SD, 16; range, 1–37) years. Three patients reported similar complaints in family members, but detailed information was not available; family history was unremarkable in 5 patients (see table 1). Mean age of the 20 patients without *SCN9A* mutations was 42.7 (SD, 15.4; median, 44; range, 7–67 years; 11 females/9 males).

Clinical Features

Pain All 8 patients complained of pain. Six (patients 1–5, 8) had VAS scores >50, and 5 (patients 2–6) had scores of >5 on at least 7 of the 10 NPS questions, indicating severe pain. Intensity and quality of pain tended to vary from patient to patient. Pain intensity and quality for the 2 patients (patients 1, 2) carrying the c.554G>A, p.R185H mutation were different from each other. Patient 1 reported less pain compared to patient 2.

Pain began in the distal extremities (feet > hands) in most patients. However, patients 3

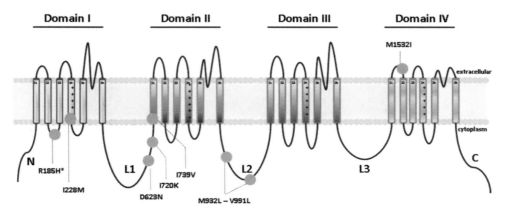

Figure 2
Schematic sodium channel showing the locations of the Na$_V$1.7 mutations found in patients with idiopathic small nerve fiber neuropathy. Mutation R185H was found in 2 patients.

Table 1
Clinical Description of Patients with Small Nerve Fiber Neuropathy and *SCN9A* Mutations

Patient	Age at Referral, yr/ Gender	Age at Onset Symptoms, yr	Initial Symptom(s)+ Location	Later Symptoms	Aggravated by Warmth/ Relieved by Cold	Family History	Medication	IENFD (corresponding normative value)	QST Impaired Modality		*SCN9A* Mutation
									Thenar	Foot	
1	54/M	24	Pain and paresthesias, feet and hand	52 years: burning feet, "electrical current" in soles, and redness feet; ↑ with exercise and interfered with walking	No/no	Brother* similar complaints; grandfather (deceased) painless burns and difficulty walking	No effect, pregabalin and amytriptyline	1.0/mm (≥3.2/ mm)	Warmth-R, cold-R, warmth-L, cold-L	Warmth-R, cold-R, heat pain-R, warmth-L, cold-L, heat pain-L	c.554G> A(R185H)
2	24/F	23	Tingling feet, lower legs, and hands	2 months later: continuous severe pain in feet; occasionally: dry mouth and orthostatic dizziness	No/no	Father similar complaints	No relief from acetaminophen, anticonvulsants, antidepressants, mexiletine, opioids	4.9/mm (≥6.7/ mm)	Warmth-L, cold-L	Warmth-R, cold-R, warmth-L, cold-L	c.554G> A(R185H)
3	63/F	22	Painful muscles persisting to present	58 years y.o.: severe burning pain, initially soles, later feet/ hands; 61 y.o.: patchy skin redness, dry eyes, dry mouth, orthostatic dizziness; 62 y.o.: tenderness and burning of scalp, burning pain of lips, mouth, and trunk	Yes/no	Sister (78 y.o.) similar complaints	Some relief from pregabalin and duloxetine	2.8/mm (≥3.3/ mm)	—	Cold-R, cold-L	c.1867G> A(D623N)

Table 1 (countined)

Patient	Age at Referral, yr/ Gender	Age at Onset Symptoms, yr	Initial Symptom(s) + Location	Later Symptoms	Aggravated by Warmth/ Relieved by Cold	Family History	Medication	IENFD (corresponding normative value)	QST Impaired Modality Thenar	Foot	SCN9A Mutation
4	51/F	14	Burning pain, hot flashes, and itching of face, lower legs, and feet	Complaints ↑ with exercise, ↓ by cooling; dry mouth, dry eyes, blurred vision, orthostatic dizziness, alternating constipation/ diarrhea, hyperhidrosis, palpitations, episodic swallowing difficulties; redness of hands; 49 y.o.: joint and muscle pain	Yes/yes	Father (deceased), sister* and 2 sons, similar complaints	Slight relief from amytriptyline	3.4/mm (≥4.1/ mm)	Warmth-L	Warmth-L, cold-L	c.2215A> G(I739V)
5	39/M	37	Stabbing pain in the whole body	2 months later: burning pain in feet/lower legs followed by lower arms; numbness in feet bilaterally; hyperhidrosis in feet, dry mouth, episodic diarrhea, blurred vision	No/no	Unremarkable	No effect from pregabalin	4.5/mm (≥4.7/ mm)	Warmth-L	Warmth-R, warmth-L	c.2 159T> A(I720K)
6	70/F	68	Stabbing pain and redness in the feet, slowly extending to lower legs, hands, and lower arms	Symptoms restrict daily activities; dry eyes and orthostatic dizziness	No/no	Unremarkable	No effect from pregabalin	2.3/mm (≥2.7/ mm)	Warmth-R, warmth-L	Cold-R, cold-L	c.4596G> A(M1532I)

Table 1 (continued)

Patient	Age at Referral, yr/ Gender	Age at Onset Symptoms, yr	Initial Symptom(s) + Location	Later Symptoms	Aggravated by Warmth/ Relieved by Cold	Family History	Medication	IENFD (corresponding normative value)	QST Impaired Modality		SCN9A Mutation
									Thenar	Foot	
7	22/M	16	Burning pain of feet and lower legs	Complaints ↑ with exercise and interfered with standing; orthostatic dizziness, dry mouth, dry eyes, constipation; sought psychiatric treatment for these symptoms	Yes/no	Unremarkable	No relief with gabapentin	4.0/mm (≥5.4/ mm)	—	Warmth-L	c.2794A> CM932L and c.2971G> T(V991L)
8	51/M	32	Excruciating pain in teeth and jaw triggered by cold + heat, sometimes radiating to temporomandib- ular joint; also, pain behind the eyes	Multiple tooth extractions did not provide pain relief; myalgia triggered by exercise, persisting 5–6 days; pain ↑ by cold and ↓ by warmth (better in summer); occasional swollen feet; for 35 years: stomach cramps and diarrhea; for several years: dry mouth, dry eyes, reduced urinary sensation, and intermittent hesitation	No/no	Sister with rheumatoid arthritis had burning hands	Pain bearable with acetaminophen; no relief antidepressants, NSAIDs	1.6/mm (≥3.2/ mm)	—	Warmth-R, cold-R	c.684C> G(I228M)

The obtained QST scores were compared with the reported normative values by Yarnitsky and Sprecher.[25] A sensory modality was classified as abnormal if the results of both method of limits and method of levels were abnormal.
↓ = reduced; ↑ = increase; * = refused participation; F = female; IENFD = intraepidermal nerve fiber density; L = left; M = male; NSAID = nonsteroidal anti-inflammatory drug; QST = quantita- tive sensory testing; R = right; y.o. = years old.

(c.1867G>A, p.D623N) and 5(c.2159T>A, p.I720K) initially experienced pain throughout the body with muscle ache, before developing distal pain. Pain was aggravated by warmth in 3 of the 8 patients, but not in the other 5. Cooling relieved pain in 1 patient, but not in the other 7. Patient 8 (c.684C>G, p.I228M) initially experienced excruciating pain in the teeth/jaw triggered by cold and heat, and pain behind both eyes, not relieved by multiple tooth extractions. He subsequently developed myalgia, aggravated by cold and relieved by warmth, which could persist for 5 to 6 days after light physical activity, and intermittent foot swelling, and was unable to work.

Autonomic Dysfunction Seven of the 8 patients reported autonomic complaints. In 5 patients, 6 or more of the 9 SFN-SIQ autonomic complaints were present. Orthostatic dizziness, palpitations, dry eyes, and dry mouth were more common (see table 2). Autonomic complaints were most prominent in patients 4 (c.2215A>G, p.I739V) and 8 (c.684C>G, p.I228M) (see table 1). Patient 4 experienced dry mouth/eyes, blurred vision, orthostatic dizziness, alternating constipation/diarrhea, hyperhidrosis, palpitations, hot flashes, and swallowing difficulties, followed by widespread joint/muscle pain. Patient 8 had a 35-year history of stomach cramps/diarrhea, and dry mouth/eyes and reduced urinary sensation/ hesitation for several years.

Autonomic symptoms were absent in 1, and much less prominent in the second, of the 2 patients with R185H mutation (see table 2).

IENFD and QST Findings

There was a decrease in IENFD below the 5th percentile for age- and sex-matched controls[22] in all 8 patients with *SCN9A* mutations (see table 1). Supplementary figure 1 shows the IENFD findings in patient 8 juxtaposed to an age- and gender-matched control subject.

On QST, 5 patients displayed abnormal warm and cold sensation, 1 patient displayed abnormal warm sensation, and 2 displayed abnormal cold sensation. One patient displayed reduced heat pain (see table 1). More abnormalities were seen in the foot (21 of 48 sensory qualities tested, 43.8%) compared with the hand (10 of 48, 20.8%).

Functional Characterization of Na$_V$1.7 Mutations

Voltage clamp analysis of the mutant channels from patients with I-SFN showed that they were all gain of function, and that they impaired slow inactivation (p.I720K, p.M1532I, p.I228M, p.I739V), depolarized slow and fast inactivation (p.D623N), or enhanced resurgent currents (p.M932L/V991L, p.R185H). None of these mutations exhibited the hyperpolarized activation or enhanced ramp currents characteristic of IEM[15] or the incomplete fast inactivation characteristic of PEPD[17] mutations of Na$_V$1.7. Current clamp analysis demonstrated that all 7 mutations rendered DRG neurons hyperexcitable. Here we present the functional profiling of 3 representative mutant channels from patients with I-SFN. Functional profiling of the other 4 mutations yielded similar results (unpublished results).

I720K: Impaired Slow Inactivation and DRG Neuron Hyperexcitability

Voltage clamp analysis of I720K mutant channels following expression in HEK293 cells demonstrated impaired slow inactivation (figure 3C). Current densities (WT: 375±68pA/pF, n=18; I720K: 228±35pA/pF, n=22), activation V$_{1/2}$ (V$_{1/2}$ represents voltage midpoint) (WT: −26.6±1.6mV, n=12; I720K: −25.8±0.9mV, n=13), fast inactivation V$_{1/2}$ (WT: −80.4±1.5mV, n=13; I720K: −79.1±1.1mV, n=13), and ramp currents (WT: 0.8±0.2%, n=9; I720K: 0.7±0.1%, n=10) for HEK293 cells transfected with WT or I720K were not significantly different. Slow inactivation was impaired for I720K mutant channels,

Table 2
SFN Symptoms Inventory Questionnaire Findings in Patients with *SCN9A* Novel Mutations

Patient	Mutation	Sweating	Diarrhea	Constipation	Micturation Problems	Dry Eyes	Dry Mouth	Orthostatic Dizziness	Palpitations	Hot Flashes	Skin Hyperesthesia	Burning Feet	Sheet Intolerance	Restless Legs
1	R185H	0[a]	0[a]	0[a]	0[a]	0[a]	0[a]	0[a]	0[a]	0[a]	1[b]	2[b]	3[b]	3[b]
2	R185H	0[a]	0[a]	0[a]	0[a]	0[a]	1[b]	1[b]	0[a]	0[a]	3[b]	3[b]	2[b]	2[b]
3	D623N	0[a]	1[b]	1[b]	0[a]	1[b]	2[b]	2[b]	2[b]	0[a]	2[b]	2[b]	2[b]	2[b]
4	I739V	3[b]	2[b]	1[b]	2[b]	2[b]	3[b]	1[b]	1[b]	3[b]	2[b]	2[b]	2[b]	2[b]
5	I720K	3[b]	1[b]	0[a]	1[b]	1[b]	2[b]	0[a]	0[a]	1[b]	2[b]	1[b]	1[b]	1[b]
6	M1532I	0[a]	0[a]	0[a]	0[a]	1[b]	0[a]	1[b]	1[b]	0[a]	3[b]	3[b]	1[b]	3[b]
7	M932L+ V991L	1[b]	0[a]	2[b]	1[b]	1[b]	1[b]	0[a]	1[b]	1[b]	1[b]	2[b]	0[a]	0[a]
8	I228M	1[b]	3[b]	1[b]	2[b]	2[b]	3[b]	1[b]	1[b]	2[b]	2[b]	2[b]	1[b]	1[b]

[a] Absence (score 0) of corresponding SFN-related symptom.
[b] Presence of SFN-related symptom, with variable intensity (score 1 = sometimes present; score 2 = often; score 3 = always present). SFN = small nerve fiber neuropathy.

with a depolarized $V_{1/2}$ (WT: -73.2 ± 2.4mV, n=6; I720K: -64.4 ± 1.5mV, n=7; $p < 0.05$; see figure 3C). Impaired slow inactivation increases the number of channels available for activation at potentials positive to -100 mV, including potentials close to resting potential of DRG neurons.

The I720K mutation had clear functional effects on DRG neurons, which were rendered hyperexcitable by the mutant channels (see figure 3). I720K produced a depolarizing shift in resting membrane potential (WT: -55.8 ± 1.7mV, n=26; I720K: -48.7 ± 1.9mV, n=29; $p < 0.05$). I720K increased excitability of DRG neurons, with a 43% reduction in current threshold to 500-millisecond stimuli (WT: 237 ± 28pA, n=26; I720K: 134 ± 30pA, n=29; $p < 0.05$). I720K significantly increased the number of action potentials evoked by 500-millisecond depolarizing stimuli at all intensities tested, from 100 to 600pA. I720K produced a trend toward an increase in the proportion of spontaneously firing cells (9 of 38 [24%] vs 2 of 28 [7%] for cells transfected with WT channels) that did not reach statistical significance ($p=0.075$); mean frequency of spontaneous activity in cells transfected with I720K was 2.6 ± 0.5Hz (n=9), with 4 of 9 spontaneously firing cells showing continuous firing at a frequency of >1Hz throughout the 30-second recording period.

D623N: Impaired Fast and Slow Inactivation and DRG Neuron Hyperexcitability

D623N mutant channels did not display gating abnormalities following expression in HEK293 cells but, when assessed by voltage clamp after expression in DRG neurons, demonstrated impaired fast inactivation and slow inactivation (figure 4A–C). Current densities (WT: 407 ± 90pA, n=12; D623N: 474 ± 121pA, n=10), activation $V_{1/2}$ (WT: -26.9 ± 2.0mV, n=12; D623N: -26.4 ± 2.3mV, n=10), and ramp currents (WT: 2.6 ± 0.4%, n=15; D623N: 2.1 ± 0.3%, n=17) were not significantly different. The $V_{1/2}$ of fast

inactivation (WT: -76.7 ± 1.4mV, n=13; D623N: -72.2 ± 1.2mV, n=13; $p < 0.05$) and slow inactivation (WT: -69.6 ± 1.4mV, n=12; D623N: -64.3 ± 2.0mV, n=11; $p < 0.05$) were depolarized for D623N mutant channels (see figure 4B, C). Impaired fast inactivation and slow inactivation increase the number of channels available for activation.

Current clamp recording showed that D623N mutant channels rendered DRG neurons hyperexcitable and produced aberrant spontaneous firing in 25% of neurons (see figure 4). D623N produced a depolarizing shift in resting membrane potential (WT: -55.0 ± 1.5mV, n=29; D623N: -45.5 ± 1.5mV, n=27; $p < 0.01$) and a 51% reduction in current threshold to 200-millisecond stimuli (WT: 256 ± 28pA, n=29; D623N: 125 ± 19pA, n=27; $p < 0.01$). D623N significantly increased the number of action potentials evoked by 500-millisecond depolarizing stimuli ranging from 100 to 275pA. D623N produced an increase in the proportion of spontaneously firing cells (9 of 36 [25%] for DRG neurons transfected with this mutant channel; 1 of 30 [3%] for cells transfected with WT channels, $p < 0.05$). Mean frequency of spontaneous activity in cells transfected with D623N was 2.4 ± 0.6Hz (n=9); 4 of 9 spontaneously firing cells showed continuous firing at a frequency of >1Hz throughout the 30-second recording period.

M932L/V991L: Increased Resurgent Currents and DRG Neuron Hyperexcitability

M932L/V991L mutant channels, assessed by voltage clamp after expression in DRG neurons (figure 5A–D), enhanced the generation of resurgent currents. Voltage clamp analysis of M932L/V991L mutant channels, both in HEK293 cells and DRG neurons, did not reveal a significant effect of the mutation on activation, fast inactivation, slow inactivation, ramp currents, or deactivation. Current densities (WT: 440 ± 49pA/pF,

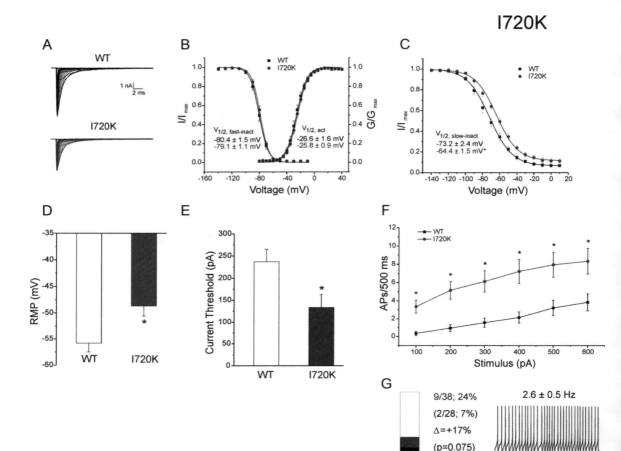

I720K

Figure 3

Electrophysiological analysis of I720K mutation. (A) Representative current traces recorded from HEK 293 cells expressing wild type (WT) (top) or I720K (bottom), evoked by voltage steps (100 milliseconds) from −80 to 40mV in 5mV increments, from a holding potential of −120mV. (B) Activation and steady state fast inactivation for WT (black squares) and I720K (red circles). Fast inactivation was examined using a series of 500-millisecond prepulses from −140 to −10mV followed by test pulses to −10mV. Left inset: midpoint values for fast inactivation ($V_{1/2, fast-inact}$) of WT (black) and I720K (red). Right inset: midpoint values for activation ($V_{1/2, act}$) of WT (black) and I720K (red). (C) Steady state slow inactivation of WT (black squares) and I720K (red circles). Slow inactivation was assessed using a 20-millisecond pulse to −10mV after a 30-second prepulse to potentials from −140 to 10mV followed by a 100-millisecond pulse to −120mV to remove fast inactivation. Inset: midpoint values of slow inactivation ($V_{1/2, slow-inact}$) (WT: black; I720K: red); *$p < 0.05$. (D) Resting membrane potential (RMP) of dorsal root ganglion (DRG) neurons expressing WT (255.8 ± 1.7, n = 26) or I720K (248.7 ± 1.9, n = 29); *$p < 0.05$. (E) Current threshold of DRG neurons expressing WT (237 ± 28, n = 26) or I720K (134 ± 30, n = 29) to 500-millisecond stimuli; $p < 0.05$. (F) Comparison of mean firing frequency in DRG neurons expressing WT and I720K across a range of current injections from 100 to 600pA; *$p < 0.05$. (G) Bar graph showing the proportion of spontaneous firing cells for DRG neurons expressing I720K (red) and WT channels (black); numbers to the right of the bar graph show mean values for WT (lower value in parentheses) and I720K (upper value). The recording on the right shows spontaneous firing (10 seconds) of representative DRG neuron expressing I720K; the numbers above the trace show average±standard deviation frequency of spontaneous action potentials. $V_{1/2}$ represents voltage midpoint, I/I represents normalized current, and G/G represents normalized conductance for fast-activation, slow-inactivation, and activation. APs, action potentials.

D623N

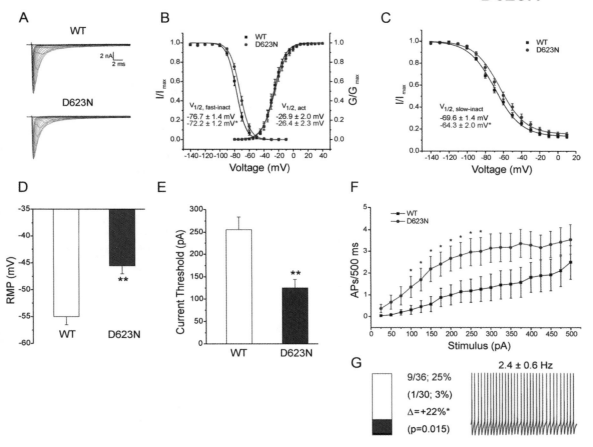

Figure 4

Electrophysiological analysis of D623N mutation. (A) Representative current traces recorded from dorsal root ganglion (DRG) neurons expressing wild type (WT) (top) or D623N (bottom), evoked by voltage steps (100 milliseconds) from −80 to 40mV in 5mV increments, from a holding potential of −100mV. (B) Activation and steady state fast inactivation for WT (black squares) and D623N (red circles). Fast inactivation was examined using a series of 500-millisecond prepulses from −140 to −10mV followed by test pulses to −10mV. Left inset: midpoint values for fast inactivation ($V_{1/2,\ \text{fast-inact}}$) of WT (black) and D623N (red). Right inset: midpoint values for activation ($V_{1/2,\ \text{act}}$) of WT (black) and D623N (red). (C) Steady state slow inactivation of WT (black squares) and D623N (red circles). Slow inactivation was assessed using a 20-millisecond pulse to −10mV after a 30-second prepulse to potentials from −140 to 10mV followed by a 100-millisecond pulse to −120mV to remove fast inactivation. Inset: midpoint values of slow inactivation ($V_{1/2,\ \text{slow-inact}}$) (WT: black; D623N: red); *$p < 0.05$. (D) Resting membrane potential (RMP) of DRG neurons expressing WT (255.0 ± 1.5, n = 29) or D623N (245.5 ± 1.5, n = 27); **$p < 0.01$. (E) Current threshold of DRG neurons expressing WT (256 ± 28, n = 29) or D623N (125 ± 19, n = 27) to 200-millisecond stimuli; **$p < 0.01$. (F) Comparison of mean firing frequency in DRG neurons expressing WT and D623N across a range of current injections from 25 to 500pA; *$p < 0.05$. (G) Bar graph showing the proportion of spontaneous firing cells for DRG neurons expressing D623N (red) and WT channels (black); numbers to the right of the bar graph show mean values for WT (lower value in parentheses) and D623N (upper value); *$p < 0.05$. The recording on the right shows spontaneous firing (10 seconds) of representative DRG neuron expressing D623N; the numbers above the trace show the average ± standard deviation frequency of spontaneous action potentials. $V_{1/2}$ represents voltage midpoint, I/I represents normalized current, and G/G represents normalized conductance for fast-activation, slow-inactivation, and activation. APs, action potentials.

n=32; M932L/ V991L: 541±86pA/pF, n=23), activation $V_{1/2}$ (WT: −20.2±0.6mV, n=16; M932L/V991L: −20.4±1.2mV, n=11), fast inactivation $V_{1/2}$ (WT: −68.5±0.6mV, n=26; M932L/V991L: −68.5±0.6mV, n=17), slow inactivation $V_{1/2}$ (WT: −66.1±1.0mV, n=24; M932L/V991L: −63.8±1.7mV, n=16), ramp currents (WT: 1.61±0.16%, n=19; M932L/V991L: 1.85±0.27%, n=14), and deactivation (no significant differences in deactivation measured between −100 and −50mV at 5mV intervals) for DRG neurons transfected with WT and M932L/V991L were not significantly different. However, a higher percentage of DRG neurons expressing M932L/V991L (5 of 10 cells, 50%; $p<0.05$) compared to cells expressing WT channels (1 of 11 cells, 9%; see figure 5D) produced resurgent currents, a change that would be expected to produce repetitive firing.

Current clamp recording showed that M932L/V991L mutant channels made DRG neurons hyperexcitable. Mean resting potential was significantly depolarized (WT: −56.9±1.9mV, n=20; M932L/V991L: −49.8±1.6mV, n=23, $p<0.01$), and threshold was significantly decreased (WT: 250±23pA, n=20; M932L/V991L: 145±22pA, n=23, $p<0.01$) in DRG neurons expressing M932L/V991L (see figure 5). The number of action potentials evoked by 500-millisecond depolarizing stimuli was increased at all stimulus strengths between 50 and 300pA for cells expressing M932L/V991L channels, compared to cells expressing WT. M932L/V991L produced a trend toward an increase in the proportion of spontaneously firing cells (4 of 27 [15%] vs 0 of 20 [0%] for cells transfected with WT channels) that did not reach statistical significance ($p=0.072$); mean frequency of spontaneous activity in cells transfected with M932L/V991L was 2.0±0.3Hz, with all 4 spontaneously firing cells showing continuous firing at a mean frequency of >1Hz throughout the 30-second recording period.

Discussion

Despite careful clinical assessment, an underlying cause cannot be found in a substantial number (24 to >90% in different series) of patients with SFN.[5,6,9] In this study we show, in 8 of 28 (28.6%) patients with skin biopsy- and QST-confirmed I-SFN, missense mutations in the SCN9A gene, which encodes a voltage-gated sodium channel, $Na_V1.7$, that is present within small peripheral nerve fibers. Electrophysiological analysis demonstrated gain of function changes in the mutant channels and showed that the mutations share the common feature of rendering DRG neurons hyperexcitable.

Our findings of gain of function mutations of $Na_V1.7$ in 28.6% of patients with I-SFN are based on an analysis of 28 Dutch Caucasian patients who met criteria that included no history or detection on screening of disorders known to cause SFN, and confirmation of the diagnosis of SFN by abnormal QST, and by reduced IENFD on skin biopsy. These patients were derived from a larger group of 248 patients referred with a clinical diagnosis of SFN for evaluation at an academic medical center. Aside from any selection bias inherent in referral to an academic medical center, and from any bias introduced by our inclusion/exclusion criteria, which yielded a study cohort of 28 patients meeting stringent criteria for I-SFN, we believe that our sample may be representative of the general Dutch Caucasian population of patients with SFN. Although there were no other distinguishing clinical characteristics, age of onset of symptoms was younger (although not statistically significant) for patients with SCN9A mutations than for patients without SCN9A mutations.

Mutations in the SCN9A gene have been previously linked to IEM, a rare inherited disorder characterized by distal burning pain,[15] and PEPD, characterized by perineal, periocular, and perimandibular pain.[17] Some of our patients with SFN also reported burning

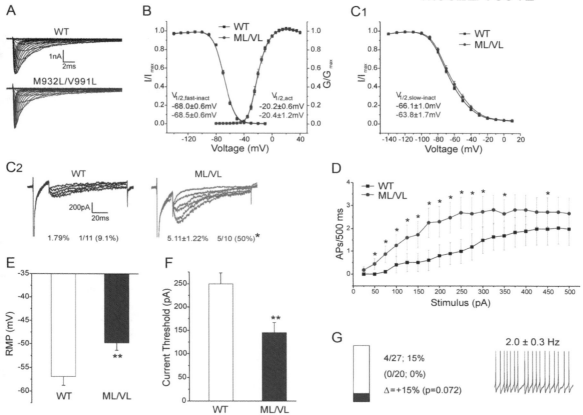

Figure 5

Electrophysiological analysis of M932L/V991L mutation. (A) Representative current traces recorded from dorsal root ganglion (DRG) neurons expressing wild type (WT) (top) or M932L/ V991L (bottom) (unless otherwise noted, protocols are the same as in figures 3 and 4). (B) Activation and steady state fast inactivation for WT (black squares) and M932L/V991L (ML/VL; red circles). Inset shows midpoint values for fast inactivation ($V_{1/2, \text{fast-inact}}$) and activation ($V_{1/2, \text{act}}$) of WT (black) and M932L/ V991L (red), respectively. (C) Steady state slow inactivation of WT (black squares) and M932L/V991L (red circles). Inset: midpoint values of slow-inactivation ($V_{1/2, \text{slow-inact}}$) (WT: black; M932L/V991L: red). (D) Resurgent currents recorded from DRG neurons expressing WT (left) or M932L/V991L (right). Resurgent currents were assessed with a 2-step protocol that initially depolarized the membrane to +30mV for 20 milliseconds before testing for resurgent sodium currents by hyperpolarizing the membrane potential in 25mV increments from 0 to −80mV for 100 milliseconds, then returning to the holding potential of −100mV. Current amplitude (normalized to peak current evoked by a +30mV depolarization) (left) and proportion of cells producing resurgent current (right) are shown below traces; *$p < 0.05$. (E) Resting membrane potential (RMP) of DRG neurons expressing WT (256.9 ± 1.9mV, n=20) or M932L/V991L (249.8 ± 1.6mV, n=23); **$p < 0.01$. (F) Current threshold of DRG neurons expressing WT (250 ± 23pA, n=20) or M932L/V991L (145 ± 22pA, n=23) to 200-millisecond stimuli; **$p < 0.01$. (G) Comparison of mean firing frequencies of DRG neurons expressing WT and M932L/V991L across the range of current injections from 25 to 500pA; *$p < 0.05$. (H) Bar graph showing the proportion of spontaneous firing cells for DRG neurons expressing M932L/V991L (red); numbers to the right of the bar graph show mean values for WT (lower value in parentheses) and M932L/ V991L (upper value); $p = 0.072$. The recording on the right shows spontaneous firing (10 seconds) of representative DRG neuron expressing M932L/V991L; the numbers above the trace show average ± standard deviation frequency of spontaneous action potentials. $V_{1/2}$ represents voltage midpoint, I/I represents normalized current, and G/G represents normalized conductance for fast-activation, slow-inactivation, and activation. APs, action potentials.

feet and hands, or pain around the eyes and jaw. However, despite this apparent similarity, our patients exhibited clinical characteristics typical for small fiber neuropathy[1-6] and differed from patients with prototypical IEM and PEPD in multiple ways: (1) Autonomic dysfunction is common in SFN, and severe autonomic symptoms were seen in almost all of our patients. Except for skin reddening, autonomic symptoms are not prominent in IEM.[15,36] (2) Location and onset of pain and related complaints were distributed throughout the body in our patients with I-SFN, whereas in IEM pain is mainly located in the distal extremities. In patient 3 (D623N), painful muscles from early childhood preceded distal complaints, whereas patient 5 (I1720K) experienced initial pain throughout the entire body, and patient 8 (I228M) initially experienced severe jaw pain. (3) Whereas IEM is characterized by erythema of the involved areas,[15] half of our patients did not display this sign. (4) Our patients did not display the aggravation of symptoms by warmth and relief by cold that are characteristic of IEM.[15,37] Five of our 8 patients denied aggravation by warmth, and 7 had no relief by cold. Patient 8 reported that cold increased symptoms and warmth relieved them. (5) The $Na_V1.7$ mutations that we profiled did not display the hyperpolarized activation and enhanced ramp responses characteristic of IEM mutations[15] or the incomplete fast inactivation[17] characteristic of PEPD mutations. The present results demonstrate that $Na_V1.7$ mutations, distinct from those that have been associated with IEM[15] and PEPD,[17] occur in a substantial proportion of patients with I-SFN.

$Na_V1.7$ is preferentially expressed within DRG and sympathetic ganglion neurons[11,12] and their axons, including small diameter ($<0.5\mu m$) intracutaneous axon terminals, where it is coexpressed with other sodium channel subtypes ($Na_V1.6/Na_V1.8/Na_V1.9$) and the sodium–calcium exchanger NCX.[13] $Na_V1.7$ channels modulate the excitability of these neurons by

opening and producing a Na^+ current in response to small depolarizations close to resting potential, thus bringing the neuron closer to the activation potential of other sodium channel isoforms.[14] The $Na_V1.7$ mutations that we found in patients with SFN impaired slow inactivation, depolarized fast and slow inactivation, or enhanced resurgent currents. Each of the mutations rendered DRG neurons hyperexcitable.

Sodium channel activity has been shown to trigger axonal degeneration via calcium-importing reverse sodium–calcium exchange in axons under conditions where the ability to extrude sodium is exceeded.[38,39] Degeneration of nonmyelinated axons has been described in hypoxic neuropathy,[40] and the distal pains reported by some of our patients are similar to the acral paresthesias that have been linked to low Na/K adenosine triphosphatase levels in peripheral nerves in chronic mountain sickness.[41] Although there is no reason to believe that the patients we have described suffered from systemic hypoxia, Na^+ influx is known to impose an energetic load on neurons and neuronal processes,[42] and increased activity of mutant $Na_V1.7$ channels would be expected to have an especially large effect on small diameter intracutaneous axons, where NCX is present,[13] due to their high surface to volume ratio and input resistance, low capacitance per unit length, and shorter wavelength.[43,44] Consistent with a role of sodium channels in I-SFN, action potential activity at physiological frequencies can sensitize axons to otherwise reversible metabolic insults, and can produce degeneration of these axons[45] that is attenuated by sodium channel blockers.[46]

In conclusion, we demonstrate the occurrence of missense mutations in the *SCN9A* gene encoding the $Na_V1.7$ sodium channel, in a substantial proportion (28.6%) of patients with biopsy- and QST-confirmed I-SFN, and show that these mutations render DRG neurons that give rise to small axons hyperexcitable. Expression of $Na_V1.7$ and NCX in small diameter axons may cause these fibers to degenerate in response to gain of function changes produced by Na$_V$1.7 mutations such as those described in this paper. Our results suggest that these mutations may predispose to the development of channelopathy-associated SFN. *SCN9A* gene analysis might be considered for patients with SFN in whom other causes are excluded, particularly patients with younger ages of onset. In terms of treatment, existing nonspecific sodium channel blockers, Na$_V$1.7-selective blockers when available, and inhibitors of NCX2 merit study as therapeutic approaches that might slow or halt axonal degeneration in I-SFN.

Acknowledgments

This work was supported in part by the Profileringsfonds of University Hospital Maastricht (C.G.F.), and by grants from the Rehabilitation Research Service and Medical Research Service, Department of Veterans Affairs (S.D.-H., S.G.W.) and Erythromelalgia Foundation (S.D.-H., S.G.W.). The Center for Neuroscience and Regeneration Research is a Collaboration of the Paralyzed Veterans of America with Yale University.

We thank D. M. L. Merckx, R. te Morsche, L. Tyrrell, L. Macala, P. Zhao, and P. Shah for dedicated assistance.

About the Authors

Catharina G. Faber, MD, PhD, Department of Neurology, University Medical Center Maastricht, Maastricht, the Netherlands

Janneke G. J. Hoeijmakers, MD, Department of Neurology, University Medical Center Maastricht, Maastricht, the Netherlands

Hye-Sook Ahn, PhD, Department of Neurology, Yale University School of Medicine, New Haven, CT; Center for Neuroscience and Regeneration Research, Veterans Affairs Medical Center, West Haven, CT

Xiaoyang Cheng, PhD, Department of Neurology, Yale University School of Medicine, New Haven, CT; Center for Neuroscience and Regeneration Research, Veterans Affairs Medical Center, West Haven, CT

Chongyang Han, PhD, Department of Neurology, Yale University School of Medicine, New Haven, CT; Center for Neuroscience and Regeneration Research, Veterans Affairs Medical Center, West Haven, CT

Jin-Sung Choi, PhD, Department of Neurology, Yale University School of Medicine, New Haven, CT; Center for Neuroscience and Regeneration Research, Veterans Affairs Medical Center, West Haven, CT

Mark Estacion, PhD, Department of Neurology, Yale University School of Medicine, New Haven, CT; Center for Neuroscience and Regeneration Research, Veterans Affairs Medical Center, West Haven, CT

Giuseppe Lauria, MD, PhD, Neuromuscular Diseases Unit, IRCCS Foundation, Carlo Besta, Milan, Italy

Els K. Vanhoutte, MD, Department of Neurology, University Medical Center Maastricht, Maastricht, the Netherlands

Monique M. Gerrits, PhD, Department of Clinical Genomics, University Medical Center Maastricht, Maastricht, the Netherlands

Sulayman Dib-Hajj, PhD, Department of Neurology, Yale University School of Medicine, New Haven, CT; Center for Neuroscience and Regeneration Research, Veterans Affairs Medical Center, West Haven, CT

Joost P. H. Drenth, MD, PhD, Department of Gastroenterology and Hepatology, Radboud University Nijmegen Medical Center, Nijmegen, the Netherlands

Stephen G. Waxman, MD, PhD, Department of Neurology, Yale University School of Medicine, New Haven, CT; Center for Neuroscience and Regeneration Research, Veterans Affairs Medical Center, West Haven, CT

Ingemar S. J. Merkies, MD, PhD, Department of Neurology, University Medical Center Maastricht, Maastricht, the Netherlands; Department of Neurology, Spaarne Hospital, Hoofddorp, the Netherlands

Authorship

C.G.F. and J.G.J.H. are first authors. S.G.W. and I.S.J.M are senior authors.

Potential Conflicts of Interest

C.G.F.: grants/grants pending, Prinses Beatrix Fonds. E.K.V.: grant, Baxter fellowship. S.D.-H.: consultancy, Regeneron Pharmaceuticals, Vertex Pharmaceuticals, Guidepoint Global; patent, sodium channel NaV1.9 (Yale holds); stock/stock options, Trans Molecular, Pfizer. S.G.W.: consultancy, Bristol Myers Squibb, Vertex Pharmaceuticals, ChromoCell, DaiNippon Sumitomo Pharm, Cardiome Pharm; grants/grants pending, Pfizer Research, Trans Molecular; patents, NaV1.9 sodium channel (Yale owns); stock/stock options, Trans Molecular. I.S.J.M.: travel support, Peripheral Nerve Society; board membership, steering committee member ICE trial that was published in 2008 plus steering committee member for CSL Behring CIDP study; grants/grants pending, GBS/CIDP International foundation grant for the PeriNomS study, Talents program grant for the PeriNomS study, Peripheral Nerve Society grant for the PeriNomS study.

References

1. Holland NR, Crawford TO, Hauer P, et al. 1998. Small-fiber sensory neuropathies: Clinical course and neuropathology of idiopathic cases. *Ann Neurol* 44: 47–59.

2. Gorson KC, Ropper AH. 1995. Idiopathic distal small fiber neuropathy. *Acta Neurol Scand* 92: 376–382.

3. Stewart JD, Low PA, Fealey RD. 1992. Distal small fiber neuropathy: Results of tests of sweating and autonomic cardiovascular reflexes. *Muscle Nerve* 15: 661–665.

4. Low PA. 1997. *Clinical autonomic disorders: Evaluation and management.* 2nd ed. Philadelphia, PA: Lippincott-Raven.

5. Lacomis D. 2002. Small-fiber neuropathy. *Muscle Nerve* 26: 173–188.

6. Devigili G, Tugnoli V, Penza P, et al. 2008. The diagnostic criteria for small fibre neuropathy: From symptoms to neuropathology. *Brain* 131: 1912–1925.

7. Tesfaye S, Boulton AJ, Dyck PJ, et al. 2010. Diabetic neuropathies: Update on definitions, diagnostic criteria, estimation of severity, and treatments. *Diabetes Care* 33: 2285–2293.

8. Lauria G. 2005. Small fibre neuropathies. *Curr Opin Neurol* 18: 591–597.

9. Bednarik J, Vlckova-Moravcova E, Bursova S, et al. 2009. Etiology of small-fiber neuropathy. *J Peripher Nerv Syst* 14: 177–183.

10. Stogbauer F, Young P, Kuhlenbaumer G, et al. 1999. Autosomal dominant burning feet syndrome. *J Neurol Neurosurg Psychiatry* 67: 78–81.

11. Toledo-Aral JJ, Moss BL, He ZJ, et al. 1997. Identification of PN1, a predominant voltage-dependent sodium channel expressed principally in peripheral neurons. *Proc Natl Acad Sci USA* 94: 1527–1532.

12. Rush AM, Dib-Hajj SD, Liu S, et al. 2006. A single sodium channel mutation produces hyper- or hypoexcitability in different types of neurons. *Proc Natl Acad Sci USA* 103: 8245–8250.

13. Persson AK, Black JA, Gasser A, et al. 2010. Sodium-calcium exchanger and multiple sodium channel isoforms in intra-epidermal nerve terminals. *Mol Pain* 6: 84.

14. Cummins TR, Howe JR, Waxman SG. 1998. Slow closed-state inactivation: A novel mechanism underlying ramp currents in cells expressing the hNE/PN1 sodium channel. *J Neurosci* 18: 9607–9619.

15. Dib-Hajj SD, Cummins TR, Black JA, Waxman SG. 2010. Sodium channels in normal and pathological pain. *Annu Rev Neurosci* 33: 325–347.

16. Dib-Hajj SD, Rush AM, Cummins TR, et al. 2005. Gain-of-function mutation in Nav1.7 in familial erythromelalgia induces bursting of sensory neurons. *Brain* 128: 1847–1854.

17. Fertleman CR, Baker MD, Parker KA, et al. 2006. SCN9A mutations in paroxysmal extreme pain disorder: Allelic variants underlie distinct channel defects and phenotypes. *Neuron* 52: 767–774.

18. Cox JJ, Reimann F, Nicholas AK, et al. 2006. An SCN9A channelopathy causes congenital inability to experience pain. *Nature* 444: 894–898.

19. Reilly MM. 2007. Sorting out the inherited neuropathies. *Pract Neurol* 7: 93–105.

20. Chamberlain JL, Pittock SJ, Oprescu AM, et al. 2010. Peripherin-IgG association with neurologic and endocrine autoimmunity. *J Autoimmun* 34: 469–477.

21. Lauria G, Hsieh ST, Johansson O, et al. 2010. European Federation of Neurological Societies/Peripheral Nerve Society Guideline on the use of skin biopsy in the diagnosis of small fiber neuropathy. Report of a joint task force of the European Federation of Neurological Societies and the Peripheral Nerve Society. *Eur J Neurol* 17: 903–912, e44–e49.

22. Bakkers M, Merkies IS, Lauria G, et al. 2009. Intraepidermal nerve fiber density and its application in sarcoidosis. *Neurology* 73: 1142–1148.

23. Shy ME, Frohman EM, So YT, et al. 2003. Quantitative sensory testing: Report of the Therapeutics and

Technology Assessment Subcommittee of the American Academy of Neurology. *Neurology* 60: 898–904.

24. Reulen JP, Lansbergen MD, Verstraete E, Spaans F. 2003. Comparison of thermal threshold tests to assess small nerve fiber function: Limits vs. levels. *Clin Neurophysiol* 114: 556–563.

25. Yarnitsky D, Sprecher E. 1994. Thermal testing: Normative data and repeatability for various test algorithms. *J Neurol Sci* 125: 39–45.

26. Hoitsma E, Drent M, Verstraete E, et al. 2003. Abnormal warm and cold sensation thresholds suggestive of small-fiber neuropathy in sarcoidosis. *Clin Neurophysiol* 114: 2326–2333.

27. Suarez GA, Opfer-Gehrking TL, Offord KP, et al. 1999. The Autonomic Symptom Profile: A new instrument to assess autonomic symptoms. *Neurology* 52: 523–528.

28. Galer BS, Jensen MP. 1997. Development and preliminary validation of a pain measure specific to neuropathic pain: The Neuropathic Pain Scale. *Neurology* 48: 332–338.

29. Maxwell C. 1978. Sensitivity and accuracy of the visual analogue scale: A psycho-physical classroom experiment. *Br J Clin Pharmacol* 6: 15–24.

30. Drenth JP, te Morsche RH, Guillet G, et al. 2005. SCN9A mutations define primary erythermalgia as a neuropathic disorder of voltage gated sodium channels. *J Invest Dermatol* 124: 1333–1338.

31. Klugbauer N, Lacinova L, Flockerzi V, Hofmann F. 1995. Structure and functional expression of a new member of the tetrodotoxin-sensitive voltage-activated sodium channel family from human neuroendocrine cells. *EMBO J* 14: 1084–1090.

32. Han C, Dib-Hajj SD, Lin Z, et al. 2009. Early- and late-onset inherited erythromelalgia: Genotype-phenotype correlation. *Brain* 132: 1711–1722.

33. Cummins TR, Rush AM, Estacion M, et al. 2009. Voltage-clamp and current-clamp recordings from mammalian DRG neurons. *Nat Protoc* 4: 1103–1112.

34. Dib-Hajj SD, Choi JS, Macala LJ, et al. 2009. Transfection of rat or mouse neurons by biolistics or electroporation. *Nat Protoc* 4: 1118–1126.

35. Jarecki BW, Piekarz AD, Jackson JO, II, Cummins TR. 2010. Human voltage-gated sodium channel mutations that cause inherited neuronal and muscle channelopathies increase resurgent sodium currents. *J Clin Invest* 120: 369–378.

36. Drenth JP, Waxman SG. 2007. Mutations in sodium-channel gene SCN9A cause a spectrum of human genetic pain disorders. *J Clin Invest* 117: 3603–3609.

37. Michiels JJ, te Morsche RH, Jansen JB, Drenth JP. 2005. Autosomal dominant erythermalgia associated with a novel mutation in the voltage-gated sodium channel alpha subunit Nav1.7. *Arch Neurol* 62: 1587–1590.

38. Stys PK, Waxman SG, Ransom BR. 1991. Na(+)-Ca2+ exchanger mediates Ca2+ influx during anoxia in mammalian central nervous system white matter. *Ann Neurol* 30: 375–380.

39. Garthwaite G, Goodwin DA, Batchelor AM, et al. 2002. Nitric oxide toxicity in CNS white matter: An in vitro study using rat optic nerve. *Neuroscience* 109: 145–155.

40. Malik RA, Masson EA, Sharma AK, et al. 1990. Hypoxic neuropathy: Relevance to human diabetic neuropathy. *Diabetologia* 33: 311–318.

41. Appenzeller O, Thomas PK, Ponsford S, et al. 2002. Acral paresthesias in the Andes and neurology at sea level. *Neurology* 59: 1532–1535.

42. Ames A, III. 2000. CNS energy metabolism as related to function. *Brain Res Brain Res Rev* 34: 42–68.

43. Waxman SG, Black JA, Kocsis JD, Ritchie JM. 1989. Low density of sodium channels supports action potential conduction in axons of neonatal rat optic nerve. *Proc Natl Acad Sci USA* 86: 1406–1410.

44. Donnelly DF. 2008. Spontaneous action potential generation due to persistent sodium channel currents in simulated carotid body afferent fibers. *J Appl Physiol* 104: 1394–1401.

45. Smith KJ, Kapoor R, Hall SM, Davies M. 2001. Electrically active axons degenerate when exposed to nitric oxide. *Ann Neurol* 49: 470–476.

46. Kapoor R, Davies M, Blaker PA, et al. 2003. Blockers of sodium and calcium entry protect axons from nitric oxide-mediated degeneration. *Ann Neurol* 53: 174–180.

NEUROPATHY-ASSOCIATED Na$_V$1.7 VARIANT I228M IMPAIRS INTEGRITY OF DORSAL ROOT GANGLION NEURON AXONS*

Anna-Karin Persson, Shujun Liu, Catharina G. Faber, Ingemar S. J. Merkies, Joel A. Black, and Stephen G. Waxman

Small-fiber neuropathy (SFN) is characterized by injury to small-diameter peripheral nerve axons and intraepidermal nerve fibers (IENF). Although mechanisms underlying loss of IENF in SFN are poorly understood, available data suggest that it results from axonal degeneration and reduced regenerative capacity. Gain-of-function variants in sodium channel Na$_V$1.7 that increase firing frequency and spontaneous firing of dorsal root ganglion (DRG) neurons have recently been identified in ~30% of patients with idiopathic SFN. In the present study, to determine whether these channel variants can impair axonal integrity, we developed an in vitro assay of DRG neurite length, and examined the effect of 3 SFN-associated variant Na$_V$1.7 channels, I228M, M932L/V991L (ML/ VL), and I720K, on DRG neurites in vitro. At 3 days after culturing, DRG neurons transfected with I228M channels exhibited ~20% reduced neurite length compared to wild-type channels; DRG neurons transfected with ML/VL and I720K variants displayed a trend toward reduced neurite length. I228M-induced reduction in neurite length was ameliorated by the use-dependent sodium channel blocker carbamazepine and by a blocker of reverse Na-Ca exchange. These in vitro observations provide evidence supporting a contribution of the I228M variant Na$_V$1.7 channel to impaired regeneration and/or degeneration of sensory axons in idiopathic SFN, and suggest that enhanced sodium channel activity and reverse Na-Ca exchange can contribute to a decrease in length of peripheral sensory axons.

Small-fiber neuropathy (SFN) is characterized by injury to unmyelinated and thinly myelinated peripheral fibers and loss of intraepidermal nerve fibers (IENF).[1–3] IENF are thought to exhibit dynamic plasticity, and although mechanisms

* Previously published in *Annals of Neurology* 73(1): 140–145, 2013. Additional supporting information can be found in the online version of this article (doi: 10.1002/ana.23725).

underlying IENF depletion in SFN are incompletely understood, available data suggest contributions from both axonal degeneration and reduced axonal regenerative capacity.[4]

An underlying cause cannot be identified in a substantial proportion of cases of SFN, which are traditionally classified as idiopathic.[1–3] Small-diameter peripheral axons and IENF are known to express voltage-gated sodium channel Na$_V$1.7.[5] Faber et al. recently identified gain-of-function Na$_V$1.7 variants (single amino acid substitutions) in ~30% of patients with biopsy-confirmed idiopathic SFN.[6] Patch-clamp studies of these Na$_V$1.7 variant channels demonstrated altered biophysical properties, resulting in gain of function at the channel level and in spontaneous firing and increased evoked firing frequency of dorsal root ganglion (DRG) neurons, which contribute to spontaneous and evoked pain. However, less is known about the molecular substrates for axonal injury and loss of IENF in idiopathic SFN.

IENF are known to express the Na-Ca exchanger-2 (NCX2) in addition to Na$_V$1.6, Na$_V$1.7, Na$_V$1.8, and Na$_V$1.9.[5] Increased Na$^+$ influx into axons expressing variant Na$_V$1.7 channels might be expected to trigger calcium influx into IENF and their small-diameter parent axons via reverse (Ca^{2+}-importing) Na-Ca exchange, particularly in view of their short length constant and high surface-to-volume ratio.[7,8] Here, we developed a tissue culture model in which we could assess the effect of SFN-associated variant Na$_V$1.7 channels on DRG neurons in vitro. We demonstrate decreased length of DRG neurites expressing variant I228M channels. We also show that a use-dependent sodium channel blocker, and blocking of reverse (Ca^{2+}-importing) operation of the Na-Ca exchanger, are protective. These observations suggest that gain-of-function variants of $Na_V1.7$ associated with SFN can contribute to impaired regeneration and/or degeneration of sensory axons through a cascade involving sodium channel activity and reverse Na-Ca exchange.

Materials and Methods

Methods for plasmid construction, isolation, culture, and transfection of DRG neurons have been described previously, and are detailed in Supplementary Material 1. Methods for live-cell imaging and quantification of neurite length are described in Supplementary Material 2.

Results

SFN-Associated $Na_V1.7$ Variants Reduce the Length of DRG Neurites in Vitro

To examine the effect of SFN-associated $Na_V1.7$ channel variants on neurites of primary sensory neurons, we transfected DRG neurons in vitro with $Na_V1.7$ wild-type (WT) and variants I228M,[9] M932L/V991L (ML/VL),[6] and I720K[6] (cotransfected with green fluorescent protein [GFP] to enable identification of transfected cells). As demonstrated in a representative 10×10 field-of-view montage image, cultures contained numerous GFP-positive neurons 3 days after transfection, with robust GFP signal in cell bodies as well as neurites (figure 1A). Examples of neurons transfected with WT, I228M, ML/VL, and I720K are shown at increased magnification in figure 1B.

Mean total neurite length/neuron was quantified from large-field images for WT-, I228M-, ML/VL-, and I720K-transfected neurons. There was an ~20% reduction ($p < 0.05$) in length of neurites of I228M-expressing neurons as compared to those transfected with WT channels (see figure 1C; WT: 1,483 neurons from n=25 large-field images; I228M: 1,436 neurons from n=25 large-field images). ML/VL- and I720K-

transfected neurons displayed a trend toward reduced neuritic length of 7% and 6%, respectively, which did not reach statistical significance (see figure 1C; ML/VL: 2,333 neurons, n=30; WT: 2,394 neurons, n=29; I720K: 1,522 neurons, n=24; WT: 1,285 cells, n=24).

I228M Channels Do Not Induce DRG Neuron Death

To determine whether I228M channels induce cell death of DRG neurons in addition to reducing neurite length, we assessed neuron viability 3 days after transfection with WT or I228M, using ethidium-homodimer 1 as a marker for dead/dying cells.[10] Within the population of transfected neurons (identified with GFP signal 1 day post-transfection), 99% of WT-channel–expressing neurons and 98% of I228M-expressing neurons remained viable in cultures at 3 days after transfection (figure 2), demonstrating that neurons expressing I228M channels in this in vitro model are not preferentially susceptible to cell death at a time (3 days in culture) when neurite length is significantly reduced.

Sodium Channel Blocker Carbamazepine Protects Neurites Expressing I228M and Has No Effect on WT-Containing Neurites

To determine whether the reduction in neurite length of I228M-transfected neurons could be attenuated by blockade of sodium channel activity, cultures were treated for 3 days with the use-dependent sodium channel blocker carbamazepine (CBZ) at a concentration (10 μM) previously shown to protect central nervous system (CNS) axons from anoxic injury.[11] After 3 days of CBZ treatment, neurites of I228M-transfected neurons exhibited increased length compared to untreated neurons in parallel cultures (figure 3A; left panel). Mean total length/neuron was increased by ~25% in CBZ-treated I228M-transfected neurons compared to untreated neurons (see figure 3A; top right), and the length of CBZ-treated neurites

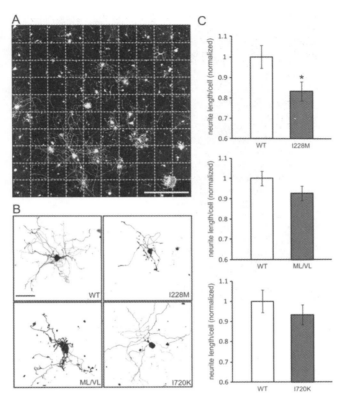

Figure 1

Neurite length of neurons expressing Na$_V$1.7 wild-type (WT) and I228M, M932L/V991L (ML/VL), and I720K channels. (A) Large-field montage image consisting of a 10×10 field-of-view montage image of a dorsal root ganglion culture 3 days after transfection with Na$_V$1.7 WT + green fluorescent protein (GFP) constructs, with GFP signal as white. Dotted lines distinguish individual field-of-view captures. Scale bar: 1,000µM. (B) Increased magnification of individual neurons transfected with Na$_V$1.7 WT, I228M, ML/VL, and I720K constructs demonstrates reduced neurite length of I228M-transfected neuron compared to WT. Scale bar: 250µM. (C) Quantifications of the total neurite length/neuron calculated from large-field images and averaged for each condition. Pairwise comparisons between neurites from neurons expressing WT channels and channel variants I228M, ML/VL, and I720K are presented. Data are normalized to WT values and presented as mean ± standard error of the mean. *$p < 0.05$.

approached that of WT-expressing neurons. As another control, we assessed the effect of CBZ on WT-transfected neurons with no mutant channels; 10 µM CBZ did not alter neurite length of WT-transfected neurons (see figure 3A; bottom right), consistent with a protective effect of CBZ through blockade of hyperactive I228M channel activity.[6]

Reverse Na-Ca Exchange Contributes to Reduced Neurite Length of I228M-Transfected Neurons

Increased axonal Na$^+$ influx has been shown to trigger reverse operation of the Na-Ca exchanger, producing injurious intra-axonal Ca^{2+} overload and axonal dysfunction in the CNS and

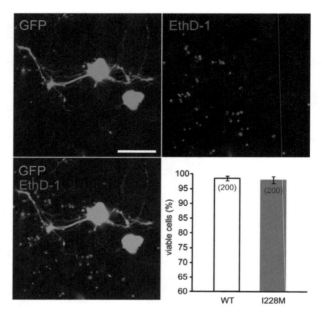

Figure 2

Cell viability of neurons 3 days after transfection with $Na_V 1.7$ wild-type (WT) or I228M channels.
Top left: Neurons 3 days after transfection with I228M + green fluorescent protein (GFP)
constructs. Top right: Same field after incubation with EthD-1, a marker for dead or dying cells.
Lower left: Merged image shows that GFP-positive cells do not colabel with EthD-1. Lower right:
Quantification of viable cells at 3 days after transfection (cells positive for GFP and negative for
EthD-1 are considered viable). Data are presented as mean±standard error of the mean, where
n=number of large-field images, and number of cells analyzed is indicated in parentheses. Scale
bar: 100μM.

Figure 3

Effect of carbamazepine (CBZ) and KB-R7943 on I228M-induced reduced neurite length. (A) Left panel: Indvidual
neurons transfected with I228M, untreated or treated with 10μM CBZ. CBZ-treated neurons display increased neurite
length compared to untreated neurons. Right panel: Quantification of the total neurite length/neuron calculated for neurons
expressing I228M (top) or wild-type (WT; bottom), untreated or treated with CBZ. CBZ significantly increases neurite
length in I228M-transfected neurons but does not alter neurite length of WT-transfected neurons. (B) Left panel: Individual
neurons transfected with I228M, untreated (top) or treated (bottom) with $0.5\mu M$ KB-R7943. KB-R7943–treated neurons
exhibit increased neurite length compared to untreated neurons. Right panel: Quantification of the total neurite length/
neuron calculated for neurons expressing I228M (top) or WT (bottom) channels, untreated or treated with KB-R7943.
KB-R7943 significantly increases neurite length in I228M-transfected neurons but does not affect neurite length of
WT-transfected neurons. Data are presented as mean ± standard error of the mean. Scale bar: 200μM. *$p < 0.05$.

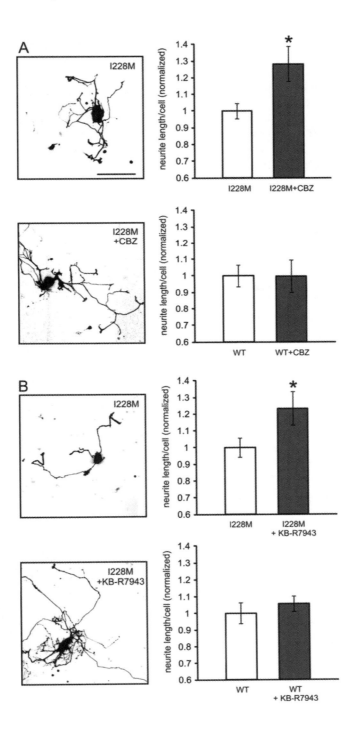

peripheral nervous system.[12,13] To investigate whether reverse Na-Ca exchange contributes to reduced neurite length in I228M-transfected neurons, we treated cultures with KB-R7943 at 0.5 μM, a concentration that inhibits reverse but not forward operation of NCX.[14] Following 3 days of treatment, I228M-transfected neurons exhibited substantially longer neurites compared to untreated I228M-transfected cells (see figure 3B; left panel). Quantification of mean total neurite length/neuron for I228M-transfected neurons demonstrated a ~25% increase with KB-R7943 treatment compared to untreated I228M-transfected neurons (see figure 3B; top right). We also assessed the effect of KB-R7943 on WT-transfected neurons with no mutant channels, as a second control. WT-transfected neurons displayed similar mean total neurite length/neuron for KB-R7943-treated and untreated cultures (see figure 3B; bottom right).

Discussion

Loss of IENF is a defining characteristic and valuable tool for diagnosis of SFN,[1-3] but molecular mechanisms underlying the axonal loss are still not understood. IENF are the distal ends of unmyelinated C- and thinly myelinated Aδ-nerve fibers that exit dermal nerve bundles and branch into fine-caliber free nerve endings within the epidermis. The epidermis is characterized by constant turnover of keratinocytes, which migrate from basal layers to the epidermal surface, so that the IENF run through a highly dynamic terrain. Substantial evidence suggests continuous axonal remodeling, regeneration, and sprouting of IENF within the mature, nonpathological epidermis.[15,16] In accordance with this schema, reduced IENF density in SFN has been proposed to result from both impaired growth or regenerative capacity of axons and axonal degeneration.[4] The present results, although based on observations of an in vitro model and not differ-

entiating between impaired regenerative capacity and axonal degeneration, show that expression of a gain-of-function Na$_V$1.7 variant associated with idiopathic SFN results in decreased length of DRG neurites in vitro, suggesting that the variant channel can injure sensory axons in one or both ways.

Faber et al. recently demonstrated gain-of-function Na$_V$1.7 variants in ~30% of patients with idiopathic SFN.[6] Na$_V$1.7 is preferentially and abundantly expressed in nociceptive DRG neurons and is, along with sodium channels Na$_V$1.6, Na$_V$1.8, and Na$_V$1.9, present in small peripheral axons and their IENF.[5] Small diameter is known to increase sensitivity to small changes in sodium conductance or influx, because it imposes a high input resistance, short electrotonic and diffusional length constant, and high surface-to-volume ratio.[7,8] Fine-caliber IENF are thus likely to be particularly vulnerable to gain-of-function changes of SFN-associated variant Na$_V$1.7 channels, and to the increased firing frequency and spontaneous firing of neurons expressing these channels.[6]

Our results demonstrate reduced length of neurites from neurons transfected with I228M variant Na$_V$1.7 channels. We also observed a trend toward shorter neurites for ML/VL and I720K variant-transfected neurons, compared to those transfected with WT channels after 3 days in vitro, implying an effect of these Na$_V$1.7 variant channels on neurite length. The significant reduction in neurite length for I228M-transfected neurons, and the trend toward reduced neurite length of ML/VL and I720K transfected neurons, may reflect differences in functional properties of DRG neurons expressing these variant channels. Electrophysiological recordings from DRG neurons in vitro showed a 29% prevalence of spontaneous firing in neurons transfected with I228M channels,[9] whereas ML/VL and I720K channels exhibited smaller proportions (15%, 17%, respectively) of spontaneous firing neurons.[6] Interestingly, the I228M variant was found in patients with proximal (face, scalp) pain at onset, whereas the I720K and ML/VL variants were identified in patients with early distal (feet) pain.[6,9]

The I228M mutation substitutes a residue within the DIS4 segment of the channel, which is invariant in all human sodium channels except Na$_V$1.9, suggesting that it may play an important role in determining the functional properties of the Na$_V$1.7 channel. Although the I228M substitution is listed as a single nucleotide polymorphism in one database (Craig Ventor Human Genome) and was reported in <0.3% of control chromosomes in another series[17] and in 0.1% of chromosomes in the 1000 Genome Project (rs71428908), Estacion et al.[9] did not find it in a control panel from 100 healthy ethnically matched controls (200 chromosomes). I228M displays substantially impaired slow inactivation, which increases the non-inactivated fraction of Na$_V$1.7 channels at potentials positive to −80mV, including resting potential.[9] At the cellular level, expression of I228M depolarizes DRG neuron resting potential by ~5mV, induces spontaneous firing in nearly 30% of these cells, and doubles the firing rate in response to graded suprathreshold stimuli.[9] Increased sodium influx into axons expressing mutant channels, and/or impaired calcium extrusion by NCX from them, would be predicted from each of these functional changes. The increased window current is predicted to produce sustained sodium influx, and spontaneous activity and increased evoked firing rates superimpose additional sodium influx associated with incremental action potentials.[18] Moreover, because the Na-Ca exchanger is electrogenic, depolarization biases exchange against calcium efflux and toward calcium influx, as has been shown in axons within the anoxic optic nerve and peripheral axons subjected to anoxia, where persistent sodium influx has been shown to trigger reverse operation of the Na-Ca exchanger, causing an injurious intra-axonal Ca^{2+} overload and axonal dysfunction.[12,13] Our results suggest that NCX (present in peripheral axons and IENF

as isoform NCX2[5]) contributes via reverse (Ca^{2+}-importing) exchange to I228M-induced reduction in neurite length.

As with all in vitro models of neurodegenerative disorders, cultured neurons do not fully recapitulate the in vivo situation. In vitro models cannot fully mimic the time-dependent (years postnatal) or length-dependent (early effect on axons approximately 1m long for length-dependent, 10cm for neuropathies with early facial involvement) patterns of axonal damage occurring in patients with SFN. Indeed, the I228M variant has been reported in a small number of unaffected control chromosomes[17] and in 2 unaffected children of a patient with I228M-associated SFN (ages younger than age of onset of neuropathy in affected individuals).[9] Nevertheless, the altered channel biophysics and proexcitatory effects of SFN-associated Na$_V$1.7 variants[6,9] suggest that, at a minimum, they act as risk factors that predispose to development of SFN. Our results show a significant reduction in neurite length for DRG neurons transfected with the I228M Na$_V$1.7 variation, and a less pronounced trend toward reduction in neurite length in DRG neurons transfected with ML/VL and I720K. One possible explanation for this effect of variant channels on neuritic length after 3 days in culture might be that higher-than-normal overall levels of WT (endogenous) and variant (transfected) Na$_V$1.7 channels offset the brief time in culture and result in an accelerated pathogenic effect.

Irrespective of whether our in vitro assay reproduces in vivo time-dependence or fully reproduces the in vivo pattern of length-dependent axonal degeneration, we observed significant protective effects of the use-dependent sodium channel blocker CBZ and of reverse Na-Ca exchange (KB-R7943) on neurite length for DRG neurons transfected with I228M. These observations suggest that, similar to their injurious role in anoxic white matter[13] and peripheral nerve[12] axons, activity of gain-of-function variant sodium channels and the Na-Ca exchanger in reverse mode may contribute to axonal injury in SFN. Assessment of IENF density, comparing progression of SFN with and without treatment with sodium channel blockers or blockers of Na-Ca exchange, might make it possible to determine whether this mechanism is at play in vivo, over years and in axons many centimeters in length, in human subjects with SFN.

Acknowledgments

This work was supported in part by grants from the Rehabilitation Research Service and Medical Research Service, Department of Veterans Affairs (S.G.W.), Maastricht University Medical Center Profileringsfonds (C.G.F.), and Erythromelalgia Foundation (S.G.W.). The Center for Neuroscience and Regeneration Research is a collaboration of the Paralyzed Veterans of America and the United Spinal Association with Yale University. A.K.P. was in part supported by a fellowship from the Swedish Research Council (K2010-78PK-21636-01-2).

We thank P. Shah and L. Tyrrell for excellent technical assistance.

About the Authors

Anna-Karin Persson, PhD, Department of Neurology, Yale University School of Medicine, New Haven, CT; Center for Neuroscience and Regeneration Research, Veterans Affairs Medical Center, West Haven, CT

Shujun Liu, MS, Department of Neurology, Yale University School of Medicine, New Haven, CT; Center for Neuroscience and Regeneration Research, Veterans Affairs Medical Center, West Haven, CT

Catharina G. Faber, MD, PhD, Department of Neurology, University Medical Center Maastricht, Maastricht, the Netherlands

Ingemar S. J. Merkies, MD, PhD, Department of Neurology, University Medical Center Maastricht, Maastricht, the Netherlands; Department of Neurology, Spaarne Hospital, Hoofddorp, the Netherlands

Joel A. Black, PhD, Department of Neurology, Yale University School of Medicine, New Haven, CT; Center for Neuroscience and Regeneration Research, Veterans Affairs Medical Center, West Haven, CT

Stephen G. Waxman, MD, PhD, Department of Neurology, Yale University School of Medicine, New Haven, CT; Center for Neuroscience and Regeneration Research, Veterans Affairs Medical Center, West Haven, CT

Potential Conflicts of Interest

C.G.F.: grants/grants pending Prinses Beatrix Fonds. I.S.J.M.: travel support, Peripheral Nerve Society; board membership, steering committee member of ICE trial and CSL Behring CIDP study (not related to current article); grants/grants pending, GBS/CIDP International foundation grant for the PeriNomS study, Talents Program grant for the PeriNomS study, Peripheral Nerve Society grant for the PeriNomS study (not related to current article). S.G.W.: consultancy, Bristol Myers Squibb, Vertex Pharmaceuticals, ChromoCell Corp, DaiNippon Sumitomo Pharm, Cardiome Pharm; grants/grants pending, Pfizer Research, Trans Molecular; patents, listed as inventor for Yale-owned patents on $Na_V1.9$ (not $Na_V1.7$, which is the topic of the current article) currently not licensed to any commercial entity; stock/stock options, Trans Molecular (not involved in work on sodium channels, pain, or neuropathies).

References

1. Bednarik J, Vlckova-Moravcova E, Bursova S, et al. 2009. Etiology of small-fiber neuropathy. *J Peripher Nerv Syst* 14: 177–183.

2. Devigili G, Tugnoli V, Penza P, et al. 2008. The diagnostic criteria for small fibre neuropathy: From symptoms to neuropathology. *Brain* 131(pt 7): 1912–1925.

3. Lacomis D. 2002. Small-fiber neuropathy. *Muscle Nerve* 26: 173–188.

4. Bursova S, Dubovy P, Vlckova-Moravcova E, et al. 2012. Expression of growth-associated protein 43 in the skin nerve fibers of patients with type 2 diabetes mellitus. *J Neurol Sci* 315: 60–63.

5. Persson AK, Black JA, Gasser A, et al. 2010. Sodium-calcium exchanger and multiple sodium channel isoforms in intra-epidermal nerve terminals. *Mol Pain* 6: 84.

6. Faber CG, Hoeijmakers JG, Ahn HS, et al. 2012. Gain of function Na$_V$1.7 mutations in idiopathic small fiber neuropathy. *Ann Neurol* 71: 26–39.

7. Donnelly DF. 2008. Spontaneous action potential generation due to persistent sodium channel currents in simulated carotid body afferent fibers. *J Appl Physiol* 104: 1394–1401.

8. Waxman SG, Black JA, Kocsis JD, Ritchie JM. 1989. Low density of sodium channels supports action potential conduction in axons of neonatal rat optic nerve. *Proc Natl Acad Sci USA* 86: 1406–1410.

9. Estacion M, Han C, Choi JS, et al. 2011. Intra- and interfamily phenotypic diversity in pain syndromes associated with a gain-of-function variant of Na$_V$1.7. *Mol Pain* 7: 92.

10. Gladman SJ, Huang W, Lim SN, et al. 2012. Improved outcome after peripheral nerve injury in mice with increased levels of endogenous omega-3 polyunsaturated fatty acids. *J Neurosci* 32: 563–571.

11. Fern R, Ransom BR, Stys PK, Waxman SG. 1993. Pharmacological protection of CNS white matter during anoxia: Actions of phenytoin, carbamazepine and diazepam. *J Pharmacol Exp Ther* 266: 1549–1555.

12. Lehning EJ, Doshi R, Isaksson N, et al. 1996. Mechanisms of injury-induced calcium entry into peripheral nerve myelinated axons: Role of reverse sodium-calcium exchange. *J Neurochem* 66: 493–500.

13. Stys PK, Waxman SG, Ransom BR. 1992. Ionic mechanisms of anoxic injury in mammalian CNS white matter: Role of Na+ channels and Na(+)-Ca2+ exchanger. *J Neurosci* 12: 430–439.

14. Watanabe Y, Koide Y, Kimura J. 2006. Topics on the Naþ/Ca2þ exchanger: Pharmacological characterization of Naþ/Ca2þ exchanger inhibitors. *J Pharmacol Sci* 102: 7–16.

15. Cheng C, Guo GF, Martinez JA, et al. 2010. Dynamic plasticity of axons within a cutaneous milieu. *J Neurosci* 30: 14735–14744.

16. Verze L, Paraninfo A, Ramieri G, et al. 1999. Immunocytochemical evidence of plasticity in the nervous structures of the rat lower lip. *Cell Tissue Res* 297: 203–211.

17. Singh NA, Pappas C, Dahle EJ, et al. 2009. A role of SCN9A in human epilepsies, as a cause of febrile seizures and as a potential modifier of Dravet syndrome. *PLoS Genet* 5: e1000649.

18. Chow CC, White JA. 1996. Spontaneous action potentials due to channel fluctuations. *Biophys J* 71: 3013–3021.

10 RIPPLES

One of the exciting things about science is that it can have an impact beyond what was expected. Research on one project can inform research on another. This can occur because *concepts* or *conclusions*, derived from one particular research effort, hold lessons for a second project; or because a new *tool* or a new *method*, developed for one project, proves to be useful in a second project; or because expertise accrued for one project turns out be relevant to a second. In some cases this ripple effect can extend from one disease to another. This was the case in the search for a gene in a 15-year-old girl. Analysis of her genes propelled us to use methods from our research on pain to help understand another disorder. Her genes were, in fact, the centerpiece of a touching story.

I am not an epileptologist. But, epilepsy and neuropathic pain share a common basis in reflecting neuronal hyperexcitability. My success studying erythromelalgia was paralleled by recognition that I had a strong toolbox for assessing neuronal hyperexcitability. In 2010 I was contacted by two geneticists interested in developmental disorders of the nervous system and epilepsy.

Miriam Meisler, professor of genetics at University of Michigan, had long-standing interests in epilepsy and intellectual disability. She had, over the years, made important contributions on the genetics of $Na_V1.6$, a sodium channel that is widely expressed in the brain. She had found mutations of $Na_V1.6$ that produce abnormalities of the brain in mice. This was an important advance. But she was still looking for a human counterpart, and was searching for $Na_V1.6$ mutations that produce human neurological disease.

Michael Hammer, the director of the Human Genomics Core at University of Arizona, was a population geneticist. He had studied the DNA of great apes, Neanderthals, and modern human beings. He had fueled popular interest in genetics by collaborating with the National Geographic Society to trace the genetic origins of hundreds of thousands of people. Combining genetic data on various groups with knowledge of their migration, he was able to look back in time at the origins of human population groups (Veeramah and Hammer 2014). For this type of work, he had amassed a powerful array of computational tools, which he used to search through the immense amount of information within the genomes of the populations he was studying.

But in 2010 Hammer had a new interest. He was working together with Meisler, trying to establish the cause of infantile epileptic encephalopathy—a syndrome marked by epilepsy, intellectual disability and autism-like behavior—by studying the DNA of a 15-year-old girl. There was no family history, and extensive medical workup had not established a cause. Hammer wanted to find the solution to a puzzle, which he felt was held somewhere within this girl's genome.

Hammer's approach was based on the "common disease/rare variant" model, which posits that rare or novel mutations can cause severe illnesses for which no other cause is apparent (Gorlov et al. 2011). As he searched for the cause of this girl's disorder, he was looking for a new or *de novo* mutation—a mistake in a gene that appeared for the first time in a single family member as a result of a mutation that occurred in an egg or sperm cell of one of the parents or in the fertilized egg itself.

Human genes are relatively stable. Only one or two mutations occur per 100 million sites (pairs of nucleotides within the DNA) per generation (Conrad et al. 2011). Mutations that cause severe disorders such as Dravet syndrome (another form of infantile epilepsy) are expected to be rare, since affected individuals tend not to reproduce. But thousands of genes participate in shaping the development of the nervous system, and each of these genes is at risk for mutations (Sepp et al. 2008). So, it was not unreasonable to expect that a neurodevelopmental disorder in this girl with no family history was due to a de novo mutation. Hammer was searching for a rare mutation, possibly one that had not previously been reported in the medical literature. He had no idea, at the outset of this work, which gene might harbor the culprit mutation. He was looking for a needle in a mountainous haystack.

To begin, Hammer performed whole-genome sequencing, which examined all of the genes within the human genome, on DNA from the patient. He compared the DNA from the patient with the DNA from her two unaffected parents and one unaffected sibling. Using the massive computational power he had built, he identified 11,292 gene variants—genes in which there was some abnormality, possibly disease-causing but possibly benign—within this family. There was initially a huge number—11,292 to be exact—of potential mutations that were candidates for further study.

To narrow the field, Hammer and his team used the powerful computational capabilities that they had to sort through these gene variants in a multitiered analysis. This filtering showed that most of these gene variants were present not only in the affected girl, but also in one or both of the parents who were unaffected; these candidate gene variants were not disease-causing and could thus be excluded. And so the field became much smaller. At this point thirty-four variants remained. These gene variants displayed a pattern that violated the rules of Mendelian inheritance—they were present in the girl with epilepsy but not in her unaffected sibling or parents. These thirty-four candidate gene variants could be considered as de novo, new mutations, and each could be considered as a suspect. But, the field still needed to be smaller. One by one, Hammer assessed the thirty-four gene variants. Ten were discarded for reasons that included their presence within the genomes of normal individuals as reported in various databases. Now a smaller group of twenty-four genes was left. Sequencing the remaining variants, one-by-one, his analysis showed that all but one were false positives.

Hammer now had a single candidate, a new de novo gene variant (Veeramah et al. 2012). It was a mutation in the *SCN8A* gene that substituted a single amino acid among the nearly 1,800 that make up the $Na_V1.6$ sodium channel. Epilepsy is produced by abnormal storms of activity in neurons within the brain, and, given the pivotal role of sodium channels in producing action potentials, a sodium channel mutation seemed to make sense. Supporting the general idea that sodium channel mutations can cause epilepsy, it was known that another type of severe epilepsy, Dravet syndrome, is in some cases caused by de novo mutations in the gene *SCN1A,* which encodes the $Na_V1.1$ sodium channel (Marini et al. 2011; Catterall, Kalume, and Oakley 2010). $Na_V1.6$ mutations had not previously been implicated in human epilepsy. Knowing that Meisler was an expert on the $Na_V1.6$ sodium channel, Hammer contacted her.

Together, Hammer and Meisler noted that $Na_V1.6$ contributes to impulse generation in most neurons within the brain. They observed that the mutation altered an amino acid that is evolutionarily conserved within the channel—the same from species to species—and they surmised that that this particular amino acid, at a specific site within the channel protein, probably was functionally important. Putting all these pieces together, they suspected that the mutation (N1768D) of $Na_V1.6$ was the culprit in the fifteen-year-old girl. This was an especially interesting prospect because $Na_V1.6$ mutations had not previously been shown to produce disease in humans.

But did the mutation actually cause epilepsy? To answer this question, a next step was to unravel the functional effects of the mutation. My research group had, by this time, completed the functional profiling for more than a dozen mutations in the $Na_V1.7$ sodium channel. Because $Na_V1.6$ contributes to the pathophysiology of multiple sclerosis, which was another focus of my laboratory (Craner et al. 2004), we were also interested in $Na_V1.6$ and had a toolbox in place to study its functional properties (Cummins et al. 2005; Herzog, Cummins, et al. 2003; Herzog, Liu, et al. 2003; Rush, Dib-Hajj, and Waxman 2005). Meisler contacted us and asked if we could functionally assess the new $Na_V1.6$ mutation. There was a lot going on in the laboratory, so we were busy, but the idea of making a contribution to research on epilepsy was appealing. We accepted the challenge.

A first step for us was to construct the mutant gene and introduce it into cells in tissue culture. Sulayman Dib-Hajj's prowess in handling large, difficult-to-work-with genes proved invaluable. Once the mutant gene had produced the mutant channels in our cells, electrophysiology expert Xiaoyang Cheng went to work. Her analysis took about ten weeks. Figure 10.1 shows the dramatic results (Veeramah et al. 2012). As a result of the functional changes caused by the mutation, more $Na_V1.6$ channels were available for operation. This change in itself would be expected to increase the excitability of neurons in the brain. But there was more. We also found (figure 10.2) that, once the mutant $Na_V1.6$ sodium channels are activated, they produce a "persistent current," which did not shut off. This change in channel function would be expected to depolarize neurons and powerfully add to their hyperexcitability. And, in addition, we observed (figure 10.3) that the mutation strongly enhanced the response of the channel to small, subtle depolarizations close to resting potential; this, too, would be expected to increase the excitability of nerve cells harboring the mutant channel. Here we had, for the

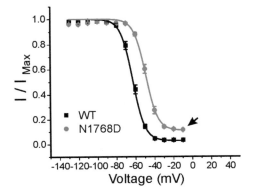

Figure 10.1
The N1768D mutation in the $Na_V1.6$ sodium channel, from a 15-year-old girl with epilepsy and a neurodevelopmental disorder, impairs channel inactivation, a process that makes channels unoperable after they open. The y-axis of this graph shows the percentage of channels that are not inactivated (and thus are available for operation) as a function of membrane potential. At membrane potentials more depolarized than –80 mV, the fraction of available channels is larger for N1768D mutant channels (red) than for normal, wild-type (WT) $Na_V1.6$ channels (black). At a membrane potential of –60 mV, close to the resting potential of neurons in the brain, only one-half of the wild-type channels are available for operation; in contrast nearly all of the mutant channels are available. At membrane potentials more depolarized than –30 mV, almost none of the wild-type channels are available and inactivation is complete, while 10% of the mutant channels are available (arrow). Thus, at the membrane potentials of most nerve cells in the brain, more of the mutant $Na_V1.6$ channels are available for operation, a change that would be expected to make neurons more excitable. Modified from Veeramah et al. (2012).

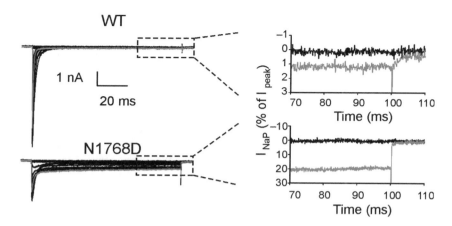

Figure 10.2

Representative transmembrane currents produced by normal wild-type (WT, top) and N1768D mutant Na$_V$1.6 channels (bottom). Cells were held at –120 mV, and step depolarizations (–80 to +60 mV in 5-mV increments) were applied every 5 sec. Insets on right show persistent currents (presented as a percentage of maximal transient peak currents) at the end of a 100-msec step depolarization to –80 mV (black) and +20 mV (red). Note the different scales for the y-axes for wild-type and mutant channels on the right. As seen in the lower right panel, the persistent current, a driver of a neuronal excitability, is more than five times larger for the mutant channels. From Veeramah et al. (2012).

first time, evidence that a mutation of Na$_V$1.6 could cause human disease. We were beginning to see that the *SCN8A* gene encoding Na$_V$1.6 might be a gene for epilepsy.

Encouraged by our finding of these pro-excitatory changes in the channel, a next step was to learn whether our prediction, that the mutated channel would cause neurons to become epileptic, was correct. To test this hypothesis, we inserted the mutant channels into neurons from the rat hippocampus, a brain region where epileptic seizures often arise, and assessed the effect of the mutant channels on excitability of these nerve cells. The results, shown in figure 10.4, were striking: The mutant channels caused hippocampal neurons to shriek when they should have been silent. In response to stimulation, the frequency of evoked firing was twice as high in cells expressing the mutant channels. Some cells expressing the mutant channels tended to fire spontaneously, without any stimulation at all. And, notably, cells expressing the mutant channel displayed "paroxysmal depolarizing shifts," or plateau-like depolarizations in membrane potential that produce inappropriately high-frequency firing, a classical hallmark of nerve cells in the epileptic brain (figure 10.4).

The paper describing these novel findings, by Hammer, Meisler, and their co-workers, and our team, was published in 2012 (Veeramah et al. 2012). Mutations of other sodium channels had been implicated in epilepsy (Catterall, Kalume, and Oakley 2010; George 2004; Oliva, Berkovic, and Petrou 2012; Veeramah et al. 2012). But this new work added a new dimension, indicting mutations in the *SCN8A* gene, which encodes the Na$_V$1.6 sodium channel—it was the first time that a mutation of Na$_V$1.6 had been linked to a human disease. Within a year or two after publication of our 2012 paper, additional mutations in the *SCN8A* gene were linked to epilepsy (de Kovel et al. 2014; Epi4K-Consortium et al. 2013; Estacion et al. 2014; Ohba et al. 2014; Vaher et al. 2013). Other mutations in the same gene followed. Hammer and Meisler continue to make *SCN8A* a focus of research.

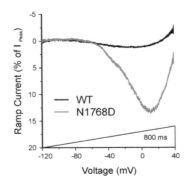

Figure 10.3
Currents generated by wild-type (WT) Na$_V$1.6 channels (top trace, black) and N1768D mutant channels (red trace) in response to a slow, ramp-like stimulus that gradually depolarizes the cell from −120 mV to +40 mV (shown at the bottom of the figure). The stimulus simulates a synaptic input. The ramp response of the mutant channels is more than ten-fold larger, indicating that the mutant channels respond more vigorously to even small, subtle inputs. From Veeramah et al. (2012).

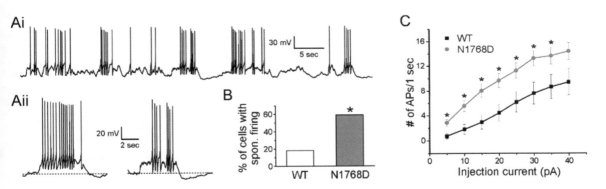

Figure 10.4
These "whole cell current-clamp" recordings show the effect of N1768D mutant channels on neurons from the rat hippocampus, a part of the brain where seizures can originate. Ai shows abnormal spontaneous firing in a hippocampal neuron transfected with N1768D mutant channels. Aii shows examples of abnormal plateau-like depolarizations, similar to the paroxysmal depolarizing shifts characteristics of epileptic neurons, in hippocampal neurons transfected with the mutant N1768D channels. Panel B shows the percentage of neurons that fired spontaneously (spon.) following transfection with mutant N1768D channels (dark bar) or with normal, wild-type (WT) Na$_V$1.6 channels (open bar). There is much more spontaneous firing in neurons containing the mutant channel. Panel C shows the number of nerve impulses (action potentials, AP) evoked by a 1-second depolarizing step stimulus at a variety of stimulation intensities, in hippocampal neurons transfected with N1768D mutant channels (red) or normal, wild-type Na$_V$1.6 channels (black). At any given stimulus intensity, neurons containing the mutant channel fire more vigorously. From Veeramah et al. (2012).

In successfully pinpointing a mutation of Na$_V$1.6, Hammer and his co-workers showed that, by strategically using whole genome sequencing, it is possible to identify—even in a small family—a novel and putatively disease-causing mutation. Hammer's identification of a single, novel mutation as a plausible disease-causing candidate was a tour de force. He had found a needle in a haystack. Our contribution was to show that the mutation, at both the ion channel level and the nerve cell level, produces functional changes that can produce epilepsy. In the aggregate the results pointed, for the first time, to mutations of Na$_V$1.6 as a cause of human disease. Another example of a successful collaboration but, in this instance, a very straightforward joint effort within the borders of our country.

There is a special postscript to this project. It was only after the Veeramah et al. paper was written and accepted for publication that I learned the identity of the girl whose DNA had taught us so much. It was Michael Hammer's daughter, Shay. Our paper appeared shortly after her death in 2011. Shay's picture can be found in the *Arizona Daily Star* (Beal 2013).

As I reflected on this, I could not help but be struck by the story behind this work. Michael Hammer had done something that most people could not have done—in offering up his own family, his own genes, and those of his daughter, and by using gene sequencing in a very powerful way, he had answered an important question and he had made a discovery that might, in the future, help other children.

Shay's genes had revealed their inner secret.

References

Beal T. 2013. "A father's search finds reason for daughter's epilepsy." *Arizona Daily Star*, June 16.

Catterall WA, Kalume F, Oakley JC. 2010. NaV1.1 channels and epilepsy. *J Physiol* 588(Pt 11): 1849–1859.

Conrad DF, Keebler JE, DePristo MA, Lindsay SJ, Zhang Y, Casals F, Idaghdour YC, et al. 2011. Variation in genome-wide mutation rates within and between human families. *Nat Genet* 43(7): 712–714.

Craner MJ, Newcombe J, Black JA, Hartle C, Cuzner ML, Waxman SG. 2004. Molecular changes in neurons in multiple sclerosis: Altered axonal expression of Nav1.2 and Nav1.6 sodium channels and Na+/Ca2+ exchanger. *Proc Natl Acad Sci USA* 101(21): 8168–8173.

Cummins TR, Dib-Hajj SD, Herzog RI, Waxman SG. 2005. Nav1.6 channels generate resurgent sodium currents in spinal sensory neurons. *FEBS Lett* 579(10): 2166–2170.

de Kovel CG, Meisler MH, Brilstra EH, van Berkestijn FM, van 't Slot R, van Lieshout S, Nijman IJ, et al. 2014. Characterization of a de novo SCN8A mutation in a patient with epileptic encephalopathy. *Epilepsy Res* 108(9): 1511–1518.

Epi4K-Consortium, Project Epilepsy Phenome/Genome, Allen AS, Berkovic SF, Cossette P, Delanty N, Dlugos D, Eichler EE, Epstein MP, et al. 2013. De novo mutations in epileptic encephalopathies. *Nature* 501(7466): 217–221.

Estacion M, O'Brien JE, Conravey A, Hammer MF, Waxman SG, Dib-Hajj SD, Meisler MH. 2014. A novel de novo mutation of SCN8A (Na1.6) with enhanced channel activation in a child with epileptic encephalopathy. *Neurobiol Dis* 69: 117–123.

George AL, Jr. 2004. Inherited channelopathies associated with epilepsy. *Epilepsy Curr* 4(2): 65–70.

Gorlov IP, Gorlova OY, Frazier ML, Spitz MR, Amos CI. 2011. Evolutionary evidence of the effect of rare variants on disease etiology. *Clin Genet* 79(3): 199–206.

Herzog RI, Cummins TR, Ghassemi F, Dib-Hajj SD, Waxman SG. 2003. Distinct repriming and closed-state inactivation kinetics of Nav1.6 and Nav1.7 sodium channels in mouse spinal sensory neurons. *J Physiol* 551(Pt 3): 741–750.

Herzog RI, Liu C, Waxman SG, Cummins TR. 2003. Calmodulin binds to the C terminus of sodium channels Nav1.4 and Nav1.6 and differentially modulates their functional properties. *J Neurosci* 23(23): 8261–8270.

Marini C, Scheffer IE, Nabbout R, Suls A, De Jonghe P, Zara F, Guerrini R. 2011. The genetics of Dravet syndrome. *Epilepsia* 52(Suppl 2): 24–29.

Ohba C, Kato M, Takahashi S, Lerman-Sagie T, Lev D, Terashima H, Kubota M, et al. 2014. Early onset epileptic encephalopathy caused by de novo SCN8A mutations. *Epilepsia* 55(7): 994–1000.

Oliva M, Berkovic SF, Petrou S. 2012. Sodium channels and the neurobiology of epilepsy. *Epilepsia* 53(11): 1849–1859.

Rush AM, Dib-Hajj SD, Waxman SG. 2005. Electrophysiological properties of two axonal sodium channels, Nav1.2 and Nav1.6, expressed in mouse spinal sensory neurones. *J Physiol* 564(Pt 3): 803–815.

Sepp KJ, Hong P, Lizarraga SB, Liu JS, Mejia LA, Walsh CA, Perrimon N. 2008. Identification of neural outgrowth genes using genome-wide RNAi. *PLoS Genet* 4(7): e1000111.

Vaher U, Noukas M, Nikopensius T, Kals M, Annilo T, Nelis M, Ounap K, et al. 2013. De novo SCN8A mutation identified by whole-exome sequencing in a boy with neonatal epileptic encephalopathy, multiple congenital anomalies, and movement disorders. *J Child Neurol* 29(12): NP202–NP206.

Veeramah KR, Hammer MF. 2014. The impact of whole-genome sequencing on the reconstruction of human population history. *Nat Rev Genet* 15(3): 149–162.

Veeramah KR, O'Brien JE, Meisler MH, Cheng X, Dib-Hajj SD, Waxman SG, Talwar D, et al. 2012. De novo pathogenic SCN8A mutation identified by whole-genome sequencing of a family quartet affected by infantile epileptic encephalopathy and SUDEP. *Am J Hum Genet* 90(3): 502–510.

IV MUTING GOD'S MEGAPHONE: FROM THE SQUID TOWARD THE CLINIC

11 SEVEN YEARS FROM THEORY TOWARD THERAPY ... VIA "PAIN IN A DISH"

Discovering that the *SCN9A* gene and its $Na_V1.7$ sodium channel play a key role in pain marked, in a sense, a successful end of the search for a pain gene. I could have finished this book at that point. But a larger quest was ahead. Science goes on and on, with the answer to each question raising new challenges and suggesting new possibilities.

Turning a target—$Na_V1.7$ in this instance—into a treatment is not easy. There is a lot of work to do in the laboratory before a potential medicine even begins to be tested in humans. Then one must define the appropriate people to test it in, and design the most informative trial. Human subjects with the disease under study have to be located and enrolled. They have to be randomized into multiple groups, one group receiving the drug under study and the other group receiving placebo pills containing an inactive substance, matched to look exactly like the drug. Specific end points—the change in size of a tumor, or the change in blood pressure, or the change in intensity or duration of pain—have to be chosen, and careful measurements have to be made. Side effects must be assessed. And, after all of the measurements have been collected, the data must be analyzed by careful statistical methods. Meticulous records must be kept at each stage. And they must be submitted to governmental regulators. There are a lot of steps: advance ... stall ... breakthrough ... advance ... setback ... and so on. All moving, one hopes, in the right direction from target toward treatment.

By 2009 I had entered a part of my quest that appeared to point toward a new treatment for pain. Progress in this "translational" work was slower than in our earlier studies, at times tortuously slow. But, as I was writing this book, we reached a milestone. While not yet at our final goal, we were moving from theory toward therapy both through clinical studies and via a stopover in the laboratory where we would study "human pain in a dish."

New Medicines: A Big Challenge

Biomedical scientists do not work in a vacuum. The development of new medications occurs not just in academia but also in the biopharmaceutical industry, which spans from start-up biotech companies (some barely large enough to be called a company) to large multinational conglomerates. These organizations have expertise in areas—high-throughput drug screening that permits assessment of thousands of candidate drugs, medicinal chemistry required for design and construction of new medicinal molecules, pharmacokinetic and pharmacodynamic expertise necessary for optimization of drug uptake, metabolism, and excretion—complementing the strengths of academic researchers. And biopharmaceutical companies have the expertise and money to do clinical trials.

But even for a large organization, the pathway to a new medication can be challenging. The correct drug molecule must be studied, at the right dose, in patients with the right disease. Even large companies with substantial resources must make strategic decisions, choosing a small number of potential new drugs from a large number of candidates for study in clinical trials. There is not enough time or money to follow up on every lead. A clinical trial of any new drug is an educated bet.

New medications for pain, for many reasons, are especially hard to find. Pain is a human experience; it is hard to measure. It does not have size like a tumor, and cannot be counted like white blood cells or measured like height or weight. There is, at this time, no validated biomarker for pain. Clinical trials depend on subjective responses of the participants who are asked to rate their pain on scales that go from 0 to 10. The responses may vary depending on the setting and can be skewed by fatigue, patient expectations, or distraction. A high rate of placebo response further confounds analysis. There is a history of candidate molecules, initially considered as promising, which were later eliminated from the development pipeline because clinical trials did not show efficacy, or because of a wrong choice of dosing, or because of safety concerns or side effects which restricted tolerability, or because, in that particular trial, there was an unusually robust response to placebo.

How, then, might the likelihood of developing a new pain medication be maximized? Organizations that choose to search for more effective pain medications are increasingly looking for demonstration *in humans* that a specific molecule in the body (a "target") plays an important role in a disease process, and that inhibiting or enhancing the function of this molecule ("targeting" it or "engaging" it) has a measureable and clinically significant effect in human beings. This is called "human validation."

Once a molecular target is identified and validated, a next step is the identification of molecules that have an action on it, hopefully in a specific way, so that side effects due to actions on other "off-target" molecules can be minimized. This part of the process often begins with high-throughput screening. To do this, cells that express the target molecule are grown in tissue culture, and robotic technology is used to screen hundreds of thousands of compounds from reference libraries. When a "hit," or a compound that has a significant effect on the target, is found, it is counterscreened against cells that express other molecules to confirm that it does not act on off-target molecules to cause unacceptable side effects such as cardiac arrhythmias due to an unwanted action on the heart. Chemists then build upon the identification of the "lead compound" by modifying it, turning to other related compounds in the library, or rationally designing compounds that even more effectively engage the target. The goal is a therapeutic compound that optimizes traits such as absorption, distribution within the body, duration of action, excretion, and side effects. Experiments are then done to screen for toxicity and deleterious side effects.

A good outcome in preclinical experiments sets the stage for clinical studies. These occur in four phases: Phase I clinical studies are carried out in a small number of healthy human subjects to assess safety, find a safe dosage range, and identify side effects. This is usually the first time that the compound has been studied within human subjects. A drop in blood pressure, nausea, headache, or a rash can halt the progress of the drug at this stage. If unacceptable side effects are not seen, studies on the compound can move to Phase II where efficacy is initially assessed in small numbers of patients. Phase II studies represent a critical proof-of-principle step in development of a new medication, and in many cases the results of these studies are used to determine whether the drug will advance to Phase III studies, in which larger numbers of human subjects are assessed to confirm efficacy, monitor side effects, and establish dose regimens. It is not uncommon for a drug to fail, that is, not to show efficacy or to cause an expected adverse effect, during Phase III; when that happens, it can be the end of the road for that compound. Finally, after successful completion of Phase III studies and approval by the appropriate regulatory agencies such as the U.S. Food and Drug Administration (FDA) or the European Medications Agency (EMA), Phase IV studies gather information on the effects of the drug in larger populations and monitor for toxicity and side effects with long-term use.

All of this takes time and money. One review (Morgan et al. 2011) reported cost estimates for development of a new medication that ranged from $161 million to $1.8 billion. The higher estimates, of more than $1 billion (DiMasi, Hansen, and Grabowski 2003; Herper 2012) factor in the research costs of drugs that do not succeed in the clinical marketplace and average them together with the research costs of drugs that are successfully licensed and manufactured. The successful drug, according to this type of analysis, pays the cost of other compounds that failed to make it through the development pipeline. Other estimates peg the cost of development of a new medication as being lower, of the order of several hundred million dollars (Klotz 2014). But, irrespective of how these costs are analyzed, the bottom line is clear: Development of new medications is risky and expensive. And the challenges are especially daunting in the search for new medications for pain.

From Theory toward Therapy

By 2007, I was receiving requests for help from people with the man on fire syndrome from around the world. The entreaties from parents were especially moving. It was clear from their stories that some of these children had erythromelalgia. I answered each call or email with a message as positive as I could make it: We had reason to be hopeful and were searching for new treatments.

My hope was based on the expectation that, by selectively blocking $Na_V1.7$ with new drugs, it might be possible to relieve pain. It was also buoyed by knowledge that more than half a dozen large pharmaceutical companies, and a cohort of smaller biotech companies, were trying to develop subtype-specific channel blockers that would inhibit the activity of $Na_V1.7$, leaving other sodium channel subtypes unblocked (Sun, Cohen, and Dehnhardt 2014). I was talking with many of them. An obvious question, as these compounds were being developed, was which patients to test them in. People on fire represented an obvious choice. Their pain was unequivocally produced by the activity of $Na_V1.7$ channels. Except for unusual families carrying rare pharmacoresponsive mutations (Fischer et al. 2009; Geha et al. 2016) there were no effective treatments for the man on fire syndrome. It represented an unmet medical need and a test bed.

In 2009 I began to talk substantively with Pfizer, a large multinational biopharmaceutical company, about a joint effort to assess the $Na_V1.7$ blockers they were developing. As our discussions moved forward, they converged on PF-05089771, one of the first subtype-specific blockers of $Na_V1.7$. PF-05089771 was originally invented by a research team headed by neuroscientist Douglas Krafte and chemist Chris West at Icagen, a young biotech company located in the North Carolina's Research Triangle Park. Pfizer was partnering with Icagen and ultimately acquired the smaller company in 2011.

PF-05089771 was designed to block $Na_V1.7$ by binding to the $Na_V1.7$ channel's voltage sensor (McCormack et al. 2013). Whether it would be "the" $Na_V1.7$ blocker with the optimal efficacy, absorption, and excretion profiles needed to take a new medication to the clinic was not clear to me. But PF-05089771 had a strong inhibitory effect on $Na_V1.7$. It was selective, with potency against $Na_V1.7$ that was 10-fold and 16-fold higher than for $Na_V1.2$ and $Na_V1.6$ (the two other members of the Na_V sodium channel family that most closely resembled $Na_V1.7$), and it was even more selective over other sodium channel isoforms (Alexandrou et al. 2016). This meant that PF-05089771 could block $Na_V1.7$ channels while leaving other sodium channels free to operate. It could be taken by mouth as a pill. At a minimum PF-05089771, which we started calling 771, presented an opportunity for a proof-of-concept trial of $Na_V1.7$ blockade in human beings.

The hub of Pfizer's pain research program was sited at the Pfizer Neusentis laboratories in Cambridge, England. After Yale and Pfizer signed a collaboration agreement, Ruth McKernan, the Neusentis chief scientific officer, flew to New Haven with her staff for a planning session. Our meetings began with a working dinner at Tre Scalini, an Italian restaurant in the shadow of the Quinnipiac Bridge that connects New Haven with the Connecticut shoreline. All of us, at Yale and at Pfizer, were excited. We were going to assess 771 in human subjects in whom we *knew* $Na_V1.7$ was the cause of pain.

On May 2, 2011, Yale issued a press release entitled "*YALE SCHOOL OF MEDICINE FORMS COLLABORATION WITH ICAGEN AND PFIZER TO INVESTIGATE POTENTIAL NOVEL PAIN TREATMENTS.*" It read, in part, "Yale School of Medicine has entered into a collaboration with Icagen, Inc. and Pfizer to explore the potential efficacy of investigational compounds as novel treatments for pain. These compounds, which were identified from an existing collaboration between Icagen and Pfizer, may be useful in treating pain in people with a rare genetic disorder called inherited erythromelalgia (IEM), or the 'man on fire syndrome'." We did not know, as this press release was published, that our studies on 771 would capitalize on stem cell technology that could provide, as a model, "pain in a dish."

Enabler

No two snowflakes are exactly alike. No two people are exactly alike. No two people with inherited erythromelalgia are exactly alike. And, to make things even more complex, for a person with inherited erythromelalgia no two days are alike. We needed to learn all we could about every person who might participate in a trial of 771. So, as a prelude to a clinical trial, we decided to do an observational study to quantitatively assess the clinical features of people with inherited erythromelalgia. This study, directed by Pfizer clinician Aoibhinn McDonnell, was designed to provide a high-resolution picture of the disease. The "in-house" evaluation was to take place at Pfizer's Clinical Research Unit in New Haven, located directly across Frontage Road from Yale Medical School. Remarkably, although the Pfizer Clinical Research Unit had been built next to Yale Medical School to foster collaborations, as we began this investigation, there was no precedent for Yale physicians or scientists to work within the Pfizer unit, and the lawyers on both sides initially argued about issues like indemnification which we, as scientists, had not considered. Multiple rounds of discussions by the Yale and Pfizer lawyers yielded offer and counteroffer, but no solution. In August, 2010, I wrote to Yale's deputy dean, "We believe that selective blockers of $Na_V1.7$ might provide novel, potent treatments for pain. Pfizer has several candidate compounds and we would like to study them in our patients with EM. ... Our plan is to carry out this study at the Pfizer CRU where the infrastructure is in place. ... Thus far we have hit a brick wall." A few weeks later, the legal agreements were signed.

For this study thirteen participants with a well-established diagnosis of inherited erythromelalgia, known in each case to be caused by a pathogenic $Na_V1.7$ mutation, were invited to travel from throughout the country to be initially evaluated in detail over a three-day period at the Clinical Research Unit, and then followed day by day during a three-month at-home phase, during which they would fill in a detailed pain record. We wanted to learn, for each participant, when pain episodes occurred, what triggered the pain, how severe the pain was, how long pain attacks lasted, and whether the pain varied from attack to attack. Since $Na_V1.7$ was known to be present in olfactory sensory neurons (Ahn et al. 2011; Weiss et al. 2011), we planned to measure olfactory thresholds in each subject. And, since we knew that $Na_V1.7$ was present within neurons within autonomic ganglia (Rush et al. 2006), we intended to assess heart rate and blood pressures. Finally, we planned to collect information about the psychological status of the subjects. Since we hoped it would help us to design our clinical trial, we called this observational investigation the Enabler study.

One challenge was how to arrange travel of subjects to New Haven. Prior to the study, one subject wrote the following:

Dear Dr. Waxman,

Flying anytime can be extremely challenging for us. Though we can use wheelchairs at airports, this does not enable us to avoid the primary culprit of our pain, the elevated temperatures (anything above 68 degrees). Waiting in long security lines and hot jetways, then boarding an airplane with warm (or no) airflow will usually start a flare that can continue for days. The rising cost of fuel discourages commercial airlines from using A/C and it seems even worse in warmer months. Probably because of six abreast seating, the back of the plane is even hotter than the front...

She continued,

_____'s last airplane trip was an emergency flight to _____ where first class was the only available seating. She said it wasn't nearly as bad as previous flights in coach, since the first-class cabin was cooler than the back, and there was space to elevate her legs. Additionally, the flight attendants had time to maintain towels wrapped ice packs for her burning feet... I am almost embarrassed to ask, knowing it's very presumptuous, but is it at all possible to get first class tickets to participate in the study?

We arranged for upgraded travel, in the front of the airplane.

It was a challenge, but all thirteen individuals, each carrying a mutation of $Na_V1.7$ that had previously been analyzed in detail, participated in Enabler. After their logs were completed, Pfizer statisticians and data analysts went to work. Viewed from 30,000 feet, our thirteen patients, considered as a whole, fit nicely within the criteria for erythromelalgia: burning pain in their limbs, symmetrical, triggered by warmth. But at a more granular level, looked at patient by patient and day by day, we saw a more complex picture. Our patients described a spectrum of triggers for their pain. Their logs displayed variability in the number and duration of attacks. The intensity of pain varied day to day, even for subjects carrying the same mutation within a family. And there was variability in the pattern of pain within single subjects. This was an important finding. It meant that for a clinical trial of PF-05089771 we would need to provoke pain with calibrated, reproducible triggers—carefully controlled warmth—so that the level of pain would be relatively constant. We would have to consider each patient individually; each subject would serve as his or her own control.

Surprisingly, despite their history of chronic pain, on psychological testing we found that only two subjects displayed signs of moderate anxiety and depression. Five of the thirteen subjects had psychological scores below the threshold for mild anxiety or depression. None of the subjects was severely anxious or depressed. These people on fire were coping well with the disease. Perhaps this was a selection artifact, since it is possible that only individuals who were feeling psychologically well opted to participate in Enabler. Alternatively, it was possible that the mere act of participating in this study could have had a positive effect on the psychological well-being of the participants, possibly even affecting the level of their pain.

Pfizer took the lead in writing up the Enabler paper (McDonnell et al. 2016). Patience is not one of my virtues, and I grumbled via telephone and email about a pace of writing that was slower than I would have liked. The paper was submitted to *Brain* in May of 2015 and was returned by the editor for revision a few months later. Revision, too, proceeded at what I felt was a snail-like pace. The paper was finally resubmitted and accepted late in 2015. It was published in the February 2016 issue of *Brain*. But regardless of the time course, it presented a day-to-day picture, not previously available in the medical literature, of the experience of people on fire.

Now, armed with the detailed picture of men on fire provided by Enabler, we were poised to move forward with a Phase II "proof-of-principle" study testing, for the first time, the hypothesis that this family of compounds—subtype-specific $Na_V1.7$ blockers, in this case built on a sulfonamide scaffold—could reduce pain that unequivocally arose from the activity on $Na_V1.7$. We had learned from Enabler that, because of day-to-day variation in pain, we would have to provoke pain attacks. We spent months discussing the pros and cons of various methods for provoking pain and even considered constructing a series of test chambers, each at a different temperature. We finally decided on a carefully calibrated blanket-like heating device. Months were spent designing a randomized, double-blind crossover study. After review and approval by an ethics review board, five subjects with inherited erythromelalgia, previously assessed in Enabler, each known to carry a $Na_V1.7$ mutation that had been characterized and shown to cause their disease, enrolled in this study. They ranged from eighteen to seventy-eight years of age. Each of these people made a second trip to Pfizer's New Haven Clinical Research Unit for the 771 study, beginning in October of 2012.

Each subject was to receive two single oral doses of 771 and two doses of placebo. To ensure blinding, the doses of 771 and placebo were precisely matched, both in appearance and in size. Neither the subjects, nor the doctors, knew whether 771 or placebo was given on any given occasion. When the study was finally "unblinded," we hoped that it would give us a glimpse of the effect of blockade of $Na_V1.7$ on pain in human beings.

Disease in a Dish

You only get to be "first" once. It is not often that one gets to do a study of this type, and we wanted to learn all we could from it. Clinical efficacy was being measured from the ratings of the subjects, who scored their pain after being heated on a scale of 0 to 10, while receiving either 771 or placebo. But it was important to know precisely how 771 did its job. As I recall, it was Ruth McKernan who suggested that we might also assess the drug's effect at the cellular site of action, on sensory neurons carrying mutant $Na_V1.7$ channels. The plan was to use newly developed stem cell technology to dedifferentiate blood cells from each subject, to turn them into pluripotent stem cells (sometimes called induced pluripotent stem cells, iPSC or iPS cells). These remarkable cells, produced by methods (Takahashi and Yamanaka 2006) that heralded the Nobel Prize in 2012, have been described as "chang(ing) biomedical research forever" (Papapetrou 2016). iPSC can be derived from a specific person and contain that person's DNA. They have the capability, if prompted by the right mix of chemicals, to redifferentiate into any desired type of cell. In this instance we would create pain-signaling nerve cells from the iPS cells from each subject, in a sense providing a replica of that subject's DRG neurons complete with the subject's DNA. These iPS cell–derived sensory neurons could then be maintained in culture for study. This would permit us to be sure that any blunting of pain by 771 was not a nonspecific effect, but rather was due to an action of the drug on pain-signaling sensory neurons, derived for each subject, that contained *his or her particular mutation* in the context of *his or her entire genome*. Four of the five subjects agreed to provide a blood sample.

The creation of sensory neurons from iPSC was going to be a major undertaking, requiring substantial effort and expertise. Pfizer had both. Using technology developed at Memorial Sloan Kettering Medical Center in New York (Chambers et al. 2012), Pfizer cell biologists carefully generated iPS cells from the blood cells of these four subjects and from controls. The iPS cells from each of the four subjects were treated over weeks with a carefully designed mixture of factors to transform them into sensory neurons (Cao et al., 2016). Week by week, the iPS cells grew in the laboratory. Within their sterile dishes, the cells slowly took on the shape of neurons and were labeled by special stains that specifically mark sensory neurons. They generated nerve impulses just like neurons and, indeed, contained $Na_V1.7$ channels at levels close to those observed in pain-signaling nerve cells from living animals. They were differentiating into sensory neurons.

Even more remarkable, the iPSC-derived sensory neurons from our subjects exhibited the hallmarks of DRG neurons in erythromelalgia: They were hyperexcitable, firing spontaneously even in the absence of stimulation. They had lower-than-normal thresholds so that they generated nerve impulses in response to small stimuli that normally would not evoke a response. And, the iPSC-derived nerve cells reproduced the hypersensitivity to warmth that is characteristic of inherited erythromelalgia. Even modest temperature increases reduced the threshold of these cells. This was "inherited erythromelalgia-in-a-dish."

Sensory neurons that recapitulated the clinical picture of inherited erythromelalgia, derived from each subject's iPSC, growing in sterile dishes and available for study, meant that it was now possible to ask whether 771 reduced the hyperexcitability that causes pain in people with the man on fire syndrome. Without even touching a patient, the effect of 771 could be assessed in "their" sensory neurons, or at least sensory neurons created in the laboratory that contained all 20,000 of their genes. The results were published in the paper that follows (Cao et al. 2016); 771 reduced the elevated excitability of these "erythromelalgia-in-a-dish" neurons, increasing their threshold and inhibiting their spontaneous firing. Another obvious question was whether a $Na_V1.7$ blocker like 771 would reverse the elevated sensitivity to warmth in iPSC-derived sensory neurons from our erythromelalgia patients.

And it did.

Waiting While Blinded

iPS cells and neurons derived from them are one thing, and intact living human beings are another. To assess the effect of 771 on pain, our subjects were randomized and asked to report the severity of their pain after an attack was provoked with a heating blanket. There were two treatment sessions. During each session each subject received 771 or a placebo and then "crossed over" to receive the other (Cao et al. 2016). The subjects did not know whether they had received 771 or placebo and were asked to rate their pain along a numerical rating scale (NRS) where 0 = no pain and 10 = the worst pain imaginable.

Because we as well as our research subjects were blinded, as the months rolled by, I did not know whether the drug had an effect. Then, in September 2013 I traveled to the UK to give a lecture at the Hodgkin–Huxley Symposium at Cambridge University. The symposium was a success, and my wife and I got to meet Karl Deisseroth, the inventor of optogenetics, whose room was next to ours in the Trinity Master's Lodge. But a highlight of the trip was a meeting at Trinity College with the Pfizer team. The trial was now complete, and the Pfizer investigators were finally unblinded. Their statisticians were still analyzing the results, carefully comparing the response to 771 with response to placebo. Preliminary indications suggested that the outcome was promising. The results of the final analysis, which took a few months more, are summarized in figure 6 of Cao et al. (2016). Pain was reduced by single doses of 771 in at least one of the treatment sessions in a majority of the subjects, and in two of the five subjects, pain was reduced by 771 during both of the two testing sessions. In four of the ten runs (two runs for each of the five patients), the difference in pain score for 771 compared to placebo was about three points on the NRS—a substantial effect. Here, from a small group of patients, we had a promising signal that blocking $Na_V1.7$ might cool the flames of the man on fire syndrome.

I could not help but smile as we discussed the relief of pain in human beings, by a new class of compounds that acted in a unique way to inhibit a specific type of sodium channel. After all, we were meeting at the college at Cambridge University where Hodgkin and Huxley had been fellows more than six decades previously when, while studying the giant axon of the squid, they discovered sodium channels.

An interesting sidenote was that 771 did not reverse the elevated sensitivity to heat in the iPSC-derived sensory neurons from one subject. For this subject, heat-evoked pain was not reduced by 771. The difference in the effect of 771 on iPSC-derived sensory neurons from the different subjects may have been trying to tell us something. The number of subjects was small, but, when we compared the severity of the clinical picture with the hyperexcitability of the iPSC-derived sensory neurons for each subject, and compared the effect of 771 as depicted by the patients' pain scores with its effect on hyperexcitability of their iPSC-derived sensory neurons, we saw a trend toward a correlation (Cao et al. 2016). This led us to suggest that the "disease-in-a-dish" model provided by iPSC-derived sensory neurons might, in the future, be used for screening putative new therapies.

Pfizer presented our clinical results in October 2014 at the 15th World Congress of the International Association for the Study of Pain in Buenos Aires (Hutchison et al. 2014). The abstract, published in the meeting's proceedings, noted that "in a subgroup of patients who were administered a potent and selective inhibitor of $Na_V1.7$ in a single dose, placebo-controlled crossover clinical trial, there was evidence of a clinical benefit with respect to maximum pain intensity." I previously had been held silent by the confidentiality clauses that appear in most university–industry agreements, but now, at least in a broad-brush way, I could talk about the trial. Shortly after the IASP meeting I gave the Soriano lecture, one of the major lectures at the annual meeting of the American Neurological Association. A day or two before my talk I inserted a new final slide, ending my lecture:

Where next?
Early clinical studies on genomically characterized human subjects have now been carried out. While the sample sizes are small, early results are beginning to provide proof-of-principle that blocking of $Na_V1.7$ can reduce pain in some subjects. These results suggest that a new, more effective class of pain medications, with minimal central side effects, devoid of addictive potential, is an *Achievable Objective*.

Altogether, it took more than six years from the time I began working with Pfizer until the Cao et al. (2016) paper was published. More than fifty Pfizer scientists worked on the project together with my team at Yale. It had taken nearly twelve years to translate from our early demonstration of the functional abnormalities in $Na_V1.7$ mutant channels and showing how they cause erythromelalgia (Cummins, Dib-Hajj, and Waxman 2004; Dib-Hajj et al. 2005) to a clinical trial that targeted $Na_V1.7$ (Cao et al.

2016). A long journey. But we now had new experimental tools capitalizing on stem cell technology. We had shown that the activity of Na$_V$1.7 channels could be inhibited with a drug. And we had evidence that pain could be reduced by blocking of Na$_V$1.7 channels. Several small-molecule blockers of Na$_V$1.7, as well as antibodies that inhibited this channel and gene therapy approaches that turned off the production of the channels, were under study. The important point was that, no matter which mode of blocking the activity of Na$_V$1.7 would prove to be optimal, we had evidence that it was possible to reduce pain in humans by targeting Na$_V$1.7 or the gene that encodes it.

Science Translational Medicine provisionally accepted the paper describing our iPSC results and clinical observations in late March 2016 with a request that we make some stylistic changes, redraw several figures, come up with a better title, and submit the final version by 5 p.m. on March 30. After much to-and-fro between New Haven and Cambridge, England, we sent in the final version fifteen minutes before the deadline. The paper was accepted a few days later, and I dashed off congratulatory notes to Ruth, Aoibhinn, and the other authors. It was published in *Science Translational Medicine* on April 20th of 2016 (Cao et al. 2016). Now I could change my response to questions from people on fire and from the parents of children on fire. I began to write back "I can't promise, and I can't predict how long it will take, but I am encouraged. We have a powerful set of tools and a target that matters, and I believe that, sooner or later, there are likely to be new treatments for your pain."

References

Ahn HS, Black JA, Zhao P, Tyrrell L, Waxman SG, Dib-Hajj SD. 2011. Nav1.7 is the predominant sodium channel in rodent olfactory sensory neurons. *Mol Pain* 7: 32.

Alexandrou AJ, Brown AR, Chapman ML, Estacion M, Turner J, Mis MA, Wilbrey A, et al. 2016. Subtype-selective small molecule inhibitors reveal a fundamental role for Nav1.7 in nociceptor electrogenesis, axonal conduction and presynaptic release. *PLoS One* 11(4): e0152405.

Cao L, McDonnell A, Nitzsche A, Alexandrou A, Saintot PP, Loucif AJ, Brown AR, et al. 2016. Pharmacological reversal of a pain phenotype in iPSC-derived sensory neurons and patients with inherited erythromelalgia. *Sci Transl Med* 8(335): 335ra56.

Chambers SM, Qi Y, Mica Y, Lee G, Zhang XJ, Niu L, Bilsland J, et al. 2012. Combined small-molecule inhibition accelerates developmental timing and converts human pluripotent stem cells into nociceptors. *Nat Biotechnol* 30(7): 715–720.

Cummins TR, Dib-Hajj SD, Waxman SG. 2004. Electrophysiological properties of mutant Nav1.7 sodium channels in a painful inherited neuropathy. *J Neurosci* 24(38): 8232–8236.

Dib-Hajj SD, Rush AM, Cummins TR, Hisama FM, Novella S, Tyrrell L, Marshall L, Waxman SG. 2005. Gain-of-function mutation in Nav1.7 in familial erythromelalgia induces bursting of sensory neurons. *Brain* 128(Pt 8): 1847–1854.

DiMasi JA, Hansen RW, Grabowski HG. 2003. The price of innovation: New estimates of drug development costs. *J Health Econ* 22(2): 151–185.

Fischer TZ, Gilmore ES, Estacion M, Eastman E, Taylor S, Melanson M, Dib-Hajj SD, Waxman SG. 2009. A novel Nav1.7 mutation producing carbamazepine-responsive erythromelalgia. *Ann Neurol* 65(6): 733–741.

Geha P, Yang Y, Estacion M, Schulman BR, Tokuno H, Apkarian AV, Dib-Hajj SD, Waxman SG. 2016. Pharmacotherapy for pain in a family with inherited erythromelalgia guided by genomic analysis and functional profiling. *JAMA Neurol* 73(6): 659–667.

Herper, M. 2012. "The truly staggering cost of inventing new drugs." *Forbes.com.*

Hutchison JB, Butt R, Dib-Hajj S, Estacion M, Kirby S, McDonnell A, Ali Z, Chapman M, Schulman B, Waxman SG. 2014. "Inherited erythromelalgia: A potential target for a personalised medicine." Presentation TW001, 15th World Congress on Pain, IASP, Beunos, Aires, Argentina.

Klotz, L. 2014. "What is the real drug development cost for very small biotech companies?" *Genetic Engineering & Biotechnology News*, epub Jan. 16.

McCormack K, Santos S, Chapman ML, Krafte DS, Marron BE, West CW, Krambis MJ, et al. 2013. Voltage sensor interaction site for selective small molecule inhibitors of voltage-gated sodium channels. *Proc Natl Acad Sci USA* 110(29): E2724–E2732.

McDonnell A, Schulman B, Ali Z, Dib-Hajj SD, Brock F, Cobain S, Mainka T, Vollert J, Tarabar S, Waxman SG. 2016. Inherited erythromelalgia due to mutations in SCN9A: Natural history, clinical phenotype and somatosensory profile. *Brain* 139(Pt 4): 1052–1065.

Morgan S, Grootendorst P, Lexchin J, Cunningham C, Greyson D. 2011. The cost of drug development: A systematic review. *Health Policy* 100(1): 4–17.

Papapetrou EP. 2016. Induced pluripotent stem cells, past and future. *Science* 353(6303): 991–992.

Rush AM, Dib-Hajj SD, Liu S, Cummins TR, Black JA, Waxman SG. 2006. A single sodium channel mutation produces hyper- or hypoexcitability in different types of neurons. *Proc Natl Acad Sci USA* 103(21): 8245–8250.

Sun S, Cohen CJ, Dehnhardt CM. 2014. Inhibitors of voltage-gated sodium channel Nav1.7: Patent applications since 2010. *Pharm Pat Anal* 3(5): 509–521.

Takahashi K, Yamanaka S. 2006. Induction of pluripotent stem cells from mouse embryonic and adult fibroblast cultures by defined factors. *Cell* 126(4): 663–676.

Weiss J, Pyrski M, Jacobi E, Bufe B, Willnecker V, Schick B, Zizzari P, et al. 2011. Loss-of-function mutations in sodium channel Nav1.7 cause anosmia. *Nature* 472(7342): 186–190.

PHARMACOLOGICAL REVERSAL OF A PAIN PHENOTYPE IN iPSC-DERIVED SENSORY NEURONS AND PATIENTS WITH INHERITED ERYTHROMELALGIA*

Lishuang Cao, Aoibhinn McDonnell, Anja Nitzsche, Aristos Alexandrou, Pierre-Philippe Saintot, Alexandre J.C. Loucif, Adam R. Brown, Gareth Young, Malgorzata Mis, Andrew Randall, Stephen G. Waxman, Philip Stanley, Simon Kirby, Sanela Tarabar, Alex Gutteridge, Richard Butt, Ruth M. McKernan, Paul Whiting, Zahid Ali, James Bilsland, and Edward B. Stevens

In common with other chronic pain conditions, there is an unmet clinical need in the treatment of inherited erythromelalgia (IEM). The *SCN9A* gene encoding the sodium channel $Na_V1.7$ expressed in the peripheral nervous system plays a critical role in IEM. A gain-of-function mutation in this sodium channel leads to aberrant sensory neuronal activity and extreme pain, particularly in response to heat. Five patients with IEM were treated with a new potent and selective compound that blocked the $Na_V1.7$ sodium channel resulting in a decrease in heat-induced pain in most of the patients. We derived induced pluripotent stem cell (iPSC) lines from four of five subjects and produced sensory neurons that emulated the clinical phenotype of hyperexcitability and aberrant responses to heat stimuli. When we compared the severity of the clinical phenotype with the hyperexcitability of the iPSC-derived sensory neurons, we saw a trend toward a correlation for individual mutations. The in vitro IEM phenotype was sensitive to $Na_V1.7$ blockers, including the clinical test agent. Given the importance of peripherally expressed sodium channels in many pain conditions, our approach may have broader utility for a wide range of pain and sensory conditions.

Introduction

Individual *SCN9A* mutations leading to a loss of channel function have been associated with congenital insensitivity to pain, whereas gain-of-function mutations in the *SCN9A* gene have been associated with chronic painful conditions including inherited erythromelalgia (IEM), paroxysmal

* Previously published in *Science Translational Medicine* 8(335): 335ra56, 2016.

extreme pain disorder, and idiopathic small fiber neuropathy. IEM is a chronic, extreme pain condition that results in burning pain sensations and erythema, particularly in the distal extremities.[1-4] The pain is often episodic and mild heat or a body temperature increase is a common major trigger for attacks of pain in IEM.[4]

The development of selective $Na_V1.7$ blockers, in common with other new analgesic drug targets, has been hampered by the lack of robust preclinical to clinical translation. In particular, a complete understanding of the role of $Na_V1.7$ in action potential firing in human sensory neurons has been limited by the reliance of electrophysiological studies on heterologous expression of the channel. For example, all reported IEM $Na_V1.7$ mutations are associated with a hyperpolarized voltage dependence of activation and/or voltage dependence of fast inactivation after heterologous expression in mammalian cell lines.[5-11] However, the absolute value and magnitude of changes in gating parameters for individual IEM mutations vary between different laboratories and may not directly translate to native $Na_V1.7$ in human sensory neurons.[5,6,10] Overexpression of IEM $Na_V1.7$ mutations in mouse dorsal root ganglion neurons has been used to understand the contribution of the changes in channel gating to action potential firing properties.[12] The interpretation is, however, compromised by the expression level of human $Na_V1.7$ relative to rodent tetrodotoxin-sensitive sodium channels and appropriate processing and assembly of the human isoform in a rodent neuronal background. Human pluripotent stem cell (PSC)–derived sensory neurons[13,14] provide an improved physiologically relevant model to investigate the relationship between a human ion channel in its native environment and neuronal excitability.

Induced PSC (iPSC) technology allows generation of cells from patients, which retain the genetic identity of the donor and can recapitulate disease pathology in differentiated progeny. This has the potential to enable new therapeutics to be tested on both individual patients and their cognate iPSC-derived cells to further understand both clinical efficacy and effects on the underlying cellular phenotype. However, to date, it is unclear to what extent the response of a therapeutic agent in an iPSC disease model translates to the clinic.

Here, we investigated the effect of a new selective Na$_V$1.7 blocker, PF-05089771, on the inhibition of heat-evoked pain in five IEM human subjects carrying four different SCN9A mutations. Simultaneously, we generated iPSC-derived sensory neurons (iPSC-SNs) from four of five IEM subjects to characterize the neuronal phenotype associated with individual mutations and the effects of selectively blocking Na$_V$1.7 channels on action potential generation.

Results

Differentiating iPSCs from IEM Patients into Functional Sensory Neurons

Five IEM subjects (three males and two females; average age of 40.2 years) (table 1) provided informed consent to participate in a double-blind, placebo-controlled clinical study. Extensive clinical phenotyping had previously been performed in these subjects.[4] Four of five subjects additionally consented to donate blood for iPSC generation (table 1).

Peripheral blood mononuclear cells were extracted from donated blood samples. The erythroid progenitor populations of the peripheral blood cells were reprogrammed into iPSCs, and up to three clonal iPSC lines per subject were established. Individual heterozygous mutations in the iPSCs were confirmed through Sanger sequencing (figure 1A). We also generated iPSCs from four independent non-IEM donors who were used as a control group in which no mutations in Na$_V$1.7 associated with paroxysmal extreme pain disorder, IEM, or congenital insensitivity to pain were identified. All iPSC clonal cell lines showed typical morphology for pluripotent cell colonies and expressed the pluripotency marker Oct4 (figure 1B). Array comparative genomic hybridization (CGH) analysis revealed a normal karyotype and comparable number or size of copy number variants between non-IEM

Table 1
Clinical Phenotype of IEM Subjects

Subject ID	SCN9A mutation	Gender	Age at onset of IEM (year)	Pain attack trigger	Consent* to donate blood for iPSC
EM1	S241T	F	17	Heat, exercise	Yes
EM2	I848T	M	4	Heat, exercise	Yes
EM3	V400M	M	>10	Heat, exercise, standing	Yes
EM4	V400M	M	4	Heat, exercise	No
EM5	F1449V	F	<2	Heat, exercise, standing	Yes

*Consent to donate blood for iPSC generation was optional for subjects in the clinical study.

donor and IEM subject iPSCs for most iPSC clones (figure S1, A and B).

We differentiated iPSCs into sensory neurons using a small molecule-based protocol as described previously.[13,14] One week after addition of neural growth factors, the differentiated cells exhibited a neuronal morphology and stained positive for the sensory neuron markers Brn3a, Islet1, and peripherin, with no obvious morphological difference between donor- and study subject–derived neurons (figure 1C). Neurons were further matured for another 8 weeks before electrophysiological recordings were obtained. The sensory neurons derived from non-IEM and IEM clonal iPSC lines all expressed *SCN9A* and other sodium channel subtypes as determined by quantitative polymerase chain reaction (qPCR) (figure S1C). To characterize the functional role of the $Na_V1.7$ channel in iPSC-SNs using a whole-cell patch-clamp technique, two selective $Na_V1.7$ blockers were exploited: the clinical compound PF-05089771 and an in vitro tool PF-05153462 (figure S2, A to C). In comparison to the slow kinetics of inhibition for PF-05089771, PF-05153462 displayed fast rates of blockade and was fully reversible within 10 min, enabling multiple concentrations to be applied to each cell and therefore allowing a more extensive and robust investigation of the contribution of $Na_V1.7$ to sensory neuron excitability.

Application of PF-05153462 reversibly inhibited the peak sodium current of iPSC-SNs, confirming the functional expression of $Na_V1.7$. Comparison of the $Na_V1.7$ current densities (as defined using inhibition by 100 nM PF-05153462) across iPSC-SN clones revealed no significant differences between the individual clones or between the IEM and non-IEM groups [example traces, figure 1D; quantification, figure 1E; non-parametric analysis of variance (ANOVA), $P > 0.05$]. In addition, there was no significant difference in the percentage of total sodium current (figure S3A; nonparametric ANOVA, $P > 0.05$) or current carried by $Na_V1.7$ (figure S3B; non-parametric ANOVA, $P > 0.05$) across iPSC-SN clones. These data suggested robust and equivalent expression of $Na_V1.7$ channels in iPSC-SNs, irrespective of the donor from which they were generated.

iPSC-SNs Derived from IEM Subjects Show Elevated Excitability

We observed spontaneous action potential firing from a subpopulation of iPSC-SNs at resting membrane potential (figure 2A, right). On average, the iPSC-SNs from IEM donors showed a significantly higher proportion of spontaneously firing cells compared to those from non-IEM donors ($P < 0.05$, linear logistic model), suggesting higher excitability (figure 2B).

Notwithstanding this, iPSC-SNs from subject EM1 (with the S241T mutation) and non-IEM donor D1 showed similar degrees of spontaneous firing, which was only moderately enhanced compared to the other non-IEM donors, suggesting some intrinsic heterogeneity among the iPSC-SNs from both the IEM and non-IEM donors (figure 2B). There was a small but statistically significant depolarization of resting membrane potential in the IEM subject cells (-57.4 ± 0.4 mV; $n = 272$ with all IEM subjects pooled together) compared to non-IEM donor cells (-60 ± 0.4 mV; $n = 158$ for all non-IEM subjects) (figure S3C; $P < 0.05$, ANOVA), which could have contributed to the observed increase in spontaneous activity.

Next, we studied rheobase, the minimal current injection required to evoke an action potential, as a measure of subthreshold contributions to excitability (figure 2C). On average, the rheobase was lower in the iPSC-SNs from IEM donors (122 ± 10 pA; $n = 270$) when compared to neurons from non-IEM donors (361 ± 20 pA; $n = 148$) (figure 2D; $P < 0.05$, nonparametric ANOVA). These data suggest that iPSC-SNs from IEM subjects have increased excitability.

Figure 1
iPSCs from IEM subjects and non-IEM donors differentiate into sensory neurons with comparable Na$_V$1.7 activity. (A) Sanger sequencing of IEM subject–derived iPSCs. The black arrow highlights the heterozygous point mutation in the pherogram. (B) Bright-field images of representative examples of IEM subject–derived and non-IEM donor–derived iPSCs with typical pluripotent-like morphology. Scale bars, 1000 mm. Panels below show immunostaining for nuclear Hoechst stain (blue) and expression of the Oct4 pluripotency marker (green). Scale bars, 100 mm. DAPI, 4′,6-diamidino-2-phenylindole. (C) Bright-field images of representative examples of IEM subject–derived and non-IEM donor–derived iPSCs after differentiation into sensory neurons (iPSC-SNs). Scale bars, 1000 mm. Panels below show immunostaining for expression of the sensory neuron marker Brn3a (blue), Islet1 (red), and peripherin (green). Scale bars, 200 mm. (D) Example sodium current traces measured in the iPSC-SNs derived from the non-IEM donor (D4) and IEM subject EM5 (carrying the F1449V mutation) showing subtracted currents sensitive to the Na$_V$1.7 blocker. iPSC-SNs were held at −110 mV and stepped to 0 mV to evoke voltage-gated currents, which were partially blocked by 100 nM PF-05153462. (E) Summary of Na$_V$1.7 current density in the non-IEM donor–derived and IEM subject–derived iPSC-SNs. No significant difference was observed among all the clones ($n = 13$ to 40).

We also measured evoked firing frequency in response to increasing amplitude of injected current (figure 2E). Although IEM iPSC-SNs gave rise to a higher number of action potentials at low levels of current injection compared to non-IEM cells (figure 2F), there was considerable variability in the firing frequency between cells for each iPSC clone; thus, this was not considered a reliable end point for statistical analysis. Therefore, we focused on spontaneous firing and rheobase to determine pharmacological effects of Na$_V$1.7 blockers.

Na$_V$1.7 Blockers Reduce Elevated Excitability of IEM iPSC-SNs

We further tested the effects of the selective Na$_V$1.7 blocker PF-05153462 on spontaneously firing iPSC-SNs (figure 3A). As shown in figure 3B, the spontaneous firing of iPSC-SNs from subjects EM2 (I848T mutation) and EM3 (V400M mutation) was reduced by PF-05153462 in a concentration-dependent manner. iPSC-SNs from EM1 (S241T mutation) rarely exhibited spontaneous firing (figure 2B); therefore, PF-05153462 was not tested. The spontaneous firing in iPSC-SNs from EM5 (F1449V mutation) was not sustained for sufficient duration to generate a concentration-response curve; therefore, a single concentration of PF-05153462 (100 nM) was tested and found to completely inhibit spontaneous firing ($n = 5$). PF-05089771, the

Na$_V$1.7 blocker evaluated in IEM subjects, was also tested on iPSC-SNs from subject EM2, where spontaneous firing was completely blocked at a concentration of 60 nM (figure 3C). These data indicate that the gain-of-function mutations present in IEM Na$_V$1.7 channels contribute to the higher incidence of spontaneous firing in iPSC-SNs from IEM subjects.

Next, we investigated the contribution of wild-type and IEM mutant Na$_V$1.7 channels to rheobase of the action potential using PF-05089771 (figure 3D). Voltage-clamp recordings of human embryonic kidney 293 cells stably expressing mutant Na$_V$1.7 resulted in similar half-maximal inhibitory concentration (IC$_{50}$) values, ranging from 11 to 36 nM (figure S2D). Whereas PF-05089771 increased the rheobase in a concentration-dependent manner for iPSC-SNs from both IEM subjects and non-IEM donors (suggesting a clear role of Na$_V$1.7 in setting threshold), the magnitude of this effect was significantly greater in iPSC-SNs derived from IEM subjects at all three concentrations (figure 3E; $P < 0.05$, ANOVA; $n = 6$ to 10 for each concentration). Similar results were obtained from the selective Na$_V$1.7 blocker PF-05153462 at concentrations greater than 10 nM (figure 3F; $P < 0.05$, ANOVA; $n = 6$ to 10 for each concentration). The greater contribution of Na$_V$1.7 to rheobase in sensory neurons from IEM subjects compared to non-IEM donors most likely reflects

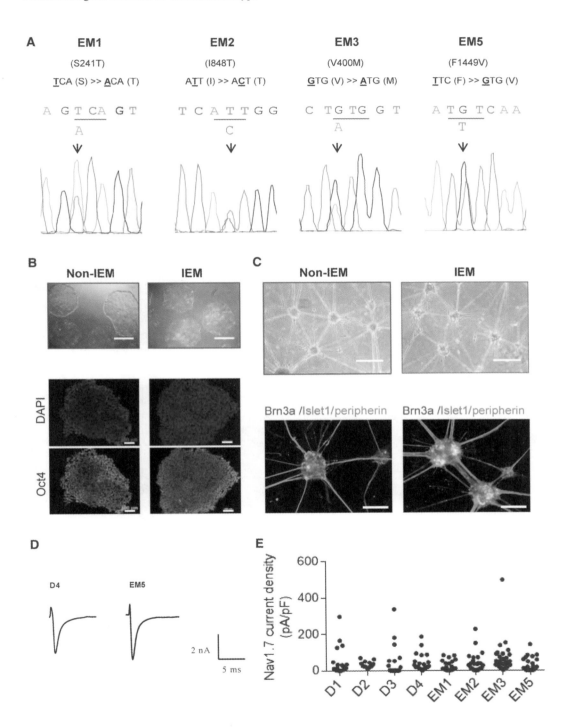

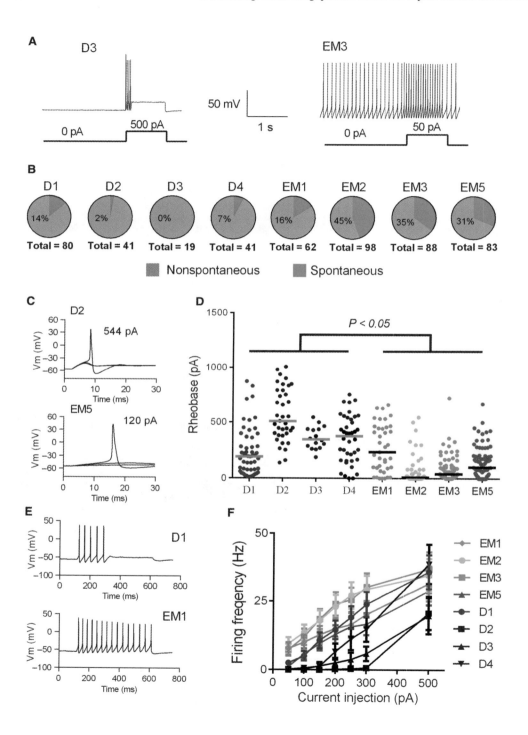

Figure 2

Excitability of iPSC-SNs from IEM and non-IEM subjects. (A) Representative traces of spontaneous firing in sensory neurons derived from iPSCs from IEM subject EM3 (V400M mutation) and non-IEM control subject D3. (B) Quantification of the number of spontaneous firing iPSC-SNs versus nonspontaneous firing iPSC-SNs from non-IEM and IEM subjects (n = 19 to 98; $P < 0.05$, linear logistic model). (C) Representative current-clamp traces showing subthreshold responses and subsequent action potentials evoked until reaching current thresholds (rheobase) of 544 pA for non-IEM subject D3 iPSC-SNs and 120 pA for IEM subject EM5 (F1449V mutation) iPSC-SNs. (D) Quantification of action potential rheobase comparing healthy control donor iPSC-SNs and IEM subject iPSC-SNs (n = 16 to 86; $P < 0.05$, nonparametric ANOVA). (E) Representative traces showing train of action potentials evoked in non-IEM control subject D1 and IEM subject EM1 (S241T mutation) iPSC-SNs after inducing depolarization by 100-pA current injection. (F) Quantification of action potential frequency induced by current injection (n = 10 to 46).

enhanced channel activity as a result of gating shifts associated with the S241T, I848T, V400M, and F1449V mutations. Together, these studies using $Na_V1.7$ blockers strongly suggest that these $Na_V1.7$ gain-of-function IEM mutations underpin the increased excitability of iPSC-SNs from IEM subjects.

Selective $Na_V1.7$ Blocker Reverses the Elevated Sensitivity to Heat in IEM iPSC-SNs

Action potential rheobase was tracked when the temperature was raised from 35° to 40°C (figure 4, A and B). In contrast to iPSC-SNs from the non-IEM donor group, the iPSC-SNs from the IEM subject group exhibited a significant decrease in rheobase in response to the modest temperature increase ($P < 0.01$, ANOVA; n = 13 to 34), indicating higher excitability of the IEM neurons upon heat stimulation. EM1 appeared to be an outlier with similar temperature sensitivity to healthy donor clones. These data suggested that the gain-of-function $Na_V1.7$ mutations in the iPSC-SNs from IEM subjects conferred an increase in excitability in response to heating at innocuous temperatures. As shown in figure 4 (C and D), 100 nM PF-0515462 was able to reverse the effect of increasing temperature on the rheobase in iPSC-SNs from subjects EM2 (I848T mutation), EM3 (V400M mutation), and EM5 (F1449V mutation) ($P < 0.05$, paired t test; n = 6 to 11) in cells with a positive rheobase response (>50 pA) to PF-05153462 at 35°C (an indication

of the functional expression of $Na_V1.7$). These data suggest that mutations in $Na_V1.7$ underlie the temperature sensitivity of IEM iPSC-SNs.

The change in temperature sensitivity after compound application was plotted against the effect of compound on rheobase at 35°C (figure 5), and a positive correlation was observed in iPSC-SNs from all EM subjects (Pearson's r = 0.22, 0.88, 0.82, and 0.77 for EM1, EM2, EM3, and EM5, respectively). The regression coefficients were significantly different from zero for iPSC-SNs from subjects EM2 (I848T mutation), EM3 (V400M mutation), and EM5 (F1449V mutation), suggesting that the amplitude of rheobase changes in response to heat was a function of available $Na_V1.7$ conductance. This effect was not evident in iPSC-SNs from subject EM1. Wild-type $Na_V1.7$ channels were also sensitive to changes in temperature (figure S4). Together, this analysis suggests that $Na_V1.7$ channels contribute to the elevated heat sensitivity of IEM iPSC-SNs.

Clinical Efficacy of the Selective $Na_V1.7$ Blocker PF-05089771

IEM subjects were randomized to participate in two independent treatment sessions (each consisting of two study periods) and to receive a single oral dose of either the $Na_V1.7$ blocker PF-05089771 or matched placebo in a crossover manner during each session. Evoked pain attacks were induced in subjects using a controlled heat stimulus applied to the extremities immediately before dosing and at intervals up to 24 hours after

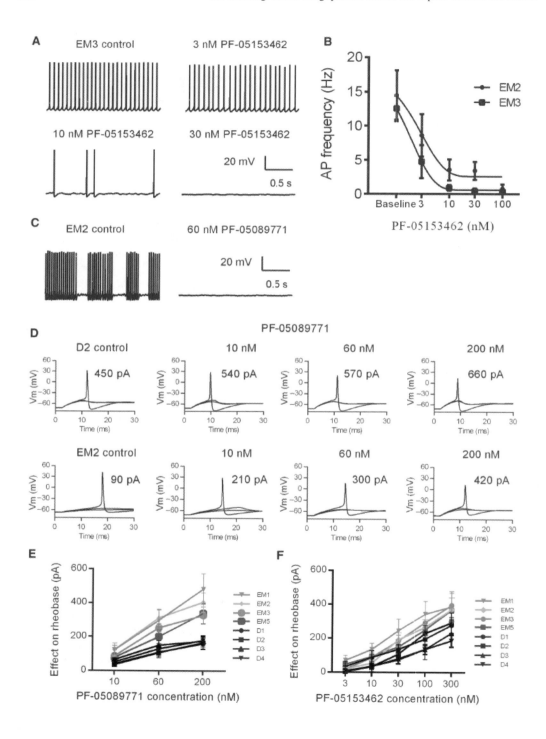

◄ ───

Figure 3

Na$_V$1.7 channel blockers reduce spontaneous firing and increase action potential rheobase in iPSC-SNs. (A) Representative traces of spontaneous action potentials in IEM subject EM3 (V400M mutation) iPSC-SNs blocked by increasing concentrations of the Na$_V$1.7 blocker PF-05153462. (B) Concentration-dependent effect of PF-05153462 on spontaneous action potential (AP) firing with a half-maximal inhibitory concentration (IC$_{50}$) of 2 nM for iPSC-SNs from IEM subjects EM2 (I848T mutation) and EM3 (V400M mutation). (C) Representative traces of spontaneous firing blocked by treatment of iPSC-SNs from IEM subject EM2 with 60 nM PF-05089771. (D) Representative current-clamp traces in iPSC-SNs from non-IEM control subject D2 and IEM subject EM2 (I848T mutation) showing an increase in rheobase after application of PF-05089771 in a concentration-dependent manner. (E) Quantification of the effect of PF-05089771 on rheobase for iPSC-SNs from non-IEM control subjects and IEM subjects (n = 6 to 10; P < 0.05, ANOVA). (F) Quantification of the effect of PF-05153462 on rheobase for iPSC-SNs from non-IEM control subjects and IEM subjects (n = 6 to 10; P < 0.05, ANOVA; comparison at each concentration greater than 10 nM).

dosing in each study period (figure 6A). Blood samples collected from subjects for pharmacokinetic analysis showed that peak plasma concentrations of PF-05089771 were obtained at 4 to 6 hours after dosing (figure S5). Mean unbound plasma concentrations of PF-05089771 at 4 and 6 hours after dosing were 166 and 161 nM, respectively.

Subjects rated their pain using a pain intensity numerical rating scale (PI-NRS) where 0 indicates no pain and 10 indicates the worst pain possible. A pain attack with a PI-NRS score of at least 5 was evoked before dosing with PF-05089771 or placebo. Efficacy end points included the average and maximum pain scores in response to evoked heat at 0 to 4, 4 to 5, 8 to 9, and 24 to 25 hours after dosing.

Individual subject maximum pain scores and change from baseline pain scores after dosing are shown in figure 6 (B and C). Maximum pain score results after dosing (figure 6D) were similar, irrespective of whether cooling rescue therapy [used by subjects EM2 (I848T mutation) and EM4 (V400M mutation)] was administered in the interval before evoking a pain attack. There was statistical significance for PF-05089771 versus placebo at the 10% level at the 4- to 5- and 8- to 9-hour time points after dosing. The P values for the comparison of PF-05089771 versus placebo were P = 0.04 at 4 to 5 hours and P = 0.08 at 8 to 9 hours when subjects who used cooling as a rescue therapy were excluded. When subjects who used cooling as a rescue therapy were

included, the corresponding P values were 0.06 and 0.03. There was no statistically significant treatment effect for PF-05089771 versus placebo at the 0- to 4-hour time point. PF-05089771 was well tolerated in all subjects, with all treatment-related adverse events classified as mild. The most common treatment-related adverse events were perioral paresthesia, facial flushing, and dizziness (table S1).

Discussion

Human iPSC-derived disease models can be used for the identification or validation of drugs to treat specific disease phenotypes,[15,16] yet the degree of translation of drug efficacy to the clinical disease state remains unexplored. Here, we show translation of a human pain phenotype and clinical effects of a new selective Na$_V$1.7 blocker to the preclinical iPSC-based disease model from a small cohort of IEM subjects harboring different mutations in the *SCN9A* gene.

The IEM subject cohort had four different mutations in *SCN9A* and exhibited pain with multiple characteristics, making it an ideal population for a qualitative, proof-of-concept translational study to assess both phenotype and its reversal through selective Na$_V$1.7 blockade. The Na$_V$1.7 blocker used, PF-05089771, shows greater selectivity for Na$_V$1.7 over all other sodium channel isoforms compared to other sodium channel blockers such as

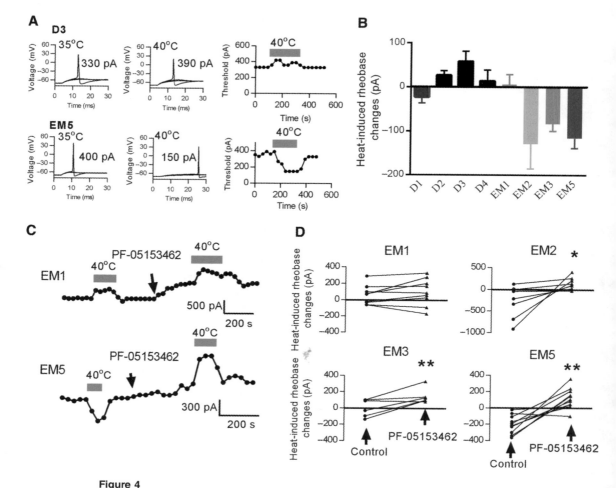

Figure 4

Na$_V$1.7 channel blocker reverses the elevated heat sensitivity of iPSC-derived sensory neurons from IEM subjects. (A) Representative traces of evoked action potentials showing a small increase in rheobase when iPSC-SNs from non-IEM control subject D3 were incubated with extracellular recording solution at an elevated temperature of 40°C (control temperature was 35°C). The rheobase for iPSC-SNs for IEM subject EM5 (F1449V mutation) was decreased relative to the D3 control. Far right panels show an example time course for rheobase changes of iPSC-SNs from non-IEM subject D3 and IEM subject EM5 (F1449V mutation) upon heating of the incubation solution. (B) Quantification of the effect of heating on rheobase for non-IEM and IEM iPSC-SNs. The heating effect was calculated as the change in the rheobase at 40°C versus 35°C ($n = 13$ to 34; $P < 0.01$, comparing non-IEM and IEM iPSC-SNs using ANOVA). (C) Representative traces of rheobase showing the effect of heating on rheobase before and after the application of the Na$_V$1.7 channel blocker PF-05153462. The heat sensitivity of rheobase was reversed by PF-05153462 on iPSC-SNs from IEM subject EM5, but no effect was seen on iPSC-SN from IEM subject EM1. (D) Quantification of the effect of PF-05153462 on heat sensitivity of iPSC-SNs from IEM subjects EM1 (S241T mutation), EM2 (I848T mutation), EM3 (V400M mutation), and EM5 (F1449V mutation) ($n = 6$ to 10; $P < 0.05$ for EM1, EM2, and EM5 and $P < 0.01$ for EM3; paired t test). Only iPSC-SNs demonstrating a positive response to PF-05153462 (where the rheobase showed sensitivity greater than 50 pA at 35°C) were included, and the number of iPSC-SNs excluded was 3 of 12 iPSC-SNs for IEM subject EM1, 2 of 10 iPSC-SNs for IEM subject EM2, 1 of 8 iPSC-SNs for IEM subject EM3, and 1 of 11 iPSC-SNs for IEM subject EM5.

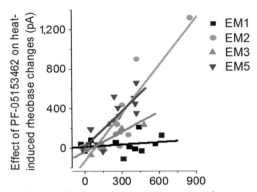

Figure 5

$Na_V1.7$ contributes to the elevated heat sensitivity of iPSC-SNs from IEM subjects. Correlation of the heat sensitivity changes to rheobase changes at 35°C induced by PF-05153462 (Pearson's $r = 0.22$, 0.88, 0.82, and for IEM subjects EM1, EM2, EM3, and EM5, respectively). The regression coefficients were significantly different from zero for IEM subjects EM2, EM3, and EM5. In contrast to figure 4D, iPSC-SNs demonstrating a positive response to PF-05153462 (rheobase changes at 35°C greater than 50 pA, indicating clear $Na_V1.7$ expression) and iPSC-SNs demonstrating a negative response to PF-05153462 (rheobase changes at 35°C less than 50 pA, indicating low or no $Na_V1.7$ expression) were included.

carbamazepine[17] and XEN402.[18,19] A well-controlled heat stimulus triggered pain attacks in the IEM subject cohort and reproduced many of the features of a natural heat-evoked pain attack.[4] The magnitude of heat-induced pain attacks at 4 to 5 and 8 to 9 hours after dosing was reduced in most of the five subjects during at least one of the treatment sessions when dosed with PF-05089771 compared to subjects who received placebo, confirming efficacy in this proof-of-concept study for the treatment of IEM with a selective $Na_V1.7$ blocker. The shorter duration of the evoked pain attacks (usually less than 1 hour compared to the longer duration recorded in the natural history study[4]) and the time of maximum concentration (T_{max}) of PF-05089771 after dosing may account for the lack of treatment response at the 0- to 4- and 24- to 25-hour time points. There appeared to be a degree of variability in response across subjects and between treatment sessions. These observations may be accounted for by the limitation of a single-dose study. iPSCs derived from these subjects provided a unique means to directly evaluate the efficacy of PF-05089771 blockade on the phenotypes of these channel mutations in human sensory neurons.

The increased excitability of iPSC-SNs from IEM subjects was not associated with increased expression of $Na_V1.7$ sodium channels; however, the mean resting membrane potential of iPSC-SNs from IEM subjects was moderately depolarized compared to neurons from the non-IEM donor group. This elevated excitability is likely to be due to an increase in $Na_V1.7$ subthreshold current as modeled by Vasylyev et al.[20] Overexpression of the F1449V, V400M, I848T, and S241T $Na_V1.7$ mutations in rodent dorsal root ganglion neurons has also been reported to reduce current threshold and increase the frequency of firing of dorsal root ganglion neurons in response to graded stimuli.[21–23] The pathophysiological consequence of IEM on neuronal excitability has been examined in clinical microneurography studies.[24,25] One subject with the I848T mutation demonstrated increased C-fiber nociceptor excitability.[26] The microneurography recordings from human nerves and the excitability measurements in iPSC-SNs from patients carrying the same $Na_V1.7$ mutation (I848T) support a role for sensory neuron hyperexcitability underlying the symptoms of IEM.

Direct proof for a role of $Na_V1.7$ in hyperexcitability of sensory neurons from IEM subjects was provided by two $Na_V1.7$ blockers. Both of these compounds have a greater effect on the rheobase of iPSC-SNs from the IEM subject group compared to the non-IEM donor group, and both compounds reduced spontaneous activity of iPSC-SNs from IEM subjects. These data demonstrate using native human $Na_V1.7$ channels in human-derived sensory neurons that $Na_V1.7$ mutations associated with IEM lead to a gain-of-function phenotype.

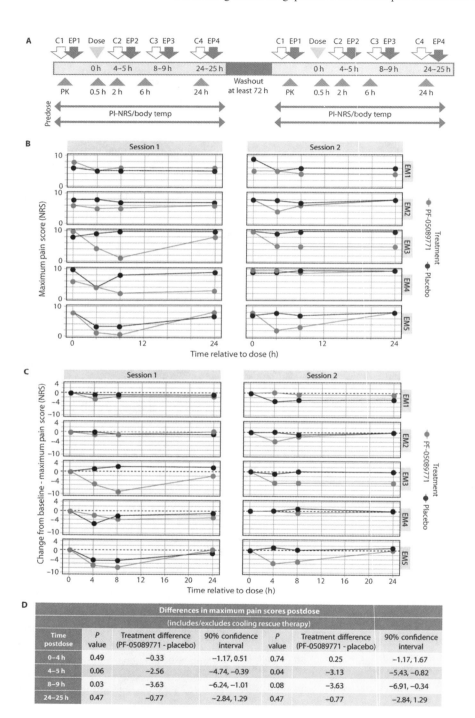

◀

Figure 6

Clinical study design overview and maximum pain scores after dosing. (A) Each treatment session consisted of two study periods separated by at least a 72-hour washout period. Subjects received either a single oral dose of the $Na_V1.7$ channel blocker PF-05089771 or placebo in a crossover manner in each study period. Pain scores were recorded every 15 min up to 10 hours after dosing. Core body temperature was measured regularly throughout the study period. The cooling paradigm (C1 to C4) was used before evoking pain (EP1 to EP4) at specific time points during the study period. Pharmacokinetic (PK) samples were collected before dosing and at 0.5, 2, 6, and 24 hours after dosing. (B) Maximum pain scores recorded by subjects using the PI-NRS after dosing with either the $Na_V1.7$ channel blocker PF-05089771 or placebo in TS1 and TS2. Individual subject results for maximum pain scores included subjects who used nonpharmacological cooling therapy to alleviate pain. IEM subject EM1 (S241T mutation) did not show any notable difference in pain scores after PF-05089771 treatment compared to placebo between TS1 and TS2. IEM subject EM2 (I848T mutation) had a reduction in pain scores in TS2 after PF-05089771 treatment compared to placebo at the 4- to 5-hour postdose time point. IEM subject EM4 (V400M mutation) had a reduction in pain score at the 4- to 5- and 8- to 10-hour postdose time point in TS1, but no difference in pain scores between drug and placebo in TS2. IEM subjects EM3 (V400M mutation) and EM5 (F1449V mutation) had a reduction in pain scores after a single dose of PF-05089771 at the 4- to 5-hour time point and the 8- to 10-hour postdose time point in both TS1 and TS2. (C) Change from baseline in maximum pain scores (PI-NRS) after PF-05089771 treatment versus placebo in individual IEM subjects. (D) Differences in maximum pain scores after dosing with PF-05089771 including and excluding IEM subjects who used cooling as "rescue" therapy.

Of particular interest is subject EM1 (S241T mutation). The iPSC-SNs from this subject were less excitable than other iPSC-SNs from the other IEM subjects in the study, yet the effect of the $Na_V1.7$ blockers on rheobase was equivalent across all IEM iPSC-SNs, confirming the $Na_V1.7$ gain-of-function phenotype. Furthermore, although most IEM patient-derived neurons were more excitable in response to heat in accordance with the clinical phenotype, PF-05153462 only blocked the heat-evoked response in EM2 (I848T mutation)-, EM3 (V400M mutation)-, and EM5 (F1449V mutation)-derived sensory neurons, demonstrating that these $Na_V1.7$ mutations contribute to enhanced temperature sensitivity. In contrast, there was no effect of temperature on EM1 (S241T mutation). It is possible that the lack of response of heat-evoked pain in EM1 (S241T mutation) to PF-05089771 in the clinical study was related to the lack of $Na_V1.7$ temperature dependence at the temperatures tested in iPSC-SNs. Age of IEM onset was delayed (17 years old) in subject EM1 (S241T mutation) compared to the other IEM subjects. Previously published studies also report that for the S241T mutation, the age of onset was between 8 and 10 years old (for four of six affected family members[27]) in comparison to early onset (from infancy until

6 years old) with mutations V400M, F1449V, and I848T.[17,21] IEM mutations in patients with delayed onset are associated with smaller shifts in channel gating and reduced hyperexcitability compared to mutations associated with onset in early childhood.[22]

The lower excitability of sensory neurons derived from iPSCs from subject EM1 carrying the S241T mutation may reflect the delayed onset of IEM, either due to differences in $Na_V1.7$ biophysics or different processing of $Na_V1.7$ during cell maturation relative to the other IEM mutant $Na_V1.7$ channels. It is not appropriate to draw a clear cause and effect relationship between the complex individual subject clinical phenotype and the phenotype of the cognate iPSC-SNs; nevertheless, it is interesting to note that subject EM1 (S241T mutation) had the mildest clinical phenotype, and the iPSC-SNs derived from this patient were the least excitable of the IEM-derived cell lines. In contrast, subject EM2 (I848T mutation) had a more severe clinical phenotype and their iPSC-SNs were highly excitable. With this apparent translation of phenotype and treatment response from clinical study subject to the cognate iPSC disease model, it will be interesting to further decipher underlying mechanisms of this variability. It is also interesting to note the range of excitability within the iPSC-SNs from the four non-IEM donors. Further studies are required to determine the degree of variation in excitability of sensory neurons across the normal human population and its biological basis.

Our data demonstrate the utility of $Na_V1.7$ blockers for the treatment of pain caused by IEM and the utility of iPSC-SNs for recapitulation of sensory nerve fiber dysfunction in vitro. Our results also highlight differences in the effect of the clinical compound in cells derived from non-IEM donors relative to IEM subjects. Thus, iPSC-SNs may further assist in the understanding of certain pain conditions and potential pharma-coresponsiveness of individuals to established and new treatments.

There are, however, some limitations to this work. IEM is a rare disease; as a result, the number of eligible subjects in the clinical study was small, representing four different mutations. Because the study involved a single dose of compound, it was not possible to gener-ate dose-response information. The free plasma concentrations of PF-05089771 in the clinical study reached magnitudes that would have been expected to fully inhibit $Na_V1.7$ activity. Given the selectivity profile of the compound, there may also have been limited activity at other peripher-ally expressed sodium channels, such as $Na_V1.6$. Prior to use in clinical practice, these results may need to be extended to additional IEM subjects, particularly those with *SCN9A* gain-of-function mutations that have not been characterized in the current study. Future studies may also look to extend these results to other *SCN9A*-associated pain conditions such as paroxysmal extreme pain disorder and idiopathic small fiber neuropathy. In addition, it may be possible to extend these results to more general chronic pain conditions in which *SCN9A* mutations associated with a gain of function of the $Na_V1.7$ channel may contribute to the pain in subgroups of subjects.

In summary, this study demonstrates the utility of iPSC technology to bridge the gap between clinical and preclinical studies, enabling an understanding of both the disease and the response to a therapeutic agent.

Materials and Methods

Study Design

The clinical study was a two-part, randomized, double-blind, third-party open, placebo-controlled exploratory crossover study conducted at a single study site. Eligible subjects were adult males or females with clinically and genetically characterized IEM. Subjects were randomized to receive a single oral dose of either PF-05089771 or placebo in a 1:1 ratio during each study period. PF-05089771 and placebo doses were closely matched to maintain the blindedness of the study. All subjects pro-vided informed consent in accordance with ethical prin-ciples originating or derived from the Declaration of Helsinki 2008 before undergoing study-related proce-dures. This study was reviewed and approved by an Inde-pendent Ethics Review Board. Because of the rarity of IEM, sample sizing for the study was originally based on enrollment of up to 14 subjects. The study was powered such that there was an 80% chance of meeting the decision criteria if the true difference in average 0- to 4-hour pain scores was 1.4. The decision criterion was a Bayesian probability of at least 0.75 of the true difference greater than 0.6.

Clinical Study

Subjects were excluded from the clinical study if they had other clinically significant illnesses or were unable to wash out of and refrain from using concomitant pain medications during the study such as carbamazepine, lamotrigine, oxcarbazepine, mexiletine and amitripty-line, capsaicin patches and local anesthetic patches, and oral/injectable corticosteroids. All subjects washed out of their concomitant pain medications before taking part in the study. To manage pain due to their IEM during the study, subjects were permitted to use nonpharmacological therapy such as cooling the extremities or acetaminophen (up to a maximum of 3000 mg/day).

The five subjects enrolled in this study had participated in a previous nondrug clinical phenotyping study in which the triggers for pain attacks and the duration, intensity, and frequency of pain attacks and ongoing pain between attacks (if any) were recorded by subjects in a pain diary on a daily basis over a 3-month period. Pain attacks occurred primarily in the feet and hands, and the principal triggers for evoking pain attacks were warmth or heat, exercise, and environmental factors (usually hot and/or humid weather).[4]

The primary objective of the drug study was to evaluate the overall pain intensity over 4 hours after a single 1600-mg oral dose of PF-05089771 against placebo in subjects experiencing either experimentally evoked (heat stimulation) pain or spontaneous pain due to IEM. The secondary objectives of the study were to evaluate the overall duration, maximum pain intensity, and duration of pain intensity (evoked or spontaneous pain) in subjects at 4 to 5, 8 to 9, and 24 to 25 hours after dosing. Use of and time to use of pharmacological therapy such as acetaminophen or nonpharmacological therapy such as cooling the extremities to relieve IEM pain during the study ("rescue therapy") were also recorded.

Part A, the first part of the study, was conducted over 1 to 2 days as an in-clinic stay to establish clinical reproducibility and reliability of evoking pain in each subject before entering part B, an extended in-clinic stay in which a single oral dose of study drug or matched placebo was administered. Subjects were randomized into part B of the study provided that they satisfied all subject selection criteria and had a self-reported spontaneous or evoked pain score of ≥5 on the PI-NRS (where 0 indicates no pain and 10 indicates worst pain possible) before dosing. Treatment session 1 (TS1) and TS2 could be run consecutively, with a minimum 72-hour washout period between the last study treatment in TS1 and the first study treatment in TS2, and a maximum period of up to 6 months between TS1 and TS2 to facilitate enrollment. The Medi-Therm III MTA 7900 (Stryker) device was used as a heating device to evoke pain, as a cooling device for the cooling paradigm part of the study, and as means to deliver nonpharmacological cooling of the extremities as rescue therapy. The Medi-Therm device supplied cold or warm water at operator-determined temperatures through the use of water-circulating thermo-regulated blankets applied to the feet and/or hands or body wraps, which were applied to the trunk. The hands and feet, including toes, were completely enclosed in the thermal blankets, which were applied in a consistent manner to each subject. Subjects rated their baseline pain score using the PI-NRS. If the subject reported any ongoing pain, attempts were made to reduce the subject's pain score to ≤3 on the PI-NRS using

a cooling paradigm. Thermal blankets were applied to the subject's extremities (feet and/or hands), and the Medi-Therm blankets cooled to 20°C (cooling paradigm) for at least 5 min (maximum of 60 min) until the subject's pain score was ≤3 on the NRS. After cooling, the thermal blankets were heated to 33°C, the starting temperature for all subjects, and the temperature was increased incrementally in 1° to 2°C steps at 10- to 15-min intervals to the device maximum of 42°C. This temperature was used for a maximum duration of 30 min, until a pain attack with a PI-NRS score of ≥5 was induced. This methodology was repeated at least one to two times in part A of the study to establish individual, standardized time and temperature parameters for evoking pain in each subject for part B, the drug phase of the study. Subjects recorded pain scores every 15 min for up to 4 hours after a pain attack was evoked.

Part B of the study had two treatment sessions (TS1 and TS2) with each treatment session consisting of two study periods (figure 6A). Subjects received a single dose of either PF-05089771 or placebo in each study period. Treatment sessions could be carried out consecutively, with a minimum washout period of at least 72 hours between study treatments, or separated by up to 6 months. In part B, subjects' extremities were cooled (C1 to C4; figure 6A) to reduce pain score to ≤3 on the NRS, followed by heat stimulation to evoke a pain attack (EP1 to EP4). Once the subject reported a pain score of ≥5 on the PI-NRS, as a result of the Medi-Therm device heat stimulus, they were randomized to one of two double-blind treatment sequences [PF-05089771/placebo or placebo/PF-05089771, each given as a single oral dose during each of the treatment sessions (TS1 and TS2)]. To maintain blinding, PF-05089771 and placebo oral doses were matched in appearance and volume. Postdose pain attacks were evoked, using individual standardized parameters established in part A with the Medi-Therm device, at 4 to 5, 8 to 9, and 24 to 25 hours after dosing. Subjects were asked to refrain from taking acetaminophen or nonpharmacological treatments (for example, Medi-Therm cooling function, ice buckets, cold water, and cool air fans) to manage pain until at least 90 min after dosing. If acetaminophen or cold therapy were requested by the subject to manage pain, the time, dose (where applicable), duration, and frequency of use were recorded. Pain scores were recorded every 5 min for the first hour after dosing and then every 15 min until 10 hours after dosing. Blood samples were collected for pharmacokinetic and safety laboratory evaluations at prespecified time points after dosing. Blood and urine samples for laboratory assessments (hematology, serum chemistry, and urinalysis) were collected 2 days before dosing, at 2 to 4 hours before dosing, and at 24 hours after dosing in each study period. Vital signs were checked 2 days before dosing, at 2 to 4 hours before dosing, and at 6 and 24 hours after dosing. Electrocardiograms were performed 2 days before dosing, at 2 to 4 hours before dosing, and at 8 and 24 hours after dosing. Adverse events were recorded at the time of occurrence from screening until follow-up (28 days after the last dose of study drug).

Collection of Blood for Generation of iPSCs

Four of five subjects (EM1, EM2, EM3, and EM5) consented to an optional procedure to donate blood for generation of iPSCs. About 60 ml of blood was collected per subject and aliquoted into six 8-ml Ficoll CPT tubes with sodium heparin (Becton Dickinson). The samples were centrifuged at room temperature, and mononuclear cells (lymphocytes and neutrophils) were harvested and further centrifuged. The centrifuged cells were aspirated and counted using a hemocytometer. Trypan blue was used to identify nonviable cells. Viable cells were resuspended in freezing solution (human AB serum plus 10% dimethyl sulfoxide) to give a final cell density of not more than 50 million cells/ml. Samples were frozen at −80°C.

Clinical Statistical Methods

The primary end point, the average heat-evoked pain score from 0 to 4 hours after dosing, was analyzed using a linear mixed model with terms for baseline, treatment period time after dosing, baseline by time after dosing interaction, treatment by time after dosing interaction, and period by time after dosing interaction. Subject was included as a random effect in this model. The secondary end points of maximum pain score following pain provocation at 4, 8, 10, and 24 hours after dosing were analyzed using a linear fixed effects model with additive terms for subject, period, and treatment. The results are summarized as estimates of treatment effects (PF-05089771 minus placebo) together with 90% confidence intervals. Maximum pain scores obtained after pain provocation following previous use of rescue therapy were included in the analyses because the rescue medication was nonpharmacological cooling,

which was also used in the study design to cool subjects if necessary before pain provocation.

Generation and Maintenance of iPSCs Derived from IEM Subjects

Blood samples from non-IEM donors were obtained from the National Health Service Blood and Transplant (NHSBT). Samples from IEM clinical trial subjects were obtained after informed consent.

Peripheral blood mononuclear cells were purified using the standard Ficoll-Paque procedure. Cells were expanded into erythroid progenitor cells and transduced with Sendai virus expressing Yamanaka factors OKSM (Life Technologies). iPSC colonies were further expanded to virus-free clonal lines that were cultured and maintained on Matrigel (BD) in TeSR1 (STEMCELL Technologies) and passaged every 6 to 7 days using dispase (Life Technologies).

Genomic DNA Isolation, Sanger Sequencing, and Array CGH

Genomic DNA of IEM subject material and iPSC clones was extracted using Qiagen RNA/DNA isolation kit. Segments containing respective mutations were PCR amplified and sequenced for mutation analysis.

Primer sequences [IDT (Integrated DNA Technologies)] used were as follows: S241T forward, 5′-CATGACT TTCTAGGAAAGCTTGTGT-3′; S241T reverse, 5′-GTC CAATTAGTGCAAACACACTCA-3′; I848T forward, 5′-ATCATTCAGACTGCTCCGAGTCTT-3′; I848T reverse, 5′-TTGCAGACACATTCTTTGTAGCTC-3′; S449N forward, 5′-GGGTTTCCTAGGATTTGGAAATGAC-3′; S449N reverse, 5′-CTGATGCTGTCCTCTGATTCTGAT-3′; V400M forward, 5′-ATTTCCATTTTTCCCTAGACG CTG-3′; V400M reverse, 5′-TACCTCAGCTTCTTCTT GCTCTTT-3′; F1449V forward, 5′-TTATAGGTAGACA AGCAGCCCAAA-3′; F1449V reverse, 5′-CCTAAATCA TAAGTTAGCCAGAACC-3′. Array CGH analysis was performed with genomic DNA of iPSC clones and corresponding subject material using CytoSure ISCA v2 4 × 180k microarrays and analyzed using CytoSure software (Oxford Gene Technology).

RNA Isolation, Complementary DNA Synthesis, and qPCR

Total RNA of cells was isolated using the RNeasy Mini Kit (Qiagen) and reverse-transcribed using SuperScript

III complementary DNA synthesis kit (Life Technologies) according to the manufacturer's protocol. qPCR was performed using the TaqMan Gene Expression system (Applied Biosystems). The TaqMan probes (Life Technologies) used were SCN1A, Hs00374696_m1; SCN2A, Hs00221379_m1; SCN3A, Hs00366902_m1; SCN4A, Hs01109480_m1; SCN8A, Hs00274075_m1; SCN9A, Hs0161567_m1; SCN10A, Hs01045149_m1; SCN11A, Hs00204222_#m1; GAPDH, Hs02758991_#g1; and HPRT, Hs02800695_m1.

Immunocytochemistry

iPSC clones or sensory neurons were fixed in 4% paraformaldehyde for 20 min at room temperature, permeabilized in 0.3% Triton X-100 in phosphate-buffered saline (PBS), and blocked with 5% donkey serum/PBS–0.1% Triton X-100 (PBS-T). iPSC clonal lines were stained with primary antibodies anti-Oct4 (sc-8628, Santa Cruz Biotechnology) and anti-Nanog (ab62734, Abcam) overnight. Sensory-like neurons were stained with anti-peripherin, anti-Brn3a, and anti-Islet1 (sc-7604, Santa Cruz Biotechnology; ab5945 and ab86501, Abcam) overnight. Cells were incubated with Alexa fluorophore secondary antibodies (Life Technologies) in PBS-T for 1 hour with intermediate washes. Nuclei were stained with Hoechst (Life Technologies). Images were acquired on the Zeiss Observer ZI with AxioVision software (Zeiss) or ImageXpress platform (Molecular Devices).

Differentiation of iPSCs into Sensory Neurons

Differentiation into sensory neurons was performed as described previously.[13,14] Differentiated neurons were maintained for 8 weeks in neural growth factor medium containing Dulbecco's modified Eagle's medium/F12 (1:1) supplemented with 10% fetal bovine serum (Life Technologies) and nerve growth factor (10 ng/ml), brain-derived neurotrophic factor (BDNF), glial cell line-derived neurotrophic factor (GDNF), neurotrophin-3 (NT-3) (PeproTech), and ascorbic acid (Sigma-Aldrich). Medium was changed twice weekly.

Electrophysiology

iPSC-SNs (typically 8 weeks after growth factor addition) were dissociated and replated as described by Chambers et al.[13] Patch-clamp experiments were performed in whole-cell configuration using a patch-clamp amplifier (200B) for voltage clamp and MultiClamp (700A or 700B) for current clamp controlled by pCLAMP 10 software (Molecular Devices). Voltage-clamp experiments were performed at room temperature, whereas current-clamp experiments were performed at 35° or 40°C using a CL-100 in-line solution heating system (Warner Instruments).

Temperature was calibrated at the outlet of the in-line heater before each experiment. Patch pipettes had resistances between 1.5 and 2 megohms. Basic extracellular solution contained 135 mM NaCl, 4.7 mM KCl, 1 mM $CaCl_2$, 1 mM $MgCl_2$, 10 mM Hepes, and 10 mM glucose (pH was adjusted to 7.4 with NaOH). The intracellular (pipette) solution for voltage clamp contained 100 mM CsF, 45 mM CsCl, 10 mM NaCl, 1 mM $MgCl_2$, 10 mM Hepes, and 5 mM EGTA (pH was adjusted to 7.3 with CsOH). For current-clamp experiments, the intracellular (pipette) solution contained 130 mM KCl, 1 mM $MgCl_2$, 5 mM MgATP, 10 mM Hepes, and 5 mM EGTA (pH was adjusted to 7.3 with KOH). The osmolarity of solutions was adjusted to 320 mosmol/liter for extracellular solution and 300 mosmol/liter for intracellular solutions. All chemicals were purchased from Sigma-Aldrich. Currents were sampled at 20 kHz and filtered at 5 kHz. In voltage-clamp recordings, between 80 and 90% of the series resistance was compensated to reduce voltage errors. The voltage protocol used to assess the effect of the compounds on voltage-gated sodium channels consisted of a step to −70 mV for 5 s from a holding potential of −110 mV, followed by a recovery step to −110 mV for 100 ms, followed by a test pulse to 0 mV lasting 20 ms. Intersweep intervals were 15 s. Current threshold (or rheobase) was measured in current-clamp mode by injecting 30-ms duration current steps of regularly increasing amplitude until a single action potential was evoked. The increasing current steps were in cycled sweeps to track the changes of current threshold (rheobase) while temperature was varied or compounds were applied to the cells. Intersweep intervals were 2 s. Two to three subclones were generated for each of the four IEM donors and four healthy donors. Excitability data were pooled from all subclones of four IEM donors (individual subclones data can be seen in figure S3D), whereas one subclone of each healthy donor was investigated.

Excitability was measured at resting membrane potential for each cell. The effect of compounds and temperature on rheobase was measured at a fixed membrane potential of −70 mV to avoid membrane potential change–induced error. Current-clamp data were analyzed using Spike2 software (Cambridge Electronic Design), Prism 6.0 (GraphPad software), and Origin 9.1 software (OriginLab). Wherever possible, the raw or derived data are presented.

Statistical Analysis

Preclinical Data   Nonparametric ANOVA was used to compare current densities, total sodium current, and rheobase between the IEM and non-IEM groups of clones. Spontaneous action potential firing was analyzed using a linear logistic model to compare the IEM and non-IEM groups. Resting membrane potential and rheobase of the action potential were analyzed using ANOVA to compare between groups. Pearson's correlation coefficients were calculated to summarize the relationships between change in temperature sensitivity and effect on rheobase. The associated regression coefficients were tested to see if they differed significantly from zero. All significance tests were one-sided and used a 5% significance level. No adjustments were made to this significance level. Distributional assumptions were checked graphically, and when violated, nonparametric tests were used. All statistical analyses were carried out using SAS 9.4 (SAS Institute Inc.).

Clinical Data   The primary end point, the average heat-evoked pain score from 0 to 4 hours after dosing, was analyzed using a linear mixed model with terms for baseline, treatment period by time after dosing, baseline by time after dosing interaction, treatment by time after dosing interaction, and period by time after dosing interaction. Subject was included as a random effect in this model. The secondary end points of maximum pain score following pain provocation at 4, 8, 10, and 24 hours after dosing were analyzed using a linear fixed effects model with additive terms for subject, period, and treatment. The results are summarized as estimates of treatment effects (PF-05089771 minus placebo) together with 90% confidence intervals. Unadjusted exact P values were given for maximum pain results, whereas a one-sided 10% significance level was used to test for a difference in the average pain from 0 to 4 hours after dosing. Distributional assumptions for the analyses were checked graphically. Maximum pain scores obtained after pain provocation following previous use of rescue therapy were included in the analyses because the rescue medication was nonpharmacological

cooling, which was also used in the study design to cool subjects if necessary before pain provocation.

Supplementary Materials

http://stm.sciencemag.org/content/suppl/2016/ 04/18/8.335.335ra56.DC1;   http://stm.sciencemag.org/ content/scitransmed/suppl/2016/04/18/8.335.335ra56 .DC1/8-335ra56_SM.pdf

Figure S1. Molecular karyotype of IEM and non-IEM iPSCs and Na_V channel subtype mRNA expression in iPSC-SNs.

Figure S2. Molecular structure and selectivity profiles of $Na_V1.7$ channel blockers.

Figure S3. Electrophysiological properties of IEM and non-IEM iPSC sensory neurons.

Figure S4. Effect of PF-05153462 on heat sensitivity of non-IEM control D3 and D4 iPSC sensory neurons.

Figure S5. Pharmacokinetic profile of PF-05089771 over time after single oral dose administration to subjects with IEM.

Table S1. Common adverse event profile for all five subjects with IEM.

Acknowledgments

We thank those subjects who participated in this study and their families. We thank F. Di Cesare for medical input into this study and S. Carolan and J. van Winkle for care of subjects and study management. We thank Z. Lin, D. Printzenhoff, M. Chapman, and N. Castle for PatchXpress characterization of PF-05089771 and PF-5153462. We thank H. Alexander and C. Campbell for help with figure design. We thank Roslin Cells Ltd. for generation of some of the iPSC lines used in this study.

About the Authors

Lishuang Cao, Pfizer Neuroscience and Pain Research Unit, Cambridge, UK

Aoibhinn McDonnell, Pfizer Neuroscience and Pain Research Unit, Cambridge, UK

Anja Nitzsche, Pfizer Neuroscience and Pain Research Unit, Cambridge, UK

Aristos Alexandrou, Pfizer Neuroscience and Pain Research Unit, Cambridge, UK

Pierre-Philippe Saintot, Pfizer Neuroscience and Pain Research Unit, Cambridge, UK

Alexandre J.C. Loucif, Pfizer Neuroscience and Pain Research Unit, Cambridge, UK

Adam R. Brown, Pfizer Neuroscience and Pain Research Unit, Cambridge, UK

Gareth Young, Pfizer Neuroscience and Pain Research Unit, Cambridge, UK

Malgorzata Mis, University of Bristol, School of Physiology, Pharmacology, and Neuroscience, Bristol, UK

Andrew Randall, Hatherly College of Life and Environmental Sciences, University of Exeter, Exeter, UK

Stephen G. Waxman, Yale Center for Neuroscience and Regeneration Research, Veterans Affairs Medical Center, West Haven, CT

Philip Stanley, Pfizer Neuroscience and Pain Research Unit, Cambridge, UK

Simon Kirby, Pfizer Neuroscience and Pain Research Unit, Cambridge, UK

Sanela Tarabar, Pfizer, New Haven, CT

Alex Gutteridge, Pfizer Neuroscience and Pain Research Unit, Cambridge, UK

Richard Butt, Pfizer Neuroscience and Pain Research Unit, Cambridge, UK

Ruth M. McKernan, Pfizer Neuroscience and Pain Research Unit, Cambridge, UK

Paul Whiting, Pfizer Neuroscience and Pain Research Unit, Cambridge, UK

Zahid Ali, Pfizer Neuroscience and Pain Research Unit, Cambridge, UK

James Bilsland, Pfizer Neuroscience and Pain Research Unit, Cambridge, UK

Edward B. Stevens, Pfizer Neuroscience and Pain Research Unit, Cambridge, UK

Funding

This study was funded by Pfizer Inc. The research leading to these results has received support from the Innovative Medicines Initiative Joint Undertaking under grant agreement no. 115439, resources of which are composed of financial contributions from the European Union's Seventh Framework Programme (FP7/2007–2013) and European Federation of Pharmaceutical Industries and Association (EFPIA) companies in kind contribution. M.M. was supported by an Industrial CASE Ph.D. studentship from the Biotechnology and Biological Sciences Research Council (BBSRC) in partnership with Pfizer. This publication reflects only the authors' views and neither the Innovative Medicines Initiative Joint Undertaking nor EFPIA nor the European Commission are liable for any use that may be made of the information contained therein.

Author Contributions

L.C., A.N., R.B., R.M.M., P.W., E.B.S., and J.B. designed the preclinical experiments. A.M. and Z.A. designed and executed the clinical study. L.C., A.A., P.-P.S., A.J.C.L., A.R.B., G.Y., and M.M. performed electrophysiological experiments. A.N. generated and differentiated iPSC lines, performed quality control, and carried out gene and protein expression. S.T. was the clinical study principal investigator. L.C., A.R., and M.M analyzed electrophysiological data. A.N. and A.G. analyzed all iPSC and iPSC-SN–related molecular data. S.K. and P.S. provided statistical analyses of clinical and preclinical data. L.C., A.M., A.N., S.T., P.W., S.G.W., S.K., Z.A., J.B., and E.B.S. wrote the paper.

Competing Interests

Na$_V$1.7 sodium channel blockers described in this study are covered by patent WO/2010/079443; International Application No. PCT/IB2010/050033; publication date, 15 July 2010; International Filing Date, 06 January 2010.

Data and Materials Availability

The ClinicalTrials.gov registration number for this study is NCT01769274.[28] Patient-derived iPSC lines are deposited in the European Bank for iPSCs (EBiSC; www.ebisc.org/) to whom initial enquiries for access should be addressed.

References and Notes

1. Drenth JPH, Waxman SG. 2007. Mutations in sodium channel gene SCN9A cause a spectrum of human genetic pain disorders. *J Clin Invest* 117: 3603–3609.

2. Dib-Hajj SD, Yang Y, Black JA, Waxman SG. 2013. The $Na_V1.7$ sodium channel: From molecule to man. *Nat Rev Neurosci* 14: 49–62.

3. Bennett DLH, Woods CG. 2014. Painful and painless channelopathies. *Lancet Neurol* 13: 587–599.

4. McDonnell A, Schulman B, Ali Z, Dib-Hajj SD, Brock F, Cobain S, Mainka T, Vollert J, Tarabar S, Waxman SG. 2016. Inherited erythromelalgia due to mutations in *SCN9A*: Natural history, clinical phenotype and somatosensory profile. *Brain* 139(Pt. 4): 1052–1065.

5. Cummins TR, Dib-Hajj SD, Waxman SG. 2004. Electrophysiological properties of mutant $Na_V1.7$ sodium channels in a painful inherited neuropathy. *J Neurosci* 24: 8232–8236.

6. Wu M-T, Huang P-Y, Yen C-T, Chen C-C, Lee M-J. 2013. A novel *SCN9A* mutation responsible for primary erythromelalgia and is resistant to the treatment of sodium channel blockers. *PLoS One* 8: e55212.

7. Estacion M, Yang Y, Dib-Hajj SD, Tyrrell L, Lin Z, Yang Y, Waxman SG. 2013. A new $Na_V1.7$ mutation in an erythromelalgia patient. *Biochem Biophys Res Commun* 432: 99–104.

8. Eberhart M, Nakajima J, Klinger AB, Neacsu C, Hühne K, O'Reilly AO, Kist AM, et al. 2014. Inherited pain: Sodium channel $Na_V1.7$ A1632T mutation causes erythromelalgia due to a shift of fast inactivation. *J Biol Chem* 289: 1971–1980.

9. Stadler T, O'Reilly AO, Lampert A. 2015. Erythromelalgia mutation Q875E stabilizes the activated state of sodium channel $Na_V1.7$. *J Biol Chem* 290: 6316–6325.

10. Emery EC, Habib AM, Cox JJ, Nicholas AK, Gribble FM, Woods CG, Reimann F. 2015. Novel *SCN9A* mutations underlying extreme pain phenotypes: Unexpected electrophysiological and clinical phenotype correlations. *J Neurosci* 35: 7674–7681.

11. Theile JW, Jarecki BW, Piekarz AD, Cummins TR. 2011. $Na_V1.7$ mutations associated with paroxysmal extreme pain disorder, but not erythromelalgia, enhance NaVb4 peptide-mediated resurgent sodium currents. *J Physiol* 589: 597–608.

12. Dib-Hajj SD, Choi JS, Macala LJ, Tyrrell L, Black JA, Cummins TR, Waxman SG. 2009. Transfection of rat or mouse neurons by biolistics or electroporation. *Nat Protoc* 4: 1118–1126.

13. Chambers SM, Qi Y, Mica Y, Gabsang L, Zhang X-J, Niu L, Bilsland J, et al. 2012. Combined small-molecule inhibition accelerates developmental timing and converts human pluripotent stem cells into nociceptors. *Nat Biotechnol* 30: 715–720.

14. Young GT, Gutteridge A, Fox HDE, Wilbrey AL, Cao L, Cho LT, Brown AR, et al. 2014. Characterizing human stem cell–derived sensory neurons at the single-cell level reveals their ion channel expression and utility in pain research. *Mol Ther* 22: 1530–1543.

15. Grskovic M, Javaherian A, Strulovici B, Daley GQ. 2011. Induced pluripotent stem cells—Opportunities for disease modelling and drug discovery. *Nat Rev Drug Discov* 10: 915–929.

16. McNeish J, Gardner JP, Wainger BJ, Woolf CJ, Eggan K. 2015. From dish to bedside: Lessons learned while translating findings from a stem cell model of disease to a clinical trial. *Cell Stem Cell* 17: 8–10.

17. Fischer TZ, Gilmore ES, Estacion M, Eastman E, Taylor S, Melanson M, Dib-Hajj SD, Waxman SG. 2009. A novel $Na_V1.7$ mutation producing carbamazepine responsive erythromelalgia. *Ann Neurol* 65: 733–741.

18. Goldberg YP, Price N, Namdari R, Cohen CJ, Lamers MH, Winters C, Price J, et al. 2012. Treatment of $Na_V1.7$-mediated pain in inherited erythromelalgia using a novel sodium channel blocker. *Pain* 153: 80–85.

19. Goldberg YP, Cohen CJ, Namdari R, Price N, Cadieux JA, Young C, Sherrington R, Pimstone SN. 2014. Letter to the Editor. *Pain* 155: 837–838.

20. Vasylyev DV, Han C, Zhao P, Dib-Hajj S, Waxman SG. 2014. Dynamic-clamp analysis of wild-type human $Na_V1.7$ and erythromelalgia mutant channel L858H. *J Neurophysiol* 111: 1429–1443.

21. Dib Hajj SD, Rush AM, Cummins TR, Hisama FM, Novella S, Tyrrell L, Marshall L, Waxman SG. 2005. Gain-of-function mutation in $Na_V1.7$ in familial erythromelalgia induces bursting of sensory neurons. *Brain* 128: 1847–1854.

22. Han C, Dib-Hajj SD, Lin Z, Li Y, Eastman EM, Tyrrell L, Cao X, Yang Y, Waxman SG. 2009. Early and late-onset inherited erythromelalgia: Genotype-phenotype correlation. *Brain* 132: 1711–1722.

23. Yang Y, Dib-Hajj SD, Zhang J, Zhang Y, Tyrrell L, Estacion M, Waxman SG. 2012. Structural modelling and mutant cycle analysis predict pharmacoresponsiveness of a $Na_V1.7$ mutant channel. *Nat Commun* 3: 1186.

24. Ørstavik K, Weidner C, Schmidit R, Schmelz M, Hilloges H, Jørum E, Handwerker H, Torebjörk E. 2003. Pathological C-fibres in patients with a chronic painful condition. *Brain* 126: 567–578.

25. Uyanik O, Quiles C, Bostock H, Dib-Hajj SD, Fischer T, Tyrrell L, Waxman SG, Serra J. 2007. Spontaneous impulse generation in C-nociceptors of familial erythromelalgia (FE) patients. *Eur J Pain* 11: S130–S293.

26. Namer B, Ørstavik K, Schmidt R, Kleggetveit I-P, Weidner C, Mørk C, Kvernebo MS, et al. 2015. Specific changes in conduction velocity recovery cycles of single nociceptors in an erythromelalgia patient with the I848T gain-of-function mutation of $Na_V1.7$. *Pain* 156: 1637–1646.

27. Michiels JJ, Te Morsche RH, Jansen JB, Drenth JP. 2005. Autosomal dominant erythermalgia associated with a novel mutation in the voltage-gated sodium channel alpha subunit $Na_V1.7$. *Arch Neurol* 62: 1587–1590.

28. ClinicalTrials.gov. [Internet]. Identifier:NCT02215252 A Clinical Trial To Evaluate PF-05089771 On Its Own And As An Add-On Therapy To Pregabalin (Lyrica) For The Treatment Of Pain Due To Diabetic Peripheral Neuropathy (DPN). Available from: https://clinicaltrials.gov/ct2/show/NCT02215252.

12 FROM TRIAL-AND-ERROR TO FIRST-TIME-AROUND: TOWARD GENOMICALLY GUIDED THERAPY

Even as $Na_V1.7$ blockers were (and are) being developed, we were also taking another approach: using the human genome to predict whether an existing medication would help a particular person. This approach, variously called "precision medicine," "personalized medicine," or "individualized medicine," uses the DNA of each specific patient to give the clinician a molecular compass that points to the most effective medication. Currently we do not have that molecular compass in pain medicine. The clinician usually begins by selecting a particular medication, based on the patient's description of the pain, the cause of the pain or its pattern, and other aspects of the patient's history. The most effective medication, the dosage, and the dosing schedule can vary from patient to patient. The choice of medication, the dose, and the dosing schedule are usually adjusted based on the patient's reports of pain relief and side effects, in a process that requires many visits to, or telephone consultations with, the clinic. There are many forms and dosages of existing medications, and many potential combinations, so in any single patient only a subset of the treatment regimens can be tried. Even when based on the best knowledge available, the process includes a degree of trial-and-error and may provide less-than-optimal relief.

Many factors—including differences in the type of injury or disease process responsible for the pain, differences in other medications that the patient may be taking, differences in diet, and environmental factors—can contribute to variability in the responses of different people to medication. In the past this added up to a sense that a given patient's response to a particular pain medication was unpredictable.

In most people with inherited erythromelalgia, pain medications other than opiates provide no relief or only minimal relief, and even opiates provide only partial relief. Yet there are exceptions to every rule. In 2009 we encountered one unusual family with inherited erythromelalgia, in whom the disorder was responsive to treatment with a medication called carbamazepine. This family was a reminder that molecular genetic analysis of very rare families can be informative.

Developed in the 1960s, carbamazepine is a nonspecific sodium channel blocker. Rather than blocking the activity of a single subtype of sodium channel, it inhibits all sodium channel subtypes. It exerts its blocking effect in an activity-dependent manner, inhibiting the channels when they are active. This medication was initially used as a treatment for epilepsy and is still used in that way. It has also proven effective in the treatment of a particular form of neuropathic pain, trigeminal neuralgia, in which patients experience attacks of severe, lancinating pain in the face. But carbamazepine is not usually effective in other forms of neuropathic pain. And, in most patients with inherited erythromelalgia, carbamazepine is not helpful. The family we encountered in 2009 was different. In this unusual family carbamazepine provided significant pain relief. The initial patient identified in this family (called the "proband" by geneticists) suffered from erythromelalgia with symptoms that began in infancy. Carbamazepine provided significant pain relief. Pain in the proband's two children was also relieved by carbamazepine. One child had approximately 56 pain attacks per week before starting carbamazepine, but only two attacks per week while being treated with this medication. The other child had a similar response. These children could not tolerate wearing socks or shoes and could not participate in athletics prior to treatment. But they were able to wear socks and shoes, to run, and to play soccer when treated.

What was this unusual family trying to tell us? Most people with inherited erythromelalgia are not helped by carbamazepine. Yet, in this unique family, carbamazepine was remarkably helpful. Their genes, we reasoned, were playing an important role in shaping their response to carbamazepine. In 2011, we made a bet that we could predict, on the basis of analysis of DNA, that a particular patient would be more, or less, responsive to a particular medication. The paper that follows (Yang et al. 2012) represents an early step toward a genomically guided "first time around" approach that will select, for each person, the most effective medication for pain.

In our initial study on the DNA from this family (Fischer et al. 2009) we found a mutation of $Na_V1.7$, V400M, which replaced a single amino acid, valine at position 400 (V400), with methionine. Voltage-clamp analysis showed us that the mutation made it easier to activate the channel, much like other inherited erythromelalgia mutations. The mutation also had an unusual pro-excitatory effect, impairing inactivation of the channel. Each of these changes would be expected to increase the excitability of DRG neurons, thereby producing pain.

To determine why carbamazepine relieved pain in this unusual family, we next examined the effect of carbamazepine on the V400M mutant channels. We observed that exposure to carbamazepine restored activation of the mutant channels to close-to-normal levels, while not affecting activation of normal, wild-type channels. These results showed us that the V400M mutation had multiple effects on the channel: First, the mutation produced gain-of-function changes in the $Na_V1.7$ channel, thereby leading to overactivity in pain-signaling neurons and to pain. Second, and unexpectedly, the mutation sensitized the channel to carbamazepine.

Each gene within our genome has many variants, even in people with no history of disease. Our studies on the V400M family showed us that there are variants within the *SCN9A* gene—small changes that substitute one out of the nearly 1,800 amino acids that make up the $Na_V1.7$ sodium channel—that alter sensitivity of the channel to a medication. Hundreds of variants—amino acid substitutions at specific sites within the channel—had been reported within various databases for the *SCN9A* gene; most had not yet been functionally studied so that their clinical implications were not yet understood. As we talked about the V400M mutation, we wanted to ask this question: Might other amino acid substitutions decrease or increase sensitivity of the channel to particular medications, as the V400M mutation did for carbamazepine? Might genomic variability, of the type that occurs in each of us, be used to guide the treatment of pain?

From Bacteria to Humans

A sodium channel is a complicated molecule: nearly 1,800 amino acids, strung together like a string of beads folded into a highly specific three-dimensional configuration. Figuring out the configuration of the protein in three dimensions, or solving the question "what is the precise pattern of folding?" can be formidable. Imagine folding up a long string of beads by crunching it up your hand. There are a multitude of folding configurations, sometimes with red bead "A" coming into close proximity to blue bead "B" located thirty beads down the line, but sometimes not.

Even our bacterial ancestors contain sodium channels. All four domains of the bacterial sodium channel share an identical structure, in contrast to mammalian sodium channels where the four domains have different structures. So, the bacterial channel provides an experimental model that is amenable to crystallographic analysis, which can provide information about the relative locations of the amino acids that make up a protein, even a protein as complex as an ion channel. Crystallography can even indicate the location of atoms within a large molecule. In 2011, William Catterall and his colleagues at the University of Washington, including crystallographer Jian Payandeh, reported the crystal structure of the bacterial sodium channel (Payandeh et al. 2011). This was an important advance; it showed how the sodium channel protein bends and folds in three dimensions, thus revealing how individual amino acids within the bacterial channel come into close contact with each other, and even signaled the locations of some of the atoms within these amino acids, inside the folded channel protein.

A few days after this report appeared, Yang Yang, a new research fellow in our group, knocked on my office door and—with his usual "we can do anything if we try" demeanor—suggested that we construct a structural model, with atomic-level resolution, of the human $Na_V1.7$ channel. His plan was to base this on the crystal structure of the bacterial channel. Tasked with doing this, he used powerful computerized algorithms to individually model each of the four transmembrane domains of the human channel, and then aligned the four domains to a structural template provided by the recently solved bacterial channel. Because the sodium channel protein is a large molecule, and weaves in and out of the cell membrane twenty-four times, there are many thousands of potential solutions to the problem, each depicting a slightly different alignment of the channel's amino acids within three-dimensional space. Yang, again using computer simulations, identified the best solution—the model with the lowest free energy. This gave us a picture of the three-dimensional structure of the folded string of amino acids within the human $Na_V1.7$ channel in a stable, biologically plausible state. We now had a model, included in Yang et al. (2012), which showed the locations of specific amino acids and some of the atoms within them in the human $Na_V1.7$ channel.

Modeling Molecules to Predict Drug Actions

A next step was to use our $Na_V1.7$ model to predict the actions of drugs on specific variants on $Na_V1.7$. The carbamazepine-sensitive V400M mutation provided a starting point. Building upon Yang's success with structural modeling, and reasoning that the location of the carbamazepine-sensitizing V400M substitution within the folded $Na_V1.7$ channel might be critical for the responsiveness of this channel variant to various medications, we reviewed our database of $Na_V1.7$ mutations. We then substituted various amino acids within the modeled channel to model these mutations, using the V400M substitution as a "seed" to search for other naturally occurring amino acid substitutions that might heighten the channel's response to carbamazepine.

Our analysis pointed to another inherited erythromelalgia mutation, S241T, as a candidate that might show increased responsiveness to carbamazepine. The site of the substituted amino acid in the S241T mutant channel is located 159 amino acids away from V400M in the linear, unfolded sequence of the channel, which is a long distance. But from our structural modeling we knew that S241T was located only 2.4 Ångstroms (Å)—less than the diameter of a water molecule from the V400M residue—within the folded three-dimensional structure. Beads 241 and 400 in the "necklace" of amino acids of $Na_V1.7$ were located right next to each other in the scrunched-up, folded configuration of the channel. To see whether this might permit us to predict the effect of carbamazepine on the S241T mutant, we next asked whether the relatively close locations of the V400M and S241T mutations within the folded channel structure reflected their working together in a coupled way during activation of the channel. Our thermodynamic analysis showed that, indeed, the V400M and S241T mutations were energetically coupled, working in tandem to effect channel activation through the same or a similar mechanism.

Based on these results, we hypothesized that the atomic proximity of these two mutations, and their mechanistic coupling, might be paralleled by pharmacological coupling. If this were the case, the two variant channels would be expected to share pharmacoresponsiveness to carbamazepine. To test this prediction, we assessed the effect of carbamazepine on the excitability of DRG neurons which we transfected with the S241T mutant channels in tissue culture, and compared the results with those obtained for cells expressing normal, wild-type $Na_V1.7$ channels. As shown in figure 5a–c of Yang et al. (Yang et al. 2012), our analysis showed that exposure to carbamazepine resulted in a doubling of current threshold for DRG neurons expressing the S241T mutant channel, making it harder to fire these cells. And carbamazepine dramatically reduced the number of action potentials produced by DRG neurons expressing the S241T mutant channel. In the aggregate, these observations demonstrated that carbamazepine can attenuate the hyperexcitability of pain-signaling neurons expressing the S241T mutant channel, as predicted by the structural modeling.

These results showed, in DRG neurons carrying the human $Na_V1.7$ channel in tissue culture, that structural modeling and thermodynamic analysis could predict the response of variant sodium channels to a pharmacotherapeutic agent. We published these results in 2012 (Yang et al. 2012). We were not yet there, but we hoped that this study would move us closer to personalized, genomically guided treatment for chronic pain.

A next step would be to study this in humans, to see whether carbamazepine would actually relieve pain in human subjects with the S241T mutation. That study (Geha et al. 2016) is described in chapter 13.

It took four years to do.

References

Fischer TZ, Gilmore ES, Estacion M, Eastman E, Taylor S, Melanson M, Dib-Hajj SD, Waxman SG. 2009. A novel $Na_V1.7$ mutation producing carbamazepine-responsive erythromelalgia. *Ann Neurol* 65(6): 733–741.

Geha P, Yang Y, Estacion M, Schulman BR, Tokuno H, Apkarian AV, Dib-Hajj SD, Waxman SG. 2016. Pharmacotherapy for pain in a family with inherited erythromelalgia guided by genomic analysis and functional profiling. *JAMA Neurol* 73(6): 659–667.

Payandeh J, Scheuer T, Zheng N, Catterall WA. 2011. The crystal structure of a voltage-gated sodium channel. *Nature* 475(7356): 353–358.

Yang Y, Dib-Hajj SD, Zhang J, Zhang Y, Tyrrell L, Estacion M, Waxman SG. 2012. Structural modelling and mutant cycle analysis predict pharmacoresponsiveness of a Na(v)1.7 mutant channel. *Nat Commun* 3: 1186.

STRUCTURAL MODELLING AND MUTANT CYCLE ANALYSIS PREDICT PHARMACORESPONSIVENESS OF A Na$_V$1.7 MUTANT CHANNEL*

Yang Yang, Sulayman D. Dib-Hajj, Jian Zhang, Yang Zhang, Lynda Tyrrell, Mark Estacion, and Stephen G. Waxman

Sodium channel Na$_V$1.7 is critical for human pain signaling. Gain-of-function mutations produce pain syndromes including inherited erythromelalgia, which is usually resistant to pharmacotherapy, but carbamazepine normalizes activation of Na$_V$1.7-V400M mutant channels from a family with carbamazepine-responsive inherited erythromelalgia. Here we show that structural modeling and thermodynamic analysis predict pharmacoresponsiveness of another mutant channel (S241T) that is located 159 amino acids distant from V400M. Structural modeling reveals that Na$_V$1.7-S241T is ~2.4 Å apart from V400M in the folded channel, and thermodynamic analysis demonstrates energetic coupling of V400M and S241T during activation. Atomic proximity and energetic coupling are paralleled by pharmacological coupling, as carbamazepine (30 µM) depolarizes S214T activation, as previously reported for V400M. Pharmacoresponsiveness of S241T to carbamazepine was further evident at a cellular level, where carbamazepine normalized the hyperexcitability of dorsal root ganglion neurons expressing S241T. We suggest that this approach might identify variants that confer enhanced pharmacoresponsiveness on a variety of channels.

Chronic pain affects more than one-quarter of Americans and pain in nearly 40% of these patients is not relieved by currently available drugs.[1] Recent studies have demonstrated that Na$_V$1.7, a voltage-gated sodium channel preferentially expressed in dorsal root ganglia (DRG) and sympathetic ganglia neurons, is essential for pain transduction.[2–5] Loss-of-function Na$_V$1.7 mutations cause congenital indifference to pain,[6] whereas gain-of-function mutations produce several painful syndromes including inherited erythromelalgia (IEM), a disorder in which, as

a result of hyperpolarized activation of Na$_V$1.7, threshold is reduced and evoked firing frequency increased in pain-signaling DRG neurons, leading to intense burning pain.[4,7,8] These studies have validated Na$_V$1.7 as a molecular target for development of new pain therapeutics.

IEM is characteristically unresponsive to existing pharmacotherapies.[7] Against this background of pharmaco-unresponsiveness, multiple-affected members of one family, carrying the Na$_V$1.7-V400M mutation, have responded favourably to carbamazepine (CBZ),[9] a state-dependent sodium channel blocker used mainly for treatment of epilepsy and trigeminal neuralgia.[10] Our previous study demonstrated that therapeutic concentrations of CBZ normalize the hyperpolarizing shift of Na$_V$1.7-V400M mutant channel activation,[9] while not affecting activation of wild-type channels. As the shift of activation voltage dependence is a strong contributor to hyperexcitability of DRG neurons expressing IEM mutations,[11] normalization of activation in V400M by CBZ seems to underlie the beneficial effect of CBZ in this family.[9] These findings suggest the feasibility of personalized pharmacotherapy based upon a pharmacogenomic approach. To achieve this goal, better understanding of structure–function relationships of human Na$_V$1.7 channel mutations that underlie drug responsiveness and development of pre-clinical assays of pharmacoresponsiveness are needed.

The first demonstration of the crystal structure of an ion channel, KcsA,[12] provided a basis for structural modeling of the ion channel superfamily. Recently, the crystal structure of the bacterial voltage-gated sodium channel NavAb has been solved, shedding new light on structural substrates for channel gating and drug

* Previously published in *Nature Communications* 3: 1186, 2012. © 2012 Macmillan Publishers Limited.

accessibility.[13] Starting from modeling of the human Na$_V$1.7 channel, we demonstrate in this study that an approach combining structural modeling, thermodynamic mutant cycle analysis and voltage- and current-clamp recording of Na$_V$1.7 mutant channels can predict pharmacoresponsiveness of a Na$_V$1.7 mutant channel (S241T) to CBZ, suggesting a novel approach to screening for amino-acid variants that enhance pharmacoresponsiveness of a variety of channels.

Results

V400 and S241 Show Atomic Proximity in Human Na$_V$1.7 Channel

Previous observations from the primary protein sequence suggest that IEM mutations of Na$_V$1.7 tend to cluster in transmembrane segments and S4–S5 linkers of domains I–III (ref. [4]) but their proximity to each other within the folded structure is not clear. To better understand structure–function relationships among IEM mutations, we constructed a structural model of transmembrane helices of human Na$_V$1.7 channel based on the recently solved crystal structure of the bacterial voltage-gated sodium channel NavAb.[13]

The human Na$_V$1.7 structural model was constructed using the GPCR-ITASSER program, an extension of the well-established I-TASSER algorithm,[14,15] incorporating a composite set of transmembrane-specific force fields and constraints.[16] Accuracy of individual domain models can be reliably estimated by the confidence score (C-score), which has a high correlation to the actual TM-score,[17] a widely used measure of similarity between two protein structures with values in the [0,1] range. Unlike RMSD (root-mean-square-deviation) score, TM-score is insensitive to local structure variation and protein size. In general, two structures with TM-scores <0.17 correspond to random similarity and those with TM-scores >0.5 indicate high similarity between the predicted model and native structure.[18,19]

Estimated TM-scores based on C-scores for our models of domains I–IV were 0.575, 0.805, 0.681 and 0.722, respectively, indicating similar folding structures to those of the bacterial sodium channel.

The linear schematic of Na$_V$1.7 channel is shown in figure 1a. Assembled folded structural models are shown in figure 1b (intramembrane side view) and figure 1c (cytosolic view). We are interested in the V400M mutation of DI/S6 helix because it is known to be pharmacoresponsive to CBZ.[9] Reasoning that location of V400M in the folded channel might be critical for its pharmacoresponsiveness, we looked for IEM mutations that are structurally close to V400M. Interestingly, our structural model revealed that the location of another IEM mutation (S241T) of DI/S4–S5 linker is close to that of V400M. The distance between S241 and V400 is only 2.4 Å measured from the closest hydrogen in the folded channel. This proximity, however, does not necessarily mean that the two residues engage in a direct interaction. Zoom-in views of DI/S6 show locations of V400 and S241 (figure 1d,e). The V400 side chain points toward the S4–S5 linker, where S241 is located (figure 1d,e). Although the effect of S241T on channel activation has been linked to increased size of the side chain at position 241 (probably through a steric hindrance effect),[20] pharmacoresponsiveness of S241T mutant channel has not been previously assessed.

Another IEM mutation (F1449V)[21] was selected for analysis because it is located at the cytoplasmic end of S6 helix, which brings it into proximity with the V400M mutation in DI/S6 (figure 1d,e). Based on homology modeling to potassium channel structure, F1449 has been suggested to contribute to a hydrophobic ring at the cytoplasmic pore opening, which acts as an activation gate.[22] Modeling of F1449 using the bacterial sodium channel structure recapitulated the hydrophobic ring. However, like the S241T mutant, the pharmacoresponsiveness of F1449V mutant channel is unknown.

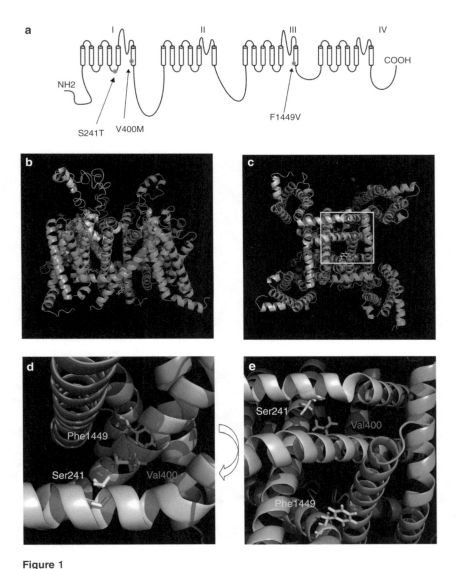

Figure 1

Structural modelling of transmembrane domains of human Na$_V$1.7 channel. (a) Schematic of the human Na$_V$1.7 channel topology showing the mutations S241T, V400M and F1449V. (b) Intra-membrane view of structural model of Na$_V$1.7 channel transmembrane domains. Domain I, light blue; Domain II, salmon; Domain III, cyan; Domain IV, lime. (c) Cytosolic view of the structural model of Na$_V$1.7 channel transmembrane domains. Boxed area containing S241, V400 and F1449 residues is enlarged in panel e. (d) Close-up intra-membrane view of the area containing S241, V400 and F1449 residues. (e) Close-up cytosolic view of the boxed area of panel c. S241, V400 and F1449 are shown as stick and coloured grey, red and yellow, respectively.

V400M and S241T Are Energetically Coupled during Activation

Previous studies show that all of these IEM mutations hyperpolarize channel activation.[4,9,20–22] However, it is not clear whether these mutations work independently or in concert to affect the same or different aspect of activation. We therefore asked whether the location of $Na_V1.7$ channel mutations demonstrated by our structural modeling might indicate mechanistic coupling during channel activation.

Thermodynamic mutant cycle analysis is a well-established approach for measuring independence or coupling of two mutations of a given protein.[23,24] We studied the coupling of V400M, a mutation located in the S6 helix, with either a structurally close mutation in the S4–S5 linker (S241T) or with a mutation in a different S6 helix (F1449V). Constructs carrying double mutations, for example, V400M and S241T or V400M and F1449V (named VM/ST and VM/FV, respectively) were created for mutant cycle analysis. Voltage dependence of activation was determined for $Na_V1.7$ WT channel, single mutations (V400M, F1449V and S241T) and double mutations (VM/ST and VM/FV) in transiently transfected HEK293 cells. If two mutations are energetically coupled (or affect channel activation through the same or shared mechanism), then the double mutation would not have an additive effect on channel activation compared with the single mutations. However, if two mutations are not energetically coupled (or affect the channel independently through distinct mechanisms), then the double mutation would have an additive effect on channel activation compared with the two single mutations.

The voltage dependence of activation for WT, the mutant pairs to be evaluated and the corresponding double mutant were fitted with the Boltzmann equation to determine the $V_{1/2}$ (half-activation voltage) and Z (proportional to the slope at half activation) (figure 2a,b). Representa-

tive traces are shown in figure 2c–h. Activation of double mutation VM/ST was rather close to that of the single mutations, indicating a non-additive effect and suggesting that V400M and S241T mutations alter activation via a common, shared mechanism (figure 2a). In contrast, activation of double mutation VM/FV was more hyperpolarized relative to the single mutations (figure 2b), indicating an additive effect and suggesting that the V400M and F1449V mutations alter activation via different, energetically independent mechanisms.

To quantitatively assess these effects, the energy change on channel activation caused by a single or double mutation was calculated. For each single or double mutation, $V_{1/2}$ and Z were used to determine free energy of activation ($\Delta G°$). The change in free energy of mutants relative to the WT channel was designated as ($\Delta\Delta G°$) and coupling free energy (magnitude of non-additivity) was ($\sum\Delta G°$). Designation and calculation of ($\Delta\Delta G°$) and ($\sum\Delta G°$) are described in Methods. Based on previous studies,[23–28] we set the following standard: if $\left|\sum\Delta G°\right| > 1\,\mathrm{kcal\,mol^{-1}}$, we accepted the two mutations as coupled (non-additive); whereas if $\left|\sum\Delta G°\right| < 1\,\mathrm{kcal\,mol^{-1}}$, we accepted the two mutations as independent (additive). We calculated $\sum\Delta G°$ for all mutation pairs and found that for the V400M: S241T mutation pair, $\left|\sum\Delta G°\right| = 2.32\,\mathrm{kcal\,mol^{-1}}$, and for V400M:F1449V mutation pair, the $\left|\sum\Delta G°\right| = 0.38\,\mathrm{kcal\,mol^{-1}}$ (supplementary table S1). These data are in good agreement with the fitted curves, and strongly suggest that V400M and S241T are energetically coupled, whereas V400M and F1449V are energetically independent during channel activation.

CBZ Depolarizes S241T Mutant Channel Activation

Structural modeling showed atomic proximity between V400 and S241, and mutant cycle analysis demonstrated that S241T is energetically

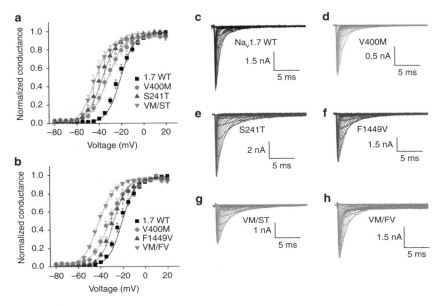

Figure 2

Mutant cycle analysis of voltage dependence of activation of $Na_V1.7$ mutations. (a) Voltage dependence of activation curves of $Na_V1.7$ WT, V400M, S241T, and V400M/S214T (VM/ST) double mutant channels. Curves were Boltzmann fits of the data. (b) Voltage dependence of activation curves of $Na_V1.7$ WT, V400M, F1449V and V400M/F1449V (VM/FV) double mutant channels. (c–h) Representative traces of current families recorded from HEK293 cells expressing WT (c), V400M (d), S241T (e), F1449V (f), VM/ST double mutant (g) and VM/FV double mutant (h) channels.

coupled with V400M during activation. Pretreatment of cells with a therapeutic concentration of CBZ (30 µM) is known to depolarize activation of V400M but not WT channels.[9]

Although residues within S4–S5 linkers of sodium channels have not been implicated in forming the local anaesthetic-binding site,[29] we hypothesized that atomic proximity and energetic coupling of V400M and S241T might be paralleled by pharmacological coupling so that they might share pharmacoresponsiveness to CBZ.

To test this hypothesis, the effect of CBZ (30 µM) pretreatment, initiated 30 min before recording,[9] on each mutant's activation was measured in HEK293 cells expressing S241T or F1449V mutant channels. Representative recordings are shown in figure 3a–d. Notably, CBZ

treatment caused a significant depolarizing shift in the $V_{1/2}$ of voltage dependence of activation of S241T mutant channels by 7.1 mV compared with dimethylsulphoxide (DMSO) treatment (DMSO: -37.6 ± 1.0 mV, $n = 10$; CBZ: -30.5 ± 1.3 mV, $n = 13$, $P < 0.01$, Student's t-test, figure 3e, supplementary table S2). In contrast, CBZ treatment of HEK293 cells expressing F1449V did not show a detectable effect on channel activation compared with DMSO treatment (activation $V_{1/2}$ for CBZ treatment: -27.1 ± 1.5 mV, $n = 8$; activation $V_{1/2}$ for DMSO treatment: -28.8 ± 1.1 mV, $n = 9$; $P > 0.05$, Student's t-test, figure 3f, supplementary table S2).

Enhancement of steady-state fast inactivation (a hyperpolarizing shift of steady-state fast inactivation $V_{1/2}$) is a classic mechanism of action

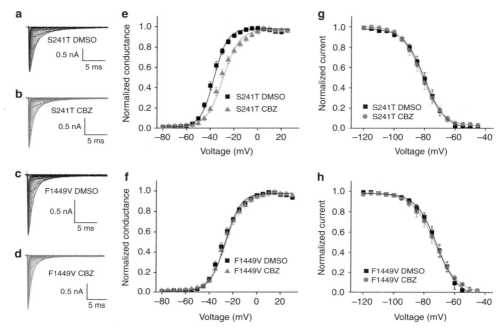

Figure 3
Voltage dependence of activation and steady-state fast inactivation of S241T and F1449V mutant
channels. (a–d) Representative traces of current families recorded from HEK293 cells expressing
S241T mutant channel treated with DMSO (a), or with CBZ (b); F1449V mutant channel treated
with DMSO (c), or with CBZ (d). (e) The averaged voltage dependence of activation of S241T
mutant channel treated with DMSO or CBZ (30 μM) was plotted and fitted with Boltzmann
equation. A depolarizing shift of activation of 7.1 mV was observed when S241T mutant channel
was treated with CBZ ($P<0.01$, Student's t-test). (f) The averaged voltage dependence of
activation of F1449V mutant channel treated with DMSO or CBZ was plotted and fitted with
Boltzmann equation. No notable shift in activation curve of F1449V mutant channel was observed.
(g–h) The voltage dependence of steady-state fast inactivation in response to 500 ms depolarizing
potential for S241T (g) or F1449V (h) mutant channel treated with DMSO or CBZ was plotted
and fitted with Boltzmann equation. No notable shift was observed.

for CBZ.[10] However, for Na$_V$1.7, a therapeutic
concentration of CBZ does not shift steady-state
fast inactivation of WT channel.[9] To determine
whether CBZ might have an effect on steady-
state fast inactivation of S241T or F1449V
mutant channels, HEK293 cells expressing
S241T or F1449V mutant channels were treated
with DMSO or CBZ (30 μM) as described earlier.
Steady-state fast inactivation was assessed in
response to a 500-ms depolarizing potential.
This protocol demonstrated a steady-state fast

inactivation $V_{1/2}$ for S241T of -79.9 ± 1.7 mV
($n=6$), and a steady-state fast inactivation $V_{1/2}$
for F1449 of -71.6 ± 1.5 mV ($n=6$) with DMSO
treatment (supplementary table S2), very close to
the values found in our previous studies without
any drug treatments.[20,22] CBZ (30 μM) did not
significantly alter the $V_{1/2}$ for either S241T or
F1449V mutant channels (-81.5 ± 2.1 mV, $n=6$;
-72.7 ± 2.2 mV, $n=8$, respectively; $P>0.05$ compared with DMSO treatment, Student's t-test,
figure 3g,h).

Expression of S241T Leads to DRG Neuron Hyperexcitability

To study the effects of S241T mutant channel on nociceptor excitability, small (20–28 μm diameter) DRG neurons from postnatal day 1–5 rats were isolated and transfected with either human $Na_V1.7$ WT or S241T mutant channels. Excitability was assessed by current-clamp recording 2 days after transfection. Current threshold, the injection current required to produce a single all-or-none action potential, was determined by applying 200 ms depolarizing currents of increasing magnitude (5 pA increments). For the neuron transfected with WT channels shown in figure 4a, current injection smaller than 225 pA generated small, graded membrane potential depolarization, with the first all-or-none action potential elicited by current injection of 230 pA. In contrast, a neuron expressing the S241T mutant channel fired the first action potential in response to current injection of 60 pA (figure 4b). On average, expression of S241T mutant caused a significant ~2.7-fold reduction of action potential threshold (83.5 ± 18.2 pA, $n = 20$) compared with DRG neurons expressing WT channel (227.6 ± 36.7 pA, $n = 19$, $P < 0.01$, Student's t-test, figure 4c).

The firing frequency of DRG neurons was also assessed by a series of 1-s current injections from 25 to 500 pA in 25-pA increments. For DRG neurons expressing WT channel, no action potentials or only a single action potential was elicited in response to depolarizing current injection, with an occasional second spike in response to stronger stimuli (figure 4d–f). In contrast, DRG neurons expressing S241T fired repetitively in response to low and high current injections (figure 4g–i). To compare firing frequency of DRG neurons expressing WT or S241T channels, the number of spikes elicited by 1-s current injection at various stimulus intensities was averaged (figure 4j). DRG neurons expressing S241T mutant channel fired significantly more spikes

than DRG neurons expressing WT channel at all stimulus intensities ≥ 125 pA (figure 4j, $P < 0.05$, Mann–Whitney test). Resting membrane potential (RMP) is known to affect DRG neuron excitability.[30] We therefore also assessed RMP of DRG neurons expressing WT or S241T mutant channels but did not observe a significant difference in RMPs (figure 4k). Taken together, these data show that expression of S241T mutant channels induces DRG neuron hyperexcitability.

CBZ Normalizes Excitability of DRG Neurons Expressing S241T

To test the prediction from our structural modeling and mutant cycle analysis, we assessed the effect of CBZ on hyperexcitability of DRG neurons expressing S241T or F1449V mutant channels using current-clamp recording. DRG neurons were treated with either DMSO or CBZ (30 μM) initiated 30 min before recording as mentioned above. Current threshold was assessed first: the response of a representative neuron expressing S241T treated with DMSO is shown in figure 5a. Current threshold for this neuron was 75 pA. In contrast, current threshold of a representative neuron expressing S241T treated with CBZ is shown in figure 5b. Current threshold for this neuron is 170 pA. On average, CBZ treatment resulted in a significant ~twofold increase in current threshold for DRG neurons expressing S241T mutant channel (CBZ treatment: 162.7 ± 24.4 pA, $n = 28$; DMSO treatment: 90.4 ± 13.2 pA, $n = 27$, $P < 0.01$, Student's t-test; figure 5c), indicating that CBZ treatment is likely to attenuate the excitability of DRG neurons expressing S241T mutant channel.

Our previous studies demonstrated that expression of F1449V mutant channel in DRG neurons reduces the current threshold and increases the firing frequency in response to sustained depolarizing stimuli.[21] As CBZ did not produce a depolarizing shift in F1449V mutant channel activation curve (figure 3f), we hypothesized

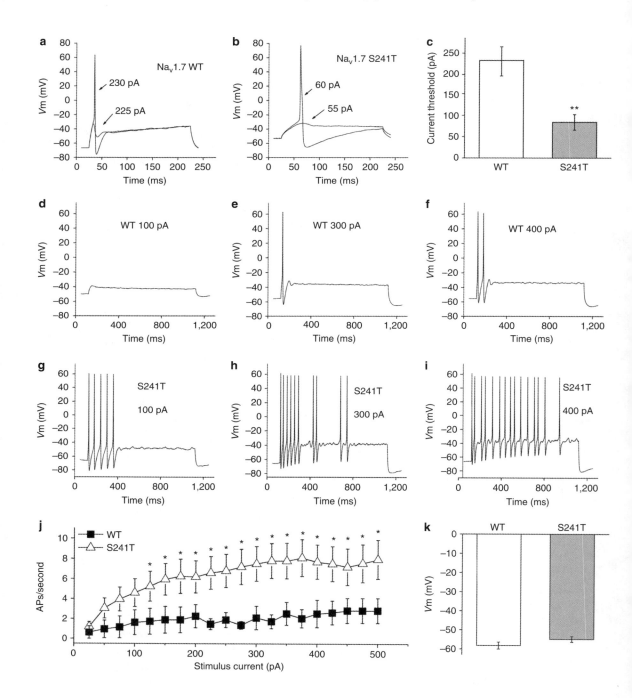

Figure 4
Current-clamp analysis of DRG neurons expressing WT or S241T mutant channel. (a) Representative DRG neuron expressing $Na_V1.7$ WT channel showed sub-threshold response to 225 pA current injection and subsequent action potential evoked by injection of 230 pA, which was the current threshold for this neuron. (b) Representative DRG neuron expressing $Na_V1.7$-S241T mutant channel showed sub-threshold response to 55 pA current injection and subsequent action potential evoked by injection of 60 pA. (c) Comparison of current threshold for DRG neurons expressing WT and S241T mutant channels. Expression of S241T channel reduced current threshold significantly (**$P<0.01$, Student's t-test). Current threshold for WT: (227.6 ± 36.7 pA, $n=19$); for S241T: (83.5 ± 18.2 pA, $n=20$). (d–f) Responses of a representative DRG neuron expressing WT channel to 1-s-long depolarizing current steps at 100 (d), 300 (e) and 400 (f) pA current injection. (g–i) Responses of a representative DRG neuron expressing S241T mutant channel to 1-s-long depolarizing current steps at 100 (g), 300 (h) and 400 (i) pA current injection. The difference in responses is apparent across this range. (j) The averaged number of action potentials between DRG neurons expressing WT and S241T mutant channel was compared. The response of DRG neurons expressing WT channel to current injection was significantly different compared with DRG neurons expressing S241T mutant channel across a range (125–500 pA) of step current injections (*$P<0.05$, Mann–Whitney test). (k) Averaged resting membrane potentials for DRG neurons expressing WT or S241T mutant channel were not statistically different. Results are presented as mean±s.e.m.

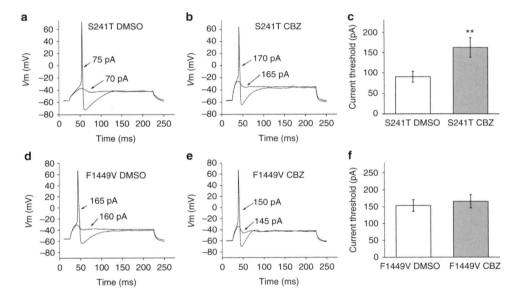

Figure 5
Current thresholds of CBZ- or DMSO-treated DRG neurons expressing S241T or F1449V mutant channels. (a,b) Sub- and supra-threshold responses of representative DRG neurons expressing S241T mutant channel treated with DMSO (a) or 30 μM CBZ (b) are shown. (c) Comparison of current threshold for DRG neurons expressing S241T mutant channel treated with DMSO or 30 μM CBZ. CBZ treatment increased the current threshold significantly (**$P<0.01$, Student's t-test). Current threshold for DMSO-treated DRG neurons: 90.4 ± 13.2 pA ($n=27$); for CBZ-treated DRG neurons: 162.7 ± 24.4 pA ($n=28$). (d,e) Sub- and supra-threshold responses of DRG neurons expressing F1449V mutant channel treated with DMSO (d) or 30 μM CBZ (e) are shown. (f) Comparison of current threshold for DRG neurons expressing F1449V mutant channel with the treatment of DMSO (153.5 ± 17.9 pA, $n=29$) or 30 μM CBZ (165.5 ± 19.7 pA, $n=28$). No significant difference was found ($P>0.05$, Student's t-test). Results are presented as mean±s.e.m.

that CBZ would not normalize firing properties of DRG neurons expressing F1449V mutant channel. Again, we assessed the current threshold first: as illustrated in figure 5d,e, current threshold of DRG neurons expressing F1449V mutant channels was similar between CBZ and DMSO treatments. For the population of neurons in these experiments, no significant difference was found for current threshold (DMSO, 153.5 ± 17.9 pA, $n = 29$; CBZ, 165.5 ± 19.7 pA, $n = 28$, $P > 0.05$, Student's t-test, figure 5f).

We further tested the effect of CBZ treatment on the firing frequency of DRG neurons expressing either the S241T or F1449V mutant channels. Robust repetitive firing was seen for neurons expressing S241T mutant channel treated with DMSO (figure 6a–c). In contrast, pretreatment with CBZ dramatically reduced the number of action potentials in DRG neurons expressing S241T mutant channel (figure 6d–f), with a statistically significant reduction of firing frequency at all stimulus intensities ≥ 100 pA ($P < 0.05$, Mann–Whitney test, figure 6g). This effect was not confounded by changes in RMPs, as CBZ did not affect RMPs of DRG neurons expressing mutant channels (figures 6h and 7h). Taken together, our data demonstrate that CBZ attenuates the hyperexcitability of DRG neurons expressing S241T mutant channel.

In contrast, CBZ did not attenuate the abnormal repetitive firing of DRG neurons expressing F1449V mutant channel. Repetitive firing was observed for neurons expressing F1449V mutant channel treated with DMSO (figure 7a–c) as well as treated with CBZ (figure 7d–f). Across a range of current injections, the firing frequency for CBZ- and DMSO-treated neurons was comparable in response to current injection ≤ 200 pA (figure 7g). Although firing frequency started to diverge with stronger injection, the effect of CBZ did not reach statistical significance even at current injection of 500 pA (figure 7g). Together with our results on V400M and S241T mutant channels, these data suggest that the effect of

CBZ is mutant specific and agrees well with our predication from structural modeling and mutant cycle analysis.

Discussion

Using structural modeling, based upon the recently solved crystal structure of a bacterial voltage-gated sodium channel,[13] we report that S241 within the DI/S4–S5 linker, while 159 amino acids distant from V400 in the channel peptide, is located close to V400 in the folded structure of the human $Na_V1.7$ sodium channel. Using mutant cycle analysis, we have demonstrated that $Na_V1.7$-V400M and -S241T mutant channels are energetically coupled during channel activation, suggesting that they contribute to the same feature of activation. As V400M mutation responds favourably to CBZ by shifting activation of V400M,[9] we reasoned that energetic coupling of V400M and S241T during channel activation might be paralleled by pharmacological coupling. Using voltage-clamp recording, we found that a therapeutic concentration of CBZ indeed normalizes the activation of S241T mutant channel. Moreover, we further show that this normalization of activation is accompanied by increased current threshold and reduced firing frequency of DRG neurons expressing S241T mutant channel. In contrast, V400M and F1449V mutants were not energetically coupled, and CBZ had no detectable effect on activation of F1449V or on the firing properties of DRG neurons expressing F1449V mutant channel. Human and rodent studies have demonstrated that the $Na_V1.7$ channel is essential for pain signaling and have validated this channel as a promising drug target for the development of novel pain therapeutics.[4] Structural and functional studies of $Na_V1.7$ mutant channels may provide insight into understanding mechanistic features of channel gating and its interaction with drugs. Previous studies of sodium channel structure and function were

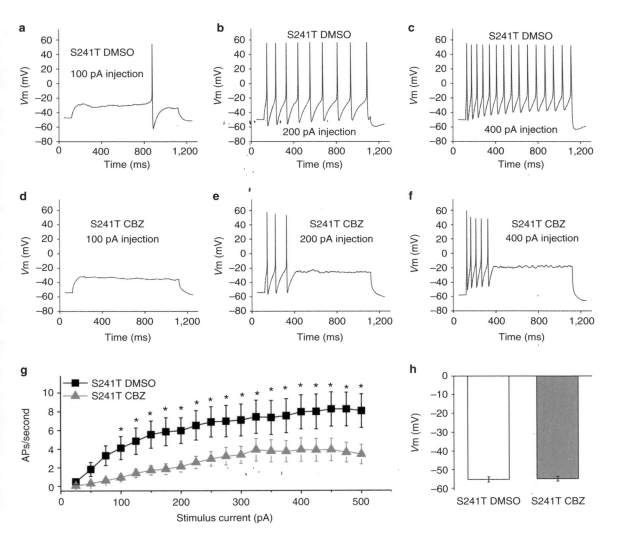

Figure 6

Firing frequencies and membrane potentials of CBZ- or DMSO-treated DRG neurons expressing S241T. (a–c) Responses of a representative DRG neuron expressing S241T mutant channel treated with DMSO to 1 s long depolarization current steps at 100 (a), 200 (b) and 400 (c) pA current injection. (d–f) Similar recordings from a representative DRG neuron expressing S241T mutant channel treated with 30 μM CBZ at 100 (d), 200 (e), and 400 (f) pA current injection. (g) Averaged response for DRG neurons expressing S241T mutant channel treated with DMSO (*n*=27) or CBZ (*n*=28) are summarized. CBZ statistically reduced firing frequency starting from 100 pA current injection (*P<0.05, Mann–Whitney test). (h) Averaged RMP between DRG neurons expressing S241T mutant channel treated with DMSO or CBZ were not statistically different (DMSO: −55.3±1.4 mV, *n*=27; CBZ: −54.9±1.3 mV, *n*=28, *P*>0.05, Student's *t*-test). Results are presented as mean±s.e.m.

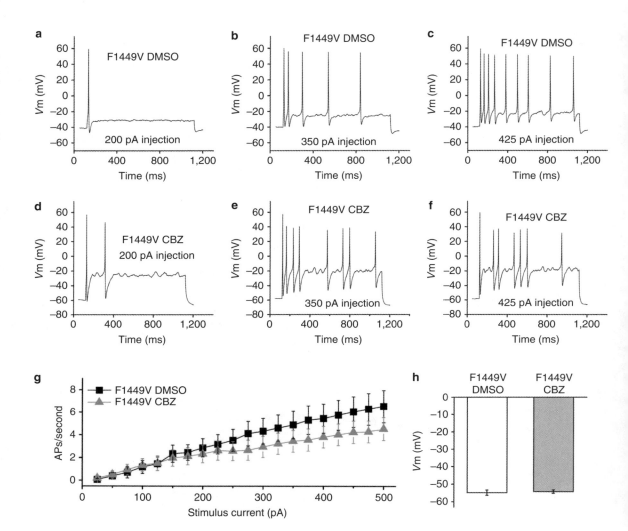

Figure 7
Firing frequencies and membrane potentials of CBZ- or DMSO-treated DRG neurons expressing
F1449V. (a–c) Responses of a representative DRG neurons expressing F1449V mutant channel
treated with DMSO to 1-s-long depolarization current steps at 200 (a), 350 (b) and 425 (c) pA
current injection. (d–f) Similar recordings from a representative DRG neuron expressing F1449V
mutant channel treated with CBZ at 200 (d), 350 (e) and 425 (f) pA current injection. (g) Averaged
firing frequencies for DRG neurons expressing F1449V mutant channel treated with DMSO
($n=29$) or CBZ ($n=28$) were compared and no statistical difference was found across the entire
range ($P>0.05$, Mann–Whitney test). (h) Averaged RMPs between DRG neurons expressing
F1449V mutant channel treated with DMSO or CBZ were not statistically different (DMSO:
-54.8 ± 1.5 mV, $n=29$; CBZ: -54.1 ± 1.0 mV, $n=28$, $P>0.05$, Student's t-test). Results are
presented as mean±s.e.m.

largely based on information obtained from the crystal structure of potassium channels.[22,25,31] Availability of the crystal structure of a bacterial voltage-gated sodium channel NavAb[13] permitted construction of a more realistic mammalian voltage-gated sodium channel model. It is worth noting that bacterial Na_V channels are four-fold symmetric, assembled from identical subunits, whereas mammalian Na_V channels have four non-identical domains encoded by a single protein. Alignment of NavAb and the four transmembrane domains of the Na_V1.7 channel is shown in supplementary table S3 and superposition of the transmembrane domains of Na_V1.7 with NavAb is shown in figure 8. Despite the difference outlined above, the bacterial Na_V

channel is the closest template for studying mammalian Na_V channel. Additionally, recent enhancements to I-TASSER,[17] a protein prediction package that has been successfully used to predict structure of many proteins including potassium channels for functional studies,[32,33] have provided improved predictions of membrane-bound proteins structure.[15,34] This method is not a simple homology modeling tool because the threading alignments from templates have been broken into pieces, which are used to reassemble the global structure of the membrane domains under the guide of a composite physics- and knowledge-based force field. As a result, it has been systematically demonstrated in community-wide CASP experiments that GPCR-

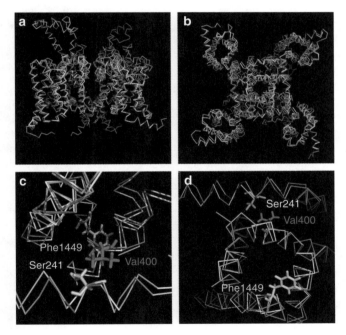

Figure 8

Alignment of Na_V1.7 structural model with NavAb structure. (a) Intra-membrane view of structural model of Na_V1.7 channel transmembrane domains aligned with NavAb structure (3RVY). Na_V1.7 Domain I, light blue; Domain II, salmon; Domain III, cyan; Domain IV, lime. NavAb, white. (b) Cytosolic view of the structural model of Na_V1.7 channel transmembrane domains aligned with NavAb structure. (c) Close-up intramembrane side view of the area containing S241 (grey), V400 (red) and F1449 (yellow) residues. (d) Close-up cytosolic view of the area containing S241, V400 and F1449 residues.

ITASSER models can be significantly closer to the target structure than the homologous modeling.[35] Taking advantage of these new developments, we constructed a structural model for the human $Na_V1.7$ channel and used it in this study to investigate the participation of different residues in channel activation, and to make predictions about drug–channel interaction.

We used thermodynamic mutant cycle analysis, a well-established tool, to quantitatively assess the energetic independence or coupling of two mutations in affecting channel activation. Mutant cycle analysis has been used to understand transition of pore elements during potassium channel gating,[23] interactions between ion channels and toxins[24,28] and identification of ion-pair-forming residues of the voltage-sensor domain in a bacterial sodium channel (NaChBac) during voltage-gated activation.[25–27] We show here that mutant cycle analysis can be used to test the hypothesis that different pathogenic IEM mutations (S241T, V400M and F1449V), all of which cause a hyperpolarizing shift of channel activation, participate in different steps of channel gating and have distinct pharmacoresponsiveness. More importantly, this analysis allowed us to predict that S241T mutant channel may interact with CBZ in a similar fashion as V400M mutant channel owing to their energetic coupling for channel activation.

Our structural model revealed that the V400 side chain points toward the DI/S4–S5 linker and is atomically close to and facing the S241 residue located in this linker, suggesting that mutations of these two residues might affect the same step in channel activation. The interaction between S4–S5 linker and S6 during channel gating has been suggested in voltage-gated K^+ (K_V) channel.[36–38] More recently, an all-atom molecular dynamics study of K_V channel gating mechanism has extended these findings by showing that channel activation imposes a pulling force on S4–S5 linker, which perturbs the interaction between S4–S5 linker and S6, leading to channel

opening.[39] Coupling of pore-forming helix to voltage sensors is also seen in Na_V channels,[40,41] most likely through S4–S5 linker.[42] A residue at the beginning of the S4–S5 linker is likely to form an interacting pair with residue at the tail end of the S6 helix,[42] further supporting the potential interaction of S4–S5 linker and S6 helix. On the other hand, F1449V may affect different steps in activation: the $Na_V1.7$ structural model places F1449 at the cytoplasmic tip of the S6 helix, suggesting that F1449 contributes to a hydrophobic ring at the cytoplasmic vestibule of the pore, consists of aromatic residues at equivalent positions in the S6 from four domains, acting as the activation gate of the channel. Taken together, our results suggest that V400M or S241T mutation may disrupt the tight packing of S4–S5 linker with S6 pore-forming helix, affecting channel activation; whereas the F1449V mutation may disrupt the hydrophobic ring and destabilize the channel preopen state, hyperpolarizing activation via a different structural action.[21,22]

Mutational analysis and functional studies have identified residues within S6 segments of domains III and IV to be important in forming drug-binding site(s) for local anesthetic and antiepileptic drugs, including CBZ (see refs [43–45] for review). The binding of a few sodium channel blockers (for example, local anesthetic drugs, anticonvulsant drugs) to the pore of voltage-gated sodium channels has been studied using structural modeling.[29,46] CBZ has been shown to interact with three key residues of $Na_V1.2$ channel (Leu1465 of DIII-S6, Phe1764 of DIV-S6 and Tyr1771 of DIV-S6).[29] In addition, N434, located near the middle of the DI/S6 helix, is also important for drug binding of $Na_V1.4$ (ref. [47]). IEM mutation N395K of $Na_V1.7$ channel, which corresponds to N434 in $Na_V1.4$, is suggested to be located within the local anesthetic-binding site of $Na_V1.7$. N395K mutation has been shown to depolarize activation of $Na_V1.7$ as well as significantly reduce use-dependent inhibition by lidocaine.[11] In addition, it has been found that the binding of local anesthetics (for example, lidocaine) to Na_V channel may lead to allosteric coupling of the binding site(s) of pore-forming helix to voltage sensors, especially in domain III and IV.[48] It is further suggested that S4–S5 linker and the intracellular end of S5 and S6 may be critical in coupling S6 helix to voltage-sensor movement in the presence of local anesthetics.[49]

These results imply that the effects of CBZ on Na_V1.7-S241T and -V400M mutant channels are not likely to be attributable to direct effects of these mutations on the drug-binding site(s). Alternatively, our data may be interpreted as suggesting a role for CBZ as a chemical chaperone for S241T and V400M mutant channels, rather than as a channel blocker. According to this hypothesis, CBZ–channel interaction may lead to stabilization of the S241T and V400M mutant channel in a WT-like conformation, and cause a depolarizing shift in activation, a biophysical change that contributes to attenuation of hyperexcitability of DRG neurons expressing mutant channels.

In summary, our results demonstrate that structural modeling and mutant cycle analysis can reveal the effect of sodium channel mutations on channel gating, and predict the responses of sodium channel mutations to a pharmacotherapeutic agent. We suggest that a similar approach, initially screening channels of interest for amino-acid variants that enhance pharmacoresponsiveness to existing agents and then using these variants as 'seeds' for further identification of other variants that enhance pharmacosensitivity, may permit identification of genomically defined subgroups of the population that are pharmacoresponsive.

Methods

Structural Modeling

Mammalian Na_V1.7 sodium channel is made up of four transmembrane domains, named I, II, III, IV linked by cyto-plasmic loops. The transmembrane helix structural model of human Na_V1.7 sodium channel was constructed in two steps. First, each of the four transmembrane domains was modeled separately using an advanced membrane-bound protein prediction algorithm GPCR-ITASSER.[16,50,51] Then, the whole channel model was built by structurally aligning four individual domain models to a global structural template of the recently solved bacterial sodium channel.

The GPCR-ITASSER algorithm is an advanced algorithm for transmembrane helical structure modeling. The program first uses a multiple threading procedure LOMETS[14] to identify the putative-related template structures in the PDB. The structural fragments (mainly α-helices) are then excised from the threading templates and assembled into full-length models by replica-exchange Monte Carlo simulations. In addition to the inherent I-TASSER force field, five transmembrane-protein-specific energy terms were also used to describe the interactions between transmembrane domain and membrane. (1) Membrane-repulsive energy is introduced for reducing the clash between intra- and extracellular domain and bilayer membrane. (2) Extracellular hydrophilic interactions for the hydrophilic interactions for residues inside and outside membrane. (3) Hydrophobic moment energy for the hydrophobic interaction between transmembrane helix and membrane. (4) Aromatic interactions for enhancing the specific interactions between aromatic–aromatic residues. (5) Cation–π interactions for specific noncovalent-binding propensities between TM helices. Finally, models of the lowest free energy are identified by clustering the simulation trajectories using SPICER,[52] and are refined at the atomic level by a fragment-guided dynamic simulation program FG-MD.[50]

We assembled the four transmembrane domains models in a clockwise order viewed from extracellular side as suggested by previous literature.[53,54] Each single domain model was aligned to the corresponding domain of the recently solved bacterial sodium channel by the structural alignment algorithm TM-align.[55] The resultant four domain complete structural model was refined again by FG-MD[50] to accommodate inter-domain steric clashes and improve the model quality.

Plasmid Preparation and HEK293 Cell Transfection

TTX-resistant human Na_V1.7 wild-type (WT) channel (hNa$_V$1.7r) was created based on the hNa$_V$1.7 (GenBank accession codes: NM_002977.3 (mRNA); NP_002968.1 (protein)). All other tested mutations were constructed on hNa$_V$1.7r background using Quick Change XL site-directed mutagenesis kit (Stratagene, La Jolla, CA, USA). WT or the mutant channels were transfected into HEK293 cells together with human β-1 and β-2 subunit[56] using Lipofectamine reagent (Invitrogen, Carlsbad, CA, USA). HEK293 cells were maintained in 1:1 Dulbecco's modified Eagle's media (DMEM)/F12 supplemented with 10% fetal bovine serum (FBS, Hyclone) in a humidified 5% CO$_2$ incubator at 37 °C. HEK293 cells were seeded onto poly-l-lysine-coated glass coverslips (BD Biosciences, San Jose, CA, USA) in a 24-well plate 1 day before transfection. Recording was performed 1 day after transfection.

Voltage-Clamp Recording of Sodium Channel in HEK Cells

Whole-cell voltage-clamp recordings were performed using the following solutions: the extracellular solution contained the following (in mM): 140 NaCl, 3 KCl, 1 MgCl$_2$, 1 CaCl$_2$, 20 Dextrose and 10 HEPES, pH = 7.3 with NaOH (320 mOsm adjusted with dextrose). The pipette solution contained the following (in mM): 140 Cs-Fluoride, 10 NaCl, 1.1 EGTA, 10 HEPES, 20 Dextrose, pH = 7.3 with CsOH (310 mOsm adjusted with dextrose). Patch pipettes had a resistance of 1–2 mΩ when filled with pipette solution. After achieving whole-cell recording configuration, the pipette and cell capacitance were manually minimized using the Axopatch 200B (Molecular Devices) compensation circuitry. Series resistance and prediction compensation (80–90%) was applied to reduce voltage errors. The recorded currents were digitized using pClamp software and a Digidata 1440A interface (Molecular Devices) at a rate of 50 kHz after passing through a low-pass Bessel filter setting of 10 kHz. Linear leak and residual capacitance artifacts were subtracted out using a P/N method provided with the Clampex software. Recording was initiated after a 5-min equilibration period after breaking in whole-cell configuration. CBZ was purchased from Sigma, dissolved in DMSO. For CBZ experiments, cells were treated with either CBZ (30 μM) or DMSO in incomplete medium without FBS for 30 min before recording and the CBZ or DMSO was maintained in the bath solution during the recording as described previously.[9]

Data analysis was performed using Clampfit (Molecular Devices) and Origin (Microcal Software). To generate activation curves, cells were held at −120 mV and stepped

to potentials of −80 to +40 mV in 5-mV increments for 100 ms. Peak inward currents were automatically extracted by Origin and fitted with BoltzIV function to determine the voltage at half activation ($V_{1/2}$), activation curve slope at half activation (Z) and reversal potential (E_{Na}) for each recording. Conductance was calculated as $G = I/(Vm - E_{Na})$ and normalized by the maximum conductance value and fit with Boltzmann equation. To generate steady-state fast-inactivation curves, cells were stepped to inactivating potentials from −120 to −40 mV for 500 ms followed by a 40-ms step to −10 mV as described previously.[21,57] Peak inward currents obtained from steady-state fast inactivation were normalized by maximum current amplitude and fitted with a Boltzmann equation.

Mutant Cycle Analysis

Double mutations (VM/ST and VM/FV) were created using site-directed mutagenesis. A total of six constructs (WT, V400M, S241T, F1449V, VM/ST, VM/FV) were expressed in HEK293 cells separately for patch-clamp analysis. The voltage dependence of activation for these mutations was analysed and a G–V curve was generated and fitted with Boltzmann equation to obtain $V_{1/2}$ and Z. Using $V_{1/2}$ and Z, the free energy to switch the channel from closed to the open state was calculated as $\Delta G°$ (C → O) (kcal/mol) = $-FZV_{1/2}$. The additional free energy required for the mutant channel to open relative to the WT channel was calculated as $\Delta\Delta G° = \Delta(FZV_{1/2}) = -F(Z_{mut}V_{1/2mut} - Z_{wt}V_{1/2wt})$. Magnitude of non-additivity (or the non-additive coupling free energy) was calculated as $\sum \Delta G° = \Delta\Delta(FZV_{1/2}) = -F[(Z_{wt}V_{1/2wt} - Z_{mut1}V_{1/2mut1}) - (Z_{mut2}V_{1/2mut2} - Z_{mut1'mut2}V_{1/2\ mut1,mut2})]$ (refs [23–28]).

Isolation and Transfection of DRG Neurons

DRG of Sprague-Dawley rat pups (postnatal day 1–5) were isolated and cultured as described previously.[58,59] Dissected ganglia were placed in ice-cold oxygenated complete saline solution (CSS), which contained the following (in mM): 137 NaCl, 5.3 KCl, 1 MgCl$_2$, 25 sorbitol, 3 CaCl$_2$ and 10 HEPES, pH 7.2. DRGs were then transferred to oxygenated 37 °C CSS solution containing 1.5 mg ml^{-1} collagenase A (Roche Applied Science) and 0.6 mM EDTA and incubated with gentle agitation at 37 °C for 20 min. This solution was exchanged with oxygenated, 37 °C CSS solution containing 1.5 mg ml^{-1} collagenase D (Roche Applied Science), 0.6 μM EDTA and 30 U ml^{-1}

papain (Worthington Biochemicals) and incubated with gentle agitation at 37 °C for 20 min. The solution was then aspirated and ganglia were triturated in DRG media: DMEM/F12 (1:1) with $100 \mu ml^{-1}$ penicillin, $0.1 mg ml^{-1}$ streptomycin (Invitrogen), and 10% FBS, which contained $1.5 mg ml^{-1}$ bovine serum albumin (Sigma-Aldrich) and $1.5 mg ml^{-1}$ trypsin inhibitor (Roche Applied Science).

WT, S241T or F1449V mutant channels were transiently transfected into the DRG neurons, respectively, along with enhanced green fluorescent protein (GFP), by electroporation with a Nucleofector II (Amaxa) system using basic Neuron SCN Nucleofector and program 'SCN basic program 6'. The ratio of sodium channel to GFP constructs was 10:1. Transfected neurons were allowed to recover for 5 min at 37 °C in 0.5 ml of Ca^{++}-free DMEM. The cell suspension was then diluted with DRG media containing $1.5 mg ml^{-1}$ bovine serum albumin and $1.5 mg ml^{-1}$ trypsin inhibitor, $80 \mu l$ mixture was placed on 12 mm circular poly-d-lysine/laminin-precoated coverslips (BD biosciences), and the cells were incubated at 37 °C in 5% CO_2 for 30 min. DRG media (1 ml per well), supplemented with $50 ng ml^{-1}$ each of mouse NGF (Alomone Labs) and glial cell line-derived neurotrophic factor (GDNF, Peprotec), was then added to cells. Cells were maintained at 37 °C in a 5% CO_2 incubator for further experiments.

Current-Clamp Recording in Transfected DRG Neurons

Whole-cell configuration was obtained in voltage-clamp mode before starting current-clamp recording. The pipette solution contained (in mM): 140 KCl, 0.5 EGTA, 3 Mg-ATP, 5 HEPES, 30 dextrose, pH=7.3 with KOH (310 mOsmol l^{-1}). The extracellular bath solution contained (in mM): 140 NaCl, 3 KCl, 2 MgCl₂, 2 CaCl₂, 15 dextrose, 10 HEPES, pH=7.3 with NaOH (315 mOsmol l^{-1}). Recording was performed on transfected nociceptive neurons, based on morphology with criteria of small diameter (20–28 mm) and round cell bodies, which also exhibited GFP fluorescence. All recordings were performed 2 days after transfection. For CBZ experiments, neurons were treated with either CBZ (30 μM) or DMSO as described above. RMP and seal stability for each neuron were evaluated during a 30-s-long period. Current threshold for action potential generation was determined by a series of 200 ms depolarizing currents in 5-pA increments. Repetitive firing frequency was examined using a series of 1-s current steps from 25 to 500 pA in 25-pA increments.

The interval between stimuli was 10 s. For firing frequency measurement, spikes with overshoot beyond 0 mV were counted as action potentials.

Data Analysis

Data were analysed with Clampfit 9.2 (Molecular Devices) and OriginPro 8.5 (Microcal Software). For statistical analysis, if samples obeyed a normal distribution, Student's t-test was used. Non-parametric Mann–Whitney test was used when samples failed the normality test. Data was presented as means±s.e.m. Statistical significance was accepted when $P < 0.05$.

Acknowledgments

We thank Dr Andrew Tan for comments on the manuscript, and Palak Shah and Bart Toftness for excellent technical assistance. This work was supported by the Medical Research Service and Rehabilitation Research Service, Department of Veterans Affairs and the Erythromelalgia Association (S.D.D-H. and S.G.W.). The Center for Neuroscience and Regeneration Research is a Collaboration of the Paralyzed Veterans of America with Yale University. J.Z. and Y.Z. are grateful for support from NSF Career Award (1027394) and NIGMS (GM083107 and GM084222).

About the Authors

Yang Yang, Department of Neurology, Yale University School of Medicine, New Haven, CT; Center for Neuroscience & Regeneration Research, Yale University School of Medicine, New Haven, CT; Rehabilitation Research Center, VA Connecticut Healthcare System, West Haven, CT

Sulayman D. Dib-Hajj, Department of Neurology, Yale University School of Medicine, New Haven, CT; Center for Neuroscience & Regeneration Research, Yale University School of Medicine, New Haven, CT; Rehabilitation Research Center, VA Connecticut Healthcare System, West Haven, CT

Jian Zhang, Center for Computational Medicine and Bioinformatics, University of Michigan

Yang Zhang, Center for Computational Medicine and Bio-informatics, University of Michigan

Lynda Tyrrell, Department of Neurology, Yale University School of Medicine, New Haven, ST.; Center for Neuro-science & Regeneration Research, Yale University School of Medicine, New Haven, CT; Rehabilitation Research Center, VA Connecticut Healthcare System, West Haven, CT

Mark Estacion, Department of Neurology, Yale University School of Medicine, New Haven, CT; Center for Neuro-science & Regeneration Research, Yale University School of Medicine, New Haven, CT; Rehabilitation Research Center, VA Connecticut Healthcare System, West Haven, CT

Stephen G. Waxman, Department of Neurology, Yale University School of Medicine, New Haven, CT; Center for Neuroscience & Regeneration Research, Yale University School of Medicine, New Haven, CT; Rehabilitation Research Center, VA Connecticut Healthcare System, West Haven, CT

Author Contributions

Y.Y., S.D.D-H., M.E. and S.G.W. designed the study. Y.Y. performed the experiments. Y.Y., S.D.D-H., and M.E. analysed the data. J.Z. and Y.Z. provided new tools. L.T. provided new reagents. S.D.D-H. and S.G.W. supervised the research. Y.Y., S.D.D-H., M.E. and S.G.W wrote the paper with inputs from all authors.

Additional Information

Supplementary Information accompanies this paper at http://www.nature.com/ naturecommunications

Competing financial interests: The authors declare no competing financial interests.

References

1. *Relieving Pain in America: A Blueprint for Transforming Prevention,* Care, Education, and Research (Washington, DC, 2011).

2. Waxman SG. 2006. Neurobiology: A channel sets the gain on pain. *Nature* 444: 831–832.

3. Dib-Hajj SD, Cummins TR, Black JA, Waxman SG. 2007. From genes to pain: Na$_V$1.7 and human pain disorders. *Trends Neurosci* 30: 555–563.

4. Dib-Hajj SD, Cummins TR, Black JA, Waxman SG. 2010. Sodium channels in normal and pathological pain. *Annu Rev Neurosci* 33: 325–347.

5. Minett MS, et al. 2012. Distinct Nav1.7-dependent pain sensations require different sets of sensory and sympathetic neurons. *Nat Commun* 3: 791.

6. Cox JJ, et al. 2006. An SCN9A channelopathy causes congenital inability to experience pain. *Nature* 444: 894–898.

7. Drenth JP, Waxman SG. 2007. Mutations in sodium-channel gene SCN9A cause a spectrum of human genetic pain disorders. *J Clin Invest* 117: 3603–3609.

8. Han C, et al. 2006. Sporadic onset of erythermalgia: A gain-of-function mutation in Nav1.7. *Ann Neurol* 59: 553–558.

9. Fischer TZ, et al. 2009. A novel Nav1.7 mutation producing carbamazepine-responsive erythromelalgia. *Ann Neurol* 65: 733–741.

10. Mantegazza M, Curia G, Biagini G, Ragsdale DS, Avoli M. 2010. Voltage-gated sodium channels as therapeutic targets in epilepsy and other neurological disorders. *Lancet Neurol* 9: 413–424.

11. Sheets PL, Jackson JO, 2nd, Waxman SG, Dib-Hajj SD, Cummins TRA. 2007. Nav1.7 channel mutation associated with hereditary erythromelalgia contributes to neuronal hyperexcitability and displays reduced lidocaine sensitivity. *J Physiol* 581: 1019–1031.

12. Doyle DA, et al. 1998. The structure of the potassium channel: Molecular basis of K+ conduction and selectivity. *Science* 280: 69–77.

13. Payandeh J, Scheuer T, Zheng N, Catterall WA. 2011. The crystal structure of a voltage-gated sodium channel. *Nature* 475: 353–358.

14. Wu S, Zhang Y. 2007. LOMETS: A local meta-threading-server for protein structure prediction. *Nucleic Acids Res* 35: 3375–3382.

15. Roy A, Kucukural A, Zhang Y. 2010. I-TASSER: A unified platform for automated protein structure and function prediction. *Nat Protoc* 5: 725–738.

16. Zhang J, Zhang Y. 2010. GPCRRD: G protein-coupled receptor spatial restraint database for 3D structure modeling and function annotation. *Bioinformatics* 26: 3004–3005.

17. Zhang Y. 2008. I-TASSER server for protein 3D structure prediction. *BMC Bioinformatics* 9: 40.

18. Xu J, Zhang Y. 2010. How significant is a protein structure similarity with TM-score = 0.5? *Bioinformatics* 26: 889–895.

19. Murzin AG, Brenner SE, Hubbard T, Chothia C. 1995. SCOP: A structural classification of proteins database for the investigation of sequences and structures. *J Mol Biol* 247: 536–540.

20. Lampert A, Dib-Hajj SD, Tyrrell L, Waxman SG. 2006. Size matters: Erythromelalgia mutation S241T in Nav1.7 alters channel gating. *J Biol Chem* 281: 36029–36035.

21. Dib-Hajj SD, et al. 2005. Gain-of-function mutation in Nav1.7 in familial erythromelalgia induces bursting of sensory neurons. *Brain* 128: 1847–1854.

22. Lampert A, et al. 2008. A pore-blocking hydrophobic motif at the cytoplasmic aperture of the closed-state Nav1.7 channel is disrupted by the erythromelalgia-associated F1449V mutation. *J Biol Chem* 283: 24118–24127.

23. Yifrach O, MacKinnon R. 2002. Energetics of pore opening in a voltage-gated K(+) channel. *Cell* 111: 231–239.

24. Ranganathan R, Lewis JH, MacKinnon R. 1996. Spatial localization of the K+ channel selectivity filter by mutant cycle-based structure analysis. *Neuron* 16: 131–139.

25. DeCaen PG, Yarov-Yarovoy V, Zhao Y, Scheuer T, Catterall WA. 2008. Disulfide locking a sodium channel voltage sensor reveals ion pair formation during activation. *Proc Natl Acad Sci USA* 105: 15142–15147.

26. DeCaen PG, Yarov-Yarovoy V, Sharp EM, Scheuer T, Catterall WA. 2009. Sequential formation of ion pairs during activation of a sodium channel voltage sensor. *Proc Natl Acad Sci USA* 106: 22498–22503.

27. Yarov-Yarovoy V, et al. 2012. Structural basis for gating charge movement in the voltage sensor of a sodium channel. *Proc Natl Acad Sci USA* 109: E93–E102.

28. Rauer H, et al. 2000. Structure-guided transformation of charybdotoxin yields an analog that selectively targets Ca(2+)-activated over voltage-gated K(+) channels. *J Biol Chem* 275: 1201–1208.

29. Lipkind GM, Fozzard HA. 2010. Molecular model of anticonvulsant drug binding to the voltage-gated sodium channel inner pore. *Mol Pharmacol* 78: 631–638.

30. Harty TP, et al. 2006. Na(V)1.7 mutant A863P in erythromelalgia: Effects of altered activation and steady-state inactivation on excitability of nociceptive dorsal root ganglion neurons. *J Neurosci* 26: 12566–12575.

31. Cestele S, et al. 2006. Structure and function of the voltage sensor of sodium channels probed by a beta-scorpion toxin. *J Biol Chem* 281: 21332–21344.

32. Yang Y, et al. 2011. Molecular basis and structural insight of vascular K(ATP) channel gating by S-glutathionylation. *J Biol Chem* 286: 9298–9307.

33. Yang Y, Shi W, Cui N, Wu Z, Jiang C. 2010. Oxidative stress inhibits vascular K(ATP) channels by S-glutathionylation. *J Biol Chem* 285: 38641–38648.

34. Roy A, Xu D, Poisson J, Zhang Y. 2011. A protocol for computer-based protein structure and function prediction. *J Vis Exp* 3: e3259.

35. Zhang Y. 2007. Template-based modeling and free modeling by I-TASSER in CASP7. *Proteins* 69(Suppl 8): 108–117.

36. Labro AJ, et al. 2011. The S4–S5 linker of KCNQ1 channels forms a structural scaffold with the S6 segment controlling gate closure. *J Biol Chem* 286: 717–725.

37. Labro AJ, et al. 2008. Kv channel gating requires a compatible S4–S5 linker and bottom part of S6, constrained by non-interacting residues. *J Gen Physiol* 132: 667–680.

38. Choveau FS, et al. 2011. KCNQ1 channels voltage dependence through a voltage-dependent binding of the S4–S5 linker to the pore domain. *J Biol Chem* 286: 707–716.

39. Jensen MO, et al. 2012. Mechanism of voltage gating in potassium channels. *Science* 336: 229–233.

40. Sheets MF, Chen T, Hanck DA. 2011. Lidocaine partially depolarizes the S4 segment in domain IV of the sodium channel. *Pflugers Arch* 461: 91–97.

41. Capes DL, Arcisio-Miranda M, Jarecki BW, French RJ, Chanda B. 2012. Gating transitions in the selectivity filter region of a sodium channel are coupled to the domain IV voltage sensor. *Proc Natl Acad Sci USA* 109: 2648–2653.

42. Muroi Y, Arcisio-Miranda M, Chowdhury S, Chanda B. 2010. Molecular determinants of coupling between the domain III voltage sensor and pore of a sodium channel. *Nat Struct Mol Biol* 17: 230–237.

43. Catterall WA. 2000. From ionic currents to molecular mechanisms: The structure and function of voltage-gated sodium channels. *Neuron* 26: 13–25.

44. Nau C, Wang GK. 2004. Interactions of local anesthetics with voltage-gated Na+ channels. *J Membr Biol* 201: 1–8.

45. Fozzard HA, Sheets MF, Hanck DA. 2011. The sodium channel as a target for local anesthetic drugs. *Front Pharmacol* 2: 68.

46. Lipkind GM, Fozzard HA. 2005. Molecular modeling of local anesthetic drug binding by voltage-gated sodium channels. *Mol Pharmacol* 68: 1611–1622.

47. Nau C, Wang SY, Strichartz GR, Wang GK. 1999. Point mutations at N434 in D1–S6 of mu1 Na(+) channels modulate binding affinity and stereoselectivity of local anesthetic enantiomers. *Mol Pharmacol* 56: 404–413.

48. Sheets MF, Hanck DA. 2003. Molecular action of lidocaine on the voltage sensors of sodium channels. *J Gen Physiol* 121: 163–175.

49. Arcisio-Miranda M, Muroi Y, Chowdhury S, Chanda B. 2010. Molecular mechanism of allosteric modification of voltage-dependent sodium channels by local anesthetics. *J Gen Physiol* 136: 541–554.

50. Zhang J, Liang Y, Zhang Y. 2011. Atomic-level protein structure refinement using fragment-guided molecular dynamics conformation sampling. *Structure* 19: 1784–1795.

51. Zhang J, Zhang Y. 2010. A novel side-chain orientation dependent potential derived from random-walk reference state for protein fold selection and structure prediction. *PLoS One* 5: e15386.

52. Zhang Y, Skolnick J. 2004. SPICKER: A clustering approach to identify near-native protein folds. *J Comput Chem* 25: 865–871.

53. Li RA, et al. 2001. Clockwise domain arrangement of the sodium channel revealed by (mu)-conotoxin (GIIIA) docking orientation. *J Biol Chem* 276: 11072–11077.

54. Dudley SC, Jr, et al. 2000. mu-conotoxin GIIIA interactions with the voltage-gated Na(+) channel predict a clockwise arrangement of the domains. *J Gen Physiol* 116: 679–690.

55. Zhang Y, Skolnick J. 2005. TM-align: A protein structure alignment algorithm based on the TM-score. *Nucleic Acids Res* 33: 2302–2309.

56. Lossin C, Wang DW, Rhodes TH, Vanoye CG, George AL, Jr. 2002. Molecular basis of an inherited epilepsy. *Neuron* 34: 877–884.

57. Cummins TR, Dib-Hajj SD, Waxman SG. 2004. Electrophysiological properties of mutant Nav1.7 sodium channels in a painful inherited neuropathy. *J Neurosci* 24: 8232–8236.

58. Estacion M, et al. 2008. NaV1.7 gain-of-function mutations as a continuum: A1632E displays physiological changes associated with erythromelalgia and paroxysmal extreme pain disorder mutations and produces symptoms of both disorders. *J Neurosci* 28: 11079–11088.

59. Han C, et al. 2009. Early- and late-onset inherited erythromelalgia: Genotype-phenotype correlation. *Brain* 132: 1711–1722.

13 PRECISION

On January 30, 2015, President Barack Obama announced details of the Precision Medicine Initiative (The White House 2015). In launching this initiative, the White House press briefing noted that "most (currently available) medical treatments have been designed for the 'average patient.'" The announcement went on to describe an "approach to disease prevention and treatment that takes into account individual differences in people's genes" as well as environment and lifestyle.

Like many colleagues in the scientific community, my team and I at Yale were pleased to learn that this initiative was moving forward. But, as we read the announcement we were bemused, for a very specific reason: As the Precision Medicine Initiative was being discussed by policy makers in Washington, we were actually doing it in New Haven.

Building upon our discovery in 2009 (Fischer et al. 2009) of a family carrying an erythromelalgia mutation that sensitized their $Na_V1.7$ channel to carbamazepine, the Yang et al. study in 2012 capitalized on powerful techniques—atomic-resolution structural modeling and thermodynamic analysis—to predict the responsiveness of another $Na_V1.7$ mutation—S241T—to this medication (Yang et al. 2012). Using patch-clamp electrophysiology, we had shown in this study that DRG neurons carrying the mutant S241T channel in tissue culture display enhanced responsiveness to carbamazepine. The results of that study, carried out at the laboratory bench, were exciting indeed. But as the Obama administration made its announcement, we were fixated on moving our precision medicine approach beyond the laboratory, to human subjects in the clinic.

We were aware of only two individuals in North America who carried the S241T mutation. Both suffered with the symptoms of the "man on fire" syndrome. One had begun to experience severe burning pain in his arms and legs, triggered by mild warmth and relieved by cooling, at age 16. He reported having up to 30 attacks per month, each lasting hours to days, in which his pain could reach as high as 9 on a 1–10 rating scale. Pain prevented him from sleeping, often waking him at night. The second individual had lived with burning pain in both feet triggered by mild warmth and relieved by cooling, beginning around age 17. She rated her pain as severe, at 8–9 on the 1–10 scale.

It had taken us nearly two years to locate these individuals and to plan a human study. Our overall objective was to assess, in human beings, whether our pharmacogenomic approach would work. This would require a complex double-blinded, placebo-controlled crossover trial. Each of the participants would receive the medication predicted to be effective, carbamazepine, or a placebo, pills containing a substance with no effect on the body. The capsules were to be prepared in the research pharmacy at the Veterans Affairs Connecticut Healthcare Center and were to be coded—identified only by a code number which did not reveal what they contained—so that neither the patients, nor the physicians who interacted with them and analyzed their reports, knew what the tablets contained. Each subject would take the pills for six weeks (a two-week "ramp-up" period, during which we would adjust the dose, a fifteen-day maintenance period, and a two-week taper-down period). Then, after a two-week wash-out period, they would "cross over." If the capsules contained placebo in the first part of the study, they would contain carbamazepine in the second part. And vice versa. For another six weeks. Blood levels would be periodically measured to be sure that the subjects were taking their pills (placebo or carba-mazepine) as prescribed and to confirm that the medications were being taken up by their bodies.

Key to the study was how we would assess the response to carbamazepine. We decided that, at home and work, each of the subjects would record his or her pain, daily, while taking placebo or carbamazepine, in a structured pain diary. This would give us a picture of our subjects' pain in their usual environment. In addition, we wanted to study the effect of carbamazepine during pain attacks, in our clinic. To do this we had to solve a problem: The pain of erythromelalgia can vary from day to day, and it is not possible to predict when an attack will occur. There was, however, a way around this problem. If we *provoked* pain attacks in the laboratory using carefully calibrated stimuli, we could assess the effect of carbamazepine on the brain's representation of pain in response to a known and reproducible trigger. Physicians don't like to inflict pain, but in this instance it was necessary if we were to carry out a conclusive study. After discussion with medical ethicists and Yale's Human Investigation Committee, we decided that, if the subjects understood the protocol and gave informed consent, we would study them at Yale Medical School where we would use a specially built heating boot to evoke painful attacks with precisely calibrated heat stimuli. Provocation of pain attacks in the laboratory in this way would give us control over the timing of the attack, and of the trigger. Built into our protocol were options for the participants to withdraw from the study at any time, or to request cooling as a "rescue therapy."

Although there was no validated biomarker for pain as we began this study, we decided to measure brain activity of the subjects. To do this, we were going to use functional magnetic resonance imaging (fMRI). This powerful methodology can noninvasively measure human brain activity as subjects carry out various tasks (for example, it can determine the part of the brain that is active when people move their fingers or when they do arithmetic calculations) or as they are subjected to various experiences (for example, it can reveal the parts of the brain that become active when one hears a happy or sad story). fMRI was already being used around the world to study brain activity in a variety of diseases. However, despite the power of fMRI to reveal the brain's secrets, people with inherited erythromelalgia are hard to find, and there had been only one prior study using functional imaging to assess the pattern of activity in the brain in inherited erythromelalgia. That study at University of Oxford (Segerdahl et al. 2012) had assessed a single subject. The Oxford study had focused on the brain's activity during pain attacks, with no attempt to treat the pain. Here, three thousand miles away at Yale, we had access to two patients with inherited erythromelalgia and a medication that we thought might be helpful.

Yale is world-renowned for research in fMRI, but in 2012 only half a dozen universities housed research programs using fMRI to study pain and Yale was not one of them. We considered partnering with Harvard, or the NIH, but distance was an issue. Then, we became aware that Paul Geha, a young psychiatrist with a special interest in pain, was finishing his residency at Yale. Paul had previously worked for five years with A. Vania Apkarian, a professor of physiology at Northwestern University who had pioneered the use of fMRI to measure brain activity related to pain. We met with Paul several times, and it was clear that he was up to the challenge. He had access to the fMRI scanners and understood the intricacies of brain imaging to study pain. And he was interested. We had our dream team.

A next step was to invite the two subjects to participate. Imagine being asked to enroll in a research study, with an explanation something like this: "We invite you to participate in a research study, which will examine the effect of an existing medication on your erythromelalgia. We cannot tell you the name of the medication. It may help you, or it may not. To participate in this study, you will have to travel to Yale for at least seven visits. During each visit, we will apply heat to your foot to evoke your pain, and we will measure your brain activity. While we do this, you will have to lie very still for more than two hours, with your head in a very large magnet. As you lie there, as still as you can be, you will hear very loud knocking noises, almost like a machine gun."

Both subjects said yes.

In late 2014 we were ready to begin. Pivotal to our success was that despite wintry conditions, the two participants each made their visits to Yale over the ensuing months. Each took carbamazepine, or placebo, for six weeks, and then, after a two-week wash out, "crossed over." Neither was told what was in the pills. Together, they completed nine fMRI scanning sessions (five for one participant; four for the other, who missed one scan).

To minimize the chance of any bias, in a double-blinded study the investigators as well as the subjects are blinded. Because we were blinded, as the study moved forward, we did not know whether carbamazepine was having an effect on our subjects' pain, or the results of the fMRI scans. It was not until the subjects had finished their trials of carbamazepine and placebo, and their scans had been formatted by computer, that we viewed the records. The results (Geha et al. 2016) were remarkable: Both subjects had filled in structured daily diaries during the entire period of the study, and these provided strong evidence for a reduction in their pain while treated with carbamazepine. Subject 1 reported a reduction of average time in pain per day from 424 minutes while on placebo to 231.9 minutes on carbamazepine, a drop of about 45%. Subject 2 reported a reduction of average time in pain per day from 61 minutes while on placebo to 9.1 minutes on carbamazepine, a drop of 85%. The diary of subject 1 revealed a reduction in the average duration of painful attacks from 615 minutes while taking placebo to 274.1 minutes while taking carbamazepine, while the diary of subject 2 documented a reduction in attack duration from 91.5 minutes while on placebo to 45.3 minutes on carbamazepine. There also was a striking improvement in sleep. Subject 1 reported 101 awakenings from pain while on placebo, and 32 awakenings from pain on carbamazepine.

The functional brain imaging results were striking as well. While untreated or during treatment with placebo, pain provoked by heat was associated with activity within parts of the brain such as the nucleus accumbens and cingulate cortex, two areas of the brain that are known to be activated in association with various chronic pain conditions. These brain areas also become active in reward-or-punishment scenarios and are thought to mediate emotional decision-making. But even more interesting were the scans during treatment with carbamazepine. These showed a change in the pattern of brain activity. In parallel with reduced pain, there was a decrease in activity in these emotional-linked brain areas. Pain reduction during treatment with carbamazepine was also paralleled by increased activity in primary and secondary sensory-motor areas of the brain as well as parietal attention areas and prefrontal cortex. So, while treated with carbamazepine, the subjects' reduction in pain was accompanied by a shift in brain resources away from areas involved in emotional decision-making and previously implicated in chronic pain, and toward brain areas that mediate sensorimotor, attention and executive function. Placebo did not produce this shift. Here we had a measure of the effect of carbamazepine which did not depend on the subjects' reports of pain but, rather, reflected a change in the activity in their brains.

The research reported in the Yang et al. (2012) and Geha et al. (2016) papers took almost five years from inception to completion. Overall, it took twelve years to advance from our initial characterization of erythromelalgia mutations and our demonstration of how they cause disease (Cummins, Dib-Hajj, and Waxman 2004; Dib-Hajj et al. 2005) to being able to show, in the Geha et al. (2016) paper, that we could use genomic information to treat pain. In moving from mutant genes and their secrets to the treatment of patients who carried these mutant genes, these studies showed us that, in principle, the goal of genomically guided, precision therapy for pain might be achievable.

In the Geha et al. paper, we pointed out that the results applied in a strict sense only to the small number of people who carry the S241T mutation, and we stressed that there was much to be done before precision pain therapy was applicable to broader populations. One approach would be to use a strategy similar to the one we used for the S241T mutation, to initially screen channels of interest to find other mutations that enhance pharmacoresponsiveness to existing agents, and then to use these as "seeds" for further identification of still other pharmacoresponsive variants; this might permit identification of genomically defined subgroups of the broad population that respond preferentially to treatment with a variety of specific medications. That strategy, if successful, could broaden the applicability of the pharmacogenomic approach to pain of many types.

The Geha et al. study was a lot of work, and we were all tired by the time it was published. In an editorial in *JAMA Neurology* that accompanied the paper, geneticist and neurologist Juan Pascual buoyed us, noting that "there are relatively few examples in medicine where molecular reasoning is rewarded with a comparable degree of success" (Pascual 2016). As this book goes to press our research team is actively pursuing the goal of pharmacologically guided pain treatment, aided by laboratory robots that multiply our human efforts. The hundreds of variants of $Na_V1.7$ that are known to exist, with others undoubtedly waiting to be identified, mean that there is a lot of work to do. But, looked at in another way, the richness of the library of gene variants provides a robust platform for the development of precision medicine. We are propelled by a vision of a future in which each person's DNA will guide his or her healthcare. In that future, as a gift from the genome, pain will be much more treatable.

References

Cummins TR, Dib-Hajj SD, Waxman SG. 2004. Electrophysiological properties of mutant Nav1.7 sodium channels in a painful inherited neuropathy. *J Neurosci* 24(38): 8232–8236.

Dib-Hajj SD, Rush AM, Cummins TR, Hisama FM, Novella S, Tyrrell L, Marshall L, Waxman SG. 2005. Gain-of-function mutation in Nav1.7 in familial erythromelalgia induces bursting of sensory neurons. *Brain* 128(Pt 8): 1847–1854.

Fischer TZ, Gilmore ES, Estacion M, Eastman E, Taylor S, Melanson M, Dib-Hajj SD, Waxman SG. 2009. A novel Nav1.7 mutation producing carbamazepine-responsive erythromelalgia. *Ann Neurol* 65(6): 733–741.

Geha P, Yang Y, Estacion M, Schulman BR, Tokuno H, Apkarian AV, Dib-Hajj SD, Waxman SG. 2016. Pharmacotherapy for pain in a family with inherited erythromelalgia guided by genomic analysis and functional profiling. *JAMA Neurol* 73(6): 659–667.

Pascual JM. 2016. Understanding atomic interactions to achieve well-being. *JAMA Neurol* 73(6): 626–627.

Segerdahl AR, Xie J, Paterson K, Ramirez JD, Tracey I, Bennett DL. 2012. Imaging the neural correlates of neuropathic pain and pleasurable relief associated with inherited erythromelalgia in a single subject with quantitative arterial spin labelling. *Pain* 153(5): 1122–1127.

The White House. 2015. "Fact Sheet: President Obama's Precision Medicine Initiative." http://www.whitehouse.gov/the -press-office/2015/01/30/fact-sheet-president-obama-s-precision-medicine-initiative/.

Yang Y, Dib-Hajj SD, Zhang J, Zhang Y, Tyrrell L, Estacion M, Waxman SG. 2012. Structural modelling and mutant cycle analysis predict pharmacoresponsiveness of a Na(v)1.7 mutant channel. *Nat Commun* 3: 1186.

PHARMACOTHERAPY FOR PAIN IN A FAMILY WITH INHERITED ERYTHROMELALGIA GUIDED BY GENOMIC ANALYSIS AND FUNCTIONAL PROFILING*

Paul Geha, Yang Yang, Mark Estacion, Betsy R. Schulman, , Hajime Tokuno, A. Vania Apkarian, Sulayman D. Dib-Hajj, and Stephen G. Waxman

Importance: There is a need for more effective pharmacotherapy for chronic pain, including pain in inherited erythromelalgia (IEM) in which gain-of-function mutations of sodium channel $Na_V1.7$ make dorsal root ganglion (DRG) neurons hyperexcitable.

Objective: To determine whether pain in IEM can be attenuated via pharmacotherapy guided by genomic analysis and functional profiling.

Design, Setting, and Participants: Pain in 2 patients with IEM due to the $Na_V1.7$ S241T mutation, predicted by structural modeling and functional analysis to be responsive to carbamazepine, was assessed in a double-blind, placebo-controlled study conducted from September 2014 to April 21, 2015. Functional magnetic resonance imaging assessed patterns of brain activity associated with pain during treatment with placebo or carbamazepine. Multielectrode array technology was used to assess the effect of carbamazepine on firing of DRG neurons carrying S241T mutant channels.

Main Outcomes and Measures: Behavioral assessment of pain; functional magnetic resonance imaging; and assessment of firing in DRG neurons carrying S241T mutant channels.

Results: This study included 2 patients from the same family with IEM and the S241T $Na_V1.7$ mutation. We showed that, as predicted by molecular modeling, thermodynamic analysis, and functional profiling, carbamazepine attenuated pain in patients with IEM due to the S241T $Na_V1.7$ mutation. Patient 1 reported a reduction in mean time in pain (TIP) per day during the 15-day maintenance period, from 424 minutes while taking placebo to 231.9 minutes while taking carbamazepine (400 mg/day), and a reduction in total TIP over the 15-day maintenance period,

* Previously published in *JAMA Neurology* 73(6): 659–667, 2016. Copyright 2016 American Medical Association.

from 6360 minutes while taking placebo to 3015 minutes while taking carbamazepine. Patient 2 reported a reduction in mean TIP per day during the maintenance period, from 61 minutes while taking placebo to 9.1 minutes while taking carbamazepine (400 mg then 200 mg/day), and a reduction in total TIP, from 915 minutes while taking placebo over the 15-day maintenance period to 136 minutes while taking carbamazepine. Patient 1 reported a reduction of mean episode duration, from 615 minutes while taking placebo to 274.1 minutes while taking carbamazepine, while patient 2 reported a reduction of the mean episode duration from 91.5 minutes while taking placebo to 45.3 minutes while taking carbamazepine. Patient 1, who had a history of night awakenings from pain, reported 101 awakenings owing to pain while taking placebo during the maintenance period and 32 awakenings while taking carbamazepine. Attenuation of pain was paralleled by a shift in brain activity from valuation and pain areas to primary and secondary somatosensory, motor, and parietal attention areas. Firing of DRG neurons expressing the S241T $Na_V1.7$ mutant channel in response to physiologically relevant thermal stimuli was reduced by carbamazepine.

Conclusions and Relevance: Our results demonstrate that pharmacotherapy guided by genomic analysis, molecular modeling, and functional profiling can attenuate neuropathic pain in patients carrying the S241T mutation.

Inherited erythromelalgia (IEM) is an autosomal dominant disorder characterized by severe burning pain in the distal extremities, triggered by warmth and relieved by cooling, caused by gain-of-function mutations of the $Na_V1.7$ sodium channel, which is encoded by the *SCN9A* gene.[1] $Na_V1.7$ is preferentially expressed within peripheral sensory dorsal root ganglion (DRG) and sympathetic ganglion neurons,[2–4] where it activates at relatively hyperpolarized potentials below the threshold for action potential generation. Na$_V$1.7 amplifies small stimuli, thereby setting the gain for firing.[2] In general, the Na$_V$1.7 mutations that cause IEM shift channel activation in a hyperpolarizing direction, making it easier to open the channel; when expressed within DRG neurons, these mutations produce hyperexcitability.[2,3] Most patients with IEM experience limited relief, if any, with available medications, and patients classically resort to cooling of the affected limbs, in some cases with prolonged ice baths that ultimately lead to tissue breakdown.[1]

While most patients with IEM do not respond to pharmacotherapy, a family with IEM, responsive to treatment with the sodium channel inhibitor carbamazepine, has been reported.[5] The mutation in this family, V400M, hyperpolarizes activation, similar to other Na$_V$1.7 mutations that cause IEM. Notably, carbamazepine at clinically relevant concentrations has a specific action on V400M mutant channels in which it normalizes activation.[5] Yang et al.[6] used this carbamazepine-responsive V400M mutation as a "seed" for atomic-level structural modeling and showed that another rare Na$_V$1.7 mutation (S241T) identified in patients with IEM, 159 amino acids distant from V400M within the linear channel sequence, is located less than 2.8Å from V400M within the folded channel protein; they used thermodynamic analysis to demonstrate energetic coupling of the S241 and V400 amino acids during channel activation. As predicted by the atomic proximity and energetic coupling to a carbamazepine-responsive mutation, carbamazepine had a specific effect, not seen in other IEM mutant channels, on S241T where it normalizes activation.[6]

In this article, we translate our in silico and in vitro analyses of the S241T mutation to a family with IEM carrying this channel variant. We hypothesized that treatment with carbamazepine would attenuate pain in patients with IEM carrying the S241T mutation and that, compared with placebo, attenuation of pain would be paralleled by a decrease in brain activity, measured with functional brain imaging (fMRI), in valuation

and pain areas previously implicated in chronic pain and modulated by treatment.[7–14]

Methods

Human Participants

The patients were 2 adults with IEM carrying the S241T mutation. Patient 1 reported onset in his teens with severe burning pain in his feet, triggered by mild warmth and relieved by cooling, followed by similar pain in his hands, knees, elbows, shoulders, and ears. He described up to 30 episodes per month, each lasting hours to days. He described his typical IEM pain episode as severe, at a 9 on the pain numerical rating scale (NRS). Venlafaxine and gabapentin did not provide relief, and lidocaine patches provided minimal relief. He reported that his IEM prevented him from sleeping through the night and that it limited physical activity. Patient 2 reported onset of burning pain in both feet, triggered by mild warmth and relieved by cooling, which began in her teens, subsequently involving her knees and ears. She rated her pain

Box 1
Key Points

Question Is genomically guided pharmacotherapy feasible in a genetic model of pain?

Findings In this study of 2 patients with inherited erythromelalgia due to the Na$_V$1.7 S241T mutation, a double-blind cross-over study showed that carbamazepine attenuated pain, as predicted by genomic/molecular analysis and functional profiling. Pain relief was paralleled by a shift in brain activity from valuation and pain areas to primary and secondary somatosensory, motor, and parietal attention areas.

Meaning Pharmacotherapy guided by genomic analysis, molecular modeling, and functional profiling reduces pain in patients with inherited erythromelalgia due to the S241T mutation. As more channel variants are linked to pain, structural and functional analyses may provide additional opportunities for genomically guided pharmacotherapy.

as severe, at 8 and 9 on the NRS pain scale. Aspirin did not provide relief.

Study Design

The Human Investigations Committees at Yale University and West Haven VAMC approved this study (NCT02214615), which was conducted from September 2014 to April 21, 2015, and written informed consent was obtained from both patients. In this double-blind crossover study, each of the 2 patients with IEM, carrying the S241T mutation, were assessed during a series of 7 hospital visits, which included 5 fMRI scans (efigure 1 in the Supplement). Details of visits, scans, drug ramp-up, maintenance, and taper-down periods are given in the eAppendix in the Supplement.

Carbamazepine Treatment and Monitoring

At each scanning visit, blood was obtained to monitor complete blood cell count and carbamazepine levels. Carbamazepine or placebo were started at 200 mg daily. Patients reported pain levels every 4 days using the NRS (0 = no pain to 10 = worst imaginable pain); if pain intensity had not improved by 2 NRS units and adverse effects were not experienced, the dose was increased by 200 mg until pain intensity improved. If pain intensity had improved, the carbamazepine dose was maintained.

Prescan Testing

Pain in IEM is triggered by warmth.[1,2] We used a calibrated warming boot to reliably elicit pain as described in the eAppendix in the Supplement.

Continuous Pain Rating

For continuous pain intensity ratings (figure 1),[7,8,11,15] patients continuously indicated their level of pain during test sessions through a linear potentiometer device attached to the dominant thumb and index finger, with voltage output displayed by a computer that indicated the extent of their finger span, providing visual feedback. Maximum thumb-finger span was used to indicate "worst imaginable pain intensity" and thumb-and-finger touching to indicate "no pain" on the generalized labeled magnitude scale. Details are provided in the eAppendix in the Supplement.

Pain Rating and Visual Magnitude Rating Tasks during fMRI

Patients were scanned while (1) rating their pain in response to thermal stimuli, (2) rating ongoing pain (no stimulation) after an episode was elicited, and (3) rating the magnitude of a moving bar using the finger-span device. The first thermal stimulation run invariably elicited an IEM episode described at session debriefing to be similar to episodes experienced during daily life. Because we were assessing the response to treatment, we titrated the thermal stimulation until the pain intensity rating reached a predetermined level during all scans (visits 2, 3, 4, 6, and 7; efigure 1 in the Supplement). During the subsequent 2 pain runs, patients rated spontaneous fluctuations of their pain collected without thermal stimulation. A visual magnitude rating was performed last as a control for visuospatial and attention components inherent in our pain rating tasks (eAppendix in the Supplement).

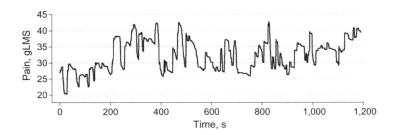

Figure 1
Inherited erythromelalgia pain rating. An example of rating of pain fluctuations after an episode is elicited with the thermal boot. The rating shown here was recorded after the thermal stimulus was switched off. gLMS indicates generalized Labeled Magnitude Scale.

fMRI Data Acquisition and Analysis

Imaging data were acquired with a Siemens 3T Trio scanner at Yale University Magnetic Resonance Research Center. Blood oxygen level–dependent images were acquired with parameters specified in the eAppendix in the Supplement. Image analysis was performed on each patient's data using FMRIB Expert Analysis Tool (http://www.fmrib.ox.ac.uk/fsl) (eAppendix in the Supplement).

Assessment of DRG Neuron Excitability

We previously showed that carbamazepine attenuates firing induced by electrical stimuli in DRG neurons expressing S241T mutant channels in experiments carried out at room temperature.[6] However, pain in IEM is triggered by warmth. To mimic the condition in human patients, we assessed the effect of carbamazepine on firing of DRG neurons expressing S241T at graded physiological temperatures (33°C, 37°C, and 40°C). Recording methods are described in the eAppendix in the Supplement.

Statistical Analysis

Multielectrode array data are expressed as mean (SEM). Statistical significance was determined by t test.

Results

Carbamazepine and Pain Attenuation in Patients Carrying the S241T Mutation

The effect of carbamazepine on S241T mutant channels[6] suggested that carbamazepine might attenuate pain in patients with IEM carrying this mutation. Both patients in this study were blinded and asked to report duration and intensity of their IEM pain and the number of pain-induced awakenings from sleep on a daily basis (figure 2).

Patient 1 reported a reduction in mean time in pain (TIP) per day during the 15-day maintenance period of the study (at 400 mg/day of carbamazepine), from 424 minutes while taking placebo to 231.9 minutes while taking carbamazepine, and a reduction in total TIP over the 15-day maintenance period, from 6360 minutes while taking placebo to 3015 minutes while

taking carbamazepine (figure 2A). Patient 2 reported a reduction in mean TIP per day during the maintenance period (at 400 and then 200 mg/day of carbamazepine), from 61 minutes while taking placebo to 9.1 minutes while taking carbamazepine, and a reduction in total TIP, from 915 minutes while taking placebo over the 15-day maintenance period to 136 minutes while taking carbamazepine (figure 2A). Patient 1 reported a reduction of mean episode duration from 615 minutes while taking placebo to 274.1 minutes while taking carbamazepine, while patient 2 reported a reduction of the mean episode duration from 91.5 minutes while taking placebo to 45.3 minutes while taking carbamazepine (figure 2B). Patient 1, who had a history of night awakenings from pain, reported 101 awakenings while taking placebo during the 15-day maintenance period and 32 awakenings while taking carbamazepine (figure 2C). Patient 2 reported 1 night awakening while taking placebo during the maintenance period and none while taking carbamazepine (figure 2C). Carbamazepine blood levels were in the therapeutic range (3.6–6.0 g/L) when patients were receiving carbamazepine (etable 1 in the Supplement).

Neither patient reported significant pain at arrival for hospital visits. Pain was provoked using a heating boot on the right foot with circulating water maintained at controlled temperatures. The empirically determined thermal stimulus in each patient invariably elicited a pain episode, which was described at session debriefing to be similar to episodes during daily life. Once pain was provoked, the thermal stimulus was terminated. Pain intensity ratings were continuously collected (figure 1; efigure 2 in the Supplement) as reported previously.[7,11,13,15] To investigate long-term effects of carbamazepine vs placebo, we compared baseline fMRI scans of chronic (4-week) carbamazepine vs placebo treatment with a triple-paired t test implemented in FMRIB toolbox across the 2 patients. We previously demonstrated that brain activity maps obtained while

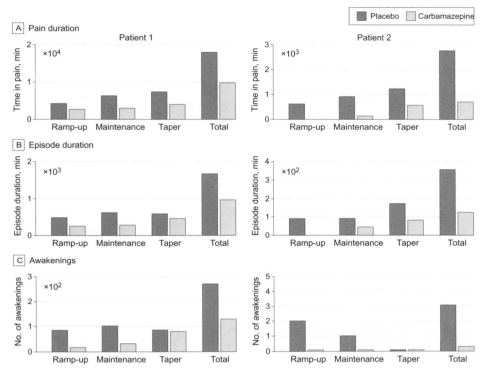

Figure 2
Pain characteristics in patients 1 and 2. Pain characteristics and effects of carbamazepine treatment vs placebo for patients 1 and 2. (A) Time in pain as reported in patients' diaries during the 3 phases of treatment ramp-up, maintenance, and taper. Histograms represent means. (B) Same as in panel A for the reported duration of inherited erythromelalgia episodes. (C) Number of awakenings due to pain during 3 phases of ramp-up, maintenance, and taper.

patients with chronic pain rate intensity of their ongoing (stimulus-free) pain are more specific to the clinical condition under study compared with brain maps obtained during application of an external stimulus.[7,11,13] This approach dissociates disease-specific ongoing fluctuations of pain, which in time shift away from sensory regions to engage valuation circuitry from acute thermal pain perception.[7,11,13,14] The analysis reported here used scans where our patients rated their pain after the stimulus was terminated. Pain ratings collected during all scans and used to derive IEM pain maps are shown for both participants in efigure 2 in the Supplement.

Association between Carbamazepine and Brain Activity

Carbamazepine treatment (carbamazepine scan < baseline; corrected for a visual control task) was associated with decreased activity in valuation areas[14,16] including the ventral striatum (nucleus accumbens), ventral pallidum, rostral anterior cingulate (rACC; Brodmann Area [BA] 32), and posterior cingulate cortex (PCC), in addition to the ventral putamen, bilateral anterior insula, right thalamus, and hypothalamus (figure 3A; efigure 3 and etable 2 in the Supplement). By contrast, treatment was associated with increased

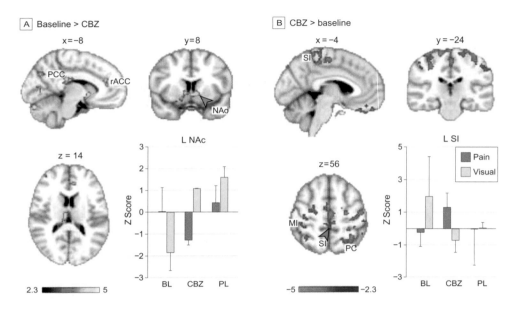

Figure 3
Brain activity modulation with carbamazepine (CBZ). Treatment effects of CBZ vs baseline. (A) Brain activity obtained when contrasting baseline to carbamazepine (baseline > CBZ) (paired t test; n = 2; fixed effects; $P < .05$, corrected for multiple comparisons). The bar plot shows mean (SEM) brain activity in z scores during pain rating (blue) and visual tracking (white) within the left (L) nucleus accumbens (NAc) (blue arrowhead) plotted for baseline (BL, left), chronic CBZ treatment (CBZ, middle), and chronic placebo (PL, right) treatment, respectively. (B) Brain activity when contrasting CBZ > baseline; the bar plot depicts mean activity within primary somatosensory area (SI) (red arrowhead). MI indicates primary motor cortex; PCC, posterior cingulate cortex; PC, parietal cortex; R, right; rACC, rostral anterior cingulate cortex; and SI, primary somatosensory cortex.

activity (carbamazepine scan > baseline) in bilateral primary and secondary somatosensory-motor areas including the medial wall foot area according to the Jüelich Histological Atlas,[17] bilateral parietal dorsal attention areas, supplementary motor area BA 6, and ventromedial prefrontal cortex (BA 11) compared with the baseline scan (figure 3B; efigure 3 and etable 2 in the Supplement; paired t test; fixed effects; n = 2, $Z > 2.3$; $P < 0.05$ corrected for multiple comparisons). However, treatment with placebo did not affect activity in the ventral striatum and had an effect opposite that of carbamazepine within the PCC, motor, and parietal areas. Placebo (baseline > placebo) decreased activity in the right dorsolat-

eral prefrontal cortex (DLPFC) (BA 44/48), right posterior insula, and left parietal and bilateral visual areas. On the other hand, it increased activity (placebo > baseline) in the medial prefrontal cortex (BA 10), right inferior frontal gyrus (BA 45/47), bilateral central opercular areas (BA 48), PCC, bilateral hippocampi, midbrain, and pons (figure 4A; efigure 4 in the Supplement). Similar to the contrast of carbamazepine and baseline, the contrast of carbamazepine vs placebo showed a shift in activity from valuation areas to primary sensory motor and attention areas with carbamazepine (figure 4B; efigure 5 in the Supplement). To confirm the latter result, we collapsed placebo and baseline sessions together; paired t test with

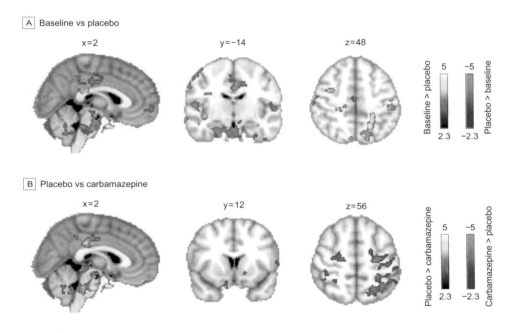

Figure 4
Brain activity modulation by placebo. (A) Treatment effects of placebo vs baseline. Areas shown in red to yellow represent the contrast (baseline > placebo) and areas shown in blue to green represent the contrast (placebo > baseline). Unlike carbamazepine, placebo decreases activity in somatosensory parietal areas and increases activity in the posterior cingulate cortex and medial prefrontal cortex, among others. (B) Contrast results between placebo scans (placebo > carbamazepine, red to yellow) and carbamazepine scans (carbamazepine > placebo, blue to green). Differences in activations are similar to those shown in figure 3 for carbamazepine and baseline.

the carbamazepine treatment scans demonstrated an increase in sensory motor/attention areas with a concomitant decrease in valuation/reward areas after carbamazepine treatment (efigure 6 in the Supplement).

Next, we asked how pain intensity modulates brain activity to compare the effects of carbamazepine and placebo. We averaged pain intensity ratings within each scanning run and regressed them against brain activity across all visits. The regression results were similar to the effects of carbamazepine and opposite to placebo treatment. Activity within valuation areas, left nucleus accumbens and rACC, in addition to the left insula, right thalamus, hypothalamus, and midbrain covaried positively with pain intensity,

whereas activity within primary and secondary sensory-motor cortices and dorsal parietal and DLPFC areas covaried negatively with pain intensity (figure 5A; efigure 7 and etable 3 in the Supplement). Additionally, activity in the left hippocampus was negatively correlated with pain intensity. Regression analysis that excluded visits when patients received carbamazepine confirmed that pain intensity covaries positively with valuation areas and negatively with primary somatosensory, motor, and parietal areas (efigure 8 in the Supplement). Hence, treatment with carbamazepine was associated with a shift of brain activity toward a pattern associated with decreased pain intensity. Using a similar analysis, we found that brain activity only in the left hippocampus,

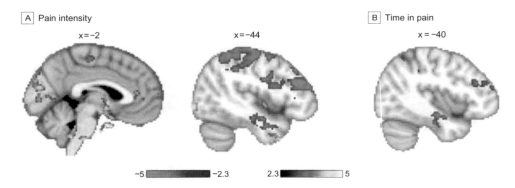

Figure 5
Brain activity associated with decreased pain. (A) Regression of brain activity during pain rating scans across all visits against pain intensity reported during scanning. (B) Regression of brain activity against time in pain as reported in patients' diaries after masking with results shown in panel A. Areas in red to yellow represent positive correlations, whereas areas in blue to green represent negative correlations.

parietal cortex, and DLPFC were inversely correlated with TIP as reported in patients' diaries (figure 5B), suggesting that there was increased activity in brain areas associated with less TIP during treatment with carbamazepine.

Carbamazepine and Warmth-Induced Firing of DRG Neurons Expressing S241T Mutant Channels

We showed previously that carbamazepine attenuates firing of DRG neurons expressing S241T mutant channels in response to graded electrical stimuli using current-clamp assays.[6] However, pain in patients with IEM, including the patients we studied, is triggered by warmth. To determine whether carbamazepine had an effect on the firing of DRG neurons expressing $Na_V1.7$ S241T channels in response to this naturally occurring stimulus, we assayed the firing of intact cultured DRG neurons using multielectrode arrays at normal skin temperature (33°C), core body temperature (37°C), and nonnoxious warmth (40°C). Firing of adult DRG neurons expressing $Na_V1.7$ S241T was evoked in a temperature-dependent manner, as reflected by a heat map (figure 6A-C), increas-

ing from a mean (SEM) frequency of 0.18 (0.03) Hz at 33°C (3 cultures using a total of 6 rats, 66 active electrodes/neurons) to 0.36 (0.04) Hz at 37°C (83 active electrodes/neurons) and to 0.56 (0.03) Hz at 40°C (98 active electrodes/neurons) (figure 7). Elevated temperature increased both the mean firing frequency and number of DRG neurons firing action potentials.

Carbamazepine at a clinically relevant concentration (30 μM)[5,6] markedly attenuated firing of DRG neurons expressing S241T mutant channels (figure 6D-F). In the presence of carbamazepine, the mean (SEM) firing frequency of neurons expressing S241T at 33°C was 0.024 (0.003) Hz ($P < 0.05$ compared with neurons before carbamazepine treatment) with 52 active electrodes/neurons, at 37°C was 0.026 (0.011) Hz ($P < 0.01$) with 48 active electrodes/neurons, and at 40°C was 0.089 (0.026) Hz ($P < 0.01$) with 44 active electrodes (figure 7). These data indicate that carbamazepine at a clinically relevant concentration inhibits warmth-evoked firing of DRG neurons expressing $Na_V1.7$ S241T across a physiological temperature range.

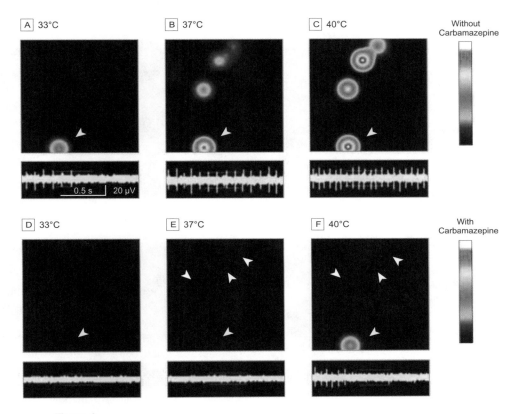

Figure 6

Carbamazepine attenuation of warmth-evoked firing in dorsal root ganglion neurons expressing Na$_V$1.7 S241T mutant channels. (A–C) Heat maps of a representative multielectrode array recording of dorsal root ganglion neurons expressing Na$_V$1.7 S241T before carbamazepine treatment (upper panels). The firing frequency of each active electrode is color coded with white/red representing high firing frequency and blue/black representing low firing frequency. Each circle corresponds to an active electrode within an 8 × 8 electrode array. There is only 1 active electrode in the heat map at 33°C (A). The number of active electrodes and firing frequency increase at 37°C (B) and 40°C (C). (D–F) Heat maps of the same multielectrode array recording well after (30-μM) carbamazepine treatment (upper panels). The number of active electrodes and firing frequency of neurons are both markedly reduced at all 3 temperatures: 33°C (D), 37°C (E), and 40°C (F). White arrowheads indicate silent neurons after carbamazepine treatment. In the lower panels in A–F, recordings from a representative neuron in the heat map indicated by yellow arrowheads are shown. Note increased firing as temperature increased in the absence of carbamazepine (A–C) and attenuation of firing by carbamazepine (D–F).

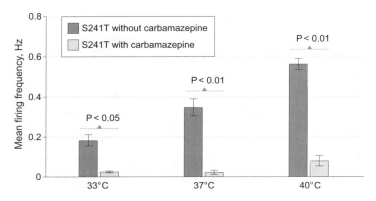

Figure 7
Firing frequency. Mean firing frequency of neurons (n = 98) expressing $Na_V1.7$ S241T before and after carbamazepine treatment at all 3 temperatures.

Discussion

Inherited erythromelalgia is caused by gain-of-function mutations of $Na_V1.7$ and is characterized clinically by severe pain, triggered by mild warmth.[1,2] Most patients with IEM do not respond to pharmacotherapy and resort to cooling, in some cases with ice or iced water that causes gangrene, to alleviate pain.[1,2] On the basis of atomic-level structural modeling and functional analysis, we predicted that carbamazepine would attenuate pain in patients with IEM due to the S241T mutation. We previously showed that within the folded channel protein, the S241 residue is located within 2.8Å of the carbamazepine-responsive V400M mutation.[6] That study demonstrated that S241T and V400M are energetically coupled during activation, a finding that predicted that carbamazepine should have a specific effect on the abnormal activation of S241T mutant channels; voltage- and current-clamp analyses showed that, indeed, carbamazepine has a specific effect, not seen in other IEM mutant channels, on S241T where it restores essentially normal activation, thereby reducing electrically induced firing of DRG neurons expressing S241T channels.[6] In the present study

using double-blind, placebo-controlled assessment, we demonstrated that carbamazepine attenuated pain induced by warmth in patients carrying the S241T mutation and showed a shift in brain activity from valuation and pain areas toward primary and secondary somatosensory-motor and parietal attention areas, a pattern of brain activity that has been associated with a shift from chronic to acute pain states.[13,18] We also showed that warmth within a physiological range triggers abnormal firing in DRG neurons carrying S241T mutant channels, recapitulating in vitro the clinical picture of sensitivity to mild increases in temperature displayed by patients with IEM, and we demonstrated that carbamazepine inhibits warmth-induced hyperactivity of DRG neurons carrying S241T mutant channels.

There were some limitations to this study. We stress that this study was based on a small number of patients and the long-term effects of carbamazepine were not assessed. Moreover, we emphasize that our results, based on study of patients with the S241T mutation, do not imply that patients with erythromelalgia due to other $Na_V1.7$ mutations will experience pain relief from carbamazepine. Rather, our results provide proof of principle, based on the S241T mutation, that genomic analysis together with molecular modeling and functional profiling can guide pain pharmacotherapy.

Carbamazepine acts on multiple sodium-channel subtypes,[19] including $Na_V1.7$,[20] and thus we cannot exclude a contribution of sodium-channel blockade within the central nervous system to the effects of carbamazepine that we observed with behavioral and fMRI measurements. While some evidence suggests an inverse association between carbamazepine levels and blood oxygen level–dependent brain activity,[21] treatment with carbamazepine was associated with increased activity in sensory/motor/attention areas, together with decreased activity in valuation areas. This shift of activity cannot be accounted for by a generalized dampening of blood oxygen level–dependent signal by carbamazepine. Importantly, the in vitro recordings in the current study demonstrated a strong attenuation of physiologically relevant warmth-induced firing of DRG neurons expressing S241T mutant channels by a clinically relevant concentration of carbamazepine. Taken together with the specific action of carbamazepine on S241T mutant channels,[6] our observations support the idea that pain in IEM reflects abnormal hyperactivity of DRG neurons carrying gain-of-function mutant $Na_V1.7$ channels[2,3,22] and suggest that carbamazepine relieves pain in human patients carrying the S241T mutation at least in part via an action on the mutant $Na_V1.7$ channel in DRG neurons.

Functional MRI revealed that brain activity shifted during carbamazepine treatment from valuation (ventral striatum, rACC, and PCC)[14,16] and pain (thalamus and insula) areas[18,23] toward primary somatosensory-motor and parietal attention areas including the medial sensory-motor cortical wall with afferent and efferent fibers to the foot. This shift in brain activity was observed during carbamazepine treatment despite the decades-long history of severe pain in these patients. Previous fMRI and clinical studies showed that placebo can reduce pain in some

patient populations while concurrently modulating activity in valuation and pain areas.[10,24–28] However, in our study, carbamazepine treatment achieved this change, whereas placebo did not.

The drop in brain activity within valuation and pain areas with carbamazepine was consistent with previous work showing decreases in the ventral striatum, rACC, and insula activity, as well as changes in their functional connectivity with successful treatment of chronic pain.[11,25] Baliki et al.[8] suggested that nucleus accumbens activity tracks the value of pain relief in chronic pain, while the ventral striatum and rACC are activated by pain and pain predictive cues.[8,29] It has also been reported that the valuation circuitry mediates reward-related decision making.[14,16] We observed a concomitant increase in activity of areas mediating somatosensory, motor, and attention tasks.[30] This observation suggests that attenuation of pain with carbamazepine may allow patients to shift brain resources from areas mediating emotional decision making and pain to sensory-motor, attention, and executive function areas mediating accurate movements and sensory perception while rating their pain experience, consistent with the suggestion that persistence of pain shifts brain activity from sensory-motor regions to emotional decision-making circuitry.[13] Activity in the parietal and DLPFC areas were particularly inversely associated with TIP as reported in patients' diaries, suggesting that the increase in activity in these areas with carbamazepine might have positive effects on attention and executive function.[31] Whether this shift is associated with improved functioning on a daily basis remains to be determined.

Segerdahl et al.[32] reported cerebral blood flow differences between states of acute thermal heating and cooling in a study that used arterial spin labeling to assess 1 patient with IEM. While some of the areas affected by carbamazepine treatment overlap with their report, mainly rACC, insula, and thalamus, methodological differences preclude direct comparisons between the 2 studies. Unlike in the study by Segerdahl et al.,[32] our patients rated the intensity of pain after a provocatory thermal stimulus was terminated. Our approach allows the identification of brain maps specific to different clinical pain conditions without the added component of ongoing stimulation,[13] which could mask differences between patients and healthy control individuals.[7]

Conclusions

In this study, genomic analysis, molecular modeling, and functional profiling provided a basis for reduction of neuropathic pain with carbamazepine in patients with IEM carrying the S241T mutation in sodium-channel Na$_V$1.7. Functional brain imaging demonstrated a change in brain activity within the pain, valuation, and somatosensory/motor/attention circuitry in patients carrying this variant, providing a potential correlate within the brain for the report of an effect of carbamazepine on pain in their home environment. As the number of sodium-channel variants linked to pain grows,[33] structural and functional analysis of other mutations may provide additional opportunities for genomically guided pain pharmacotherapy.

Acknowledgments

Author Contributions: Drs. Geha and Waxman had full access to all of the data in the study and take responsibility for the integrity of the data and the accuracy of the data analysis. *Study concept and design:* Geha, Tokuno, Dib-Hajj, Waxman. *Acquisition, analysis, or interpretation of data:* All authors. *Drafting of the manuscript:* Geha, Waxman. *Critical revision of the manuscript for important intellectual content:* All authors. *Statistical analysis:* Geha, Yang, Apkarian. *Obtained funding:* Waxman. *Administrative, technical, or material support:* Geha, Yang, Estacion, Schulman, Dib-Hajj. *Study supervision:* Waxman.

Conflict of Interest Disclosures: None reported.

Funding/Support: This work was supported in part by grants from the Rehabilitation Research Service and Medical Research Service, Department of Veterans Affairs, the Erythromelalgia Association, and the Kenneth Rainin Foundation (Dr Waxman). Dr Geha was supported by grant 1K08DA037525-01 from the National Institute on Drug Abuse and the Yale University Department of Psychiatry.

Role of the Funder/Sponsor: The funders had no role in the design and conduct of the study; collection, management, analysis, and interpretation of the data; preparation, review, or approval of the manuscript; and decision to submit the manuscript for publication.

About the Authors

Paul Geha, MD, Department of Psychiatry, Yale University School of Medicine, New Haven, CT; The John B. Pierce Laboratory, New Haven, CT

Yang Yang, PhD, Department of Neurology, Yale University School of Medicine, New Haven, CT; Neurorehabilitation Research Center, Department of Neurology, Veterans Affairs Medical Center, West Haven, CT

Mark Estacion, PhD, Department of Neurology, Yale University School of Medicine, New Haven, CT; Neurorehabilitation Research Center, Department of Neurology, Veterans Affairs Medical Center, West Haven, CT

Betsy R. Schulman, PhD, Department of Neurology, Yale University School of Medicine, New Haven, CT; Neurorehabilitation Research Center, Department of Neurology, Veterans Affairs Medical Center, West Haven, CT

Hajime Tokuno, MD, Department of Neurology, Yale University School of Medicine, New Haven, CT; Neurorehabilitation Research Center, Department of Neurology, Veterans Affairs Medical Center, West Haven, CT

A. Vania Apkarian, PhD, Department of Physiology, Northwestern University, Chicago, IL

Sulayman D. Dib-Hajj, PhD, Department of Neurology, Yale University School of Medicine, New Haven, CT; Neurorehabilitation Research Center, Department of Neurology, Veterans Affairs Medical Center, West Haven, CT

Stephen G. Waxman, MD, PhD, Department of Neurology, Yale University School of Medicine, New Haven, CT;

Neurorehabilitation Research Center, Department of Neurology, Veterans Affairs Medical Center, West Haven, CT

References

1. Drenth JP, Waxman SG. 2007. Mutations in sodium-channel gene SCN9A cause a spectrum of human genetic pain disorders. *J Clin Invest* 117(12): 3603–3609.

2. Dib-Hajj SD, Yang Y, Black JA, Waxman SG. 2013. The Na(V)1.7 sodium channel: From molecule to man. *Nat Rev Neurosci* 14(1): 49–62.

3. Rush AM, Dib-Hajj SD, Liu S, Cummins TR, Black JA, Waxman SG. 2006. A single sodium channel mutation produces hyper- or hypoexcitability in different types of neurons. *Proc Natl Acad Sci USA* 103(21): 8245–8250.

4. Toledo-Aral JJ, Moss BL, He ZJ, et al. 1997. Identification of PN1, a predominant voltage-dependent sodium channel expressed principally in peripheral neurons. *Proc Natl Acad Sci USA* 94(4): 1527–1532.

5. Fischer TZ, Gilmore ES, Estacion M, et al. 2009. A novel Nav1.7 mutation producing carbamazepine-responsive erythromelalgia. *Ann Neurol* 65(6): 733–741.

6. Yang Y, Dib-Hajj SD, Zhang J, et al. 2012. Structural modelling and mutant cycle analysis predict pharmacoresponsiveness of a Na(V)1.7 mutant channel. *Nat Commun* 3: 1186.

7. Baliki MN, Chialvo DR, Geha PY, et al. 2006. Chronic pain and the emotional brain: Specific brain activity associated with spontaneous fluctuations of intensity of chronic back pain. *J Neurosci* 26(47): 12165–12173.

8. Baliki MN, Geha PY, Fields HL, Apkarian AV. 2010. Predicting value of pain and analgesia: Nucleus accumbens response to noxious stimuli changes in the presence of chronic pain. *Neuron* 66(1): 149–160.

9. Baliki MN, Petre B, Torbey S, et al. 2012. Corticostriatal functional connectivity predicts transition to chronic back pain. *Nat Neurosci* 15(8): 1117–1119.

10. Ellingsen DM, Wessberg J, Eikemo M, et al. 2013. Placebo improves pleasure and pain through opposite modulation of sensory processing. *Proc Natl Acad Sci USA* 110(44): 17993–17998.

11. Geha PY, Baliki MN, Chialvo DR, Harden RN, Paice JA, Apkarian AV. 2007. Brain activity for spontaneous pain of postherpetic neuralgia and its modulation by lidocaine patch therapy. *Pain* 128(1–2): 88–100.

12. Geha PY, Baliki MN, Harden RN, Bauer WR, Parrish TB, Apkarian AV. 2008. The brain in chronic CRPS pain: Abnormal gray-white matter interactions in emotional and autonomic regions. *Neuron* 60(4): 570–581.

13. Hashmi JA, Baliki MN, Huang L, et al. 2013. Shape shifting pain: Chronification of back pain shifts brain representation from nociceptive to emotional circuits. *Brain* 136(pt 9): 2751–2768.

14. Kable JW, Glimcher PW. 2007. The neural correlates of subjective value during intertemporal choice. *Nat Neurosci* 10(12): 1625–1633.

15. Foss JM, Apkarian AV, Chialvo DR. 2006. Dynamics of pain: Fractal dimension of temporal variability of spontaneous pain differentiates between pain states. *J Neurophysiol* 95(2): 730–736.

16. Levy DJ, Glimcher PW. 2012. The root of all value: A neural common currency for choice. *Curr Opin Neurobiol* 22(6): 1027–1038.

17. Eickhoff SB, Stephan KE, Mohlberg H, et al. 2005. A new SPM toolbox for combining probabilistic cytoarchitectonic maps and functional imaging data. *Neuroimage* 25(4): 1325–1335.

18. Apkarian AV, Bushnell MC, Treede RD, Zubieta JK. 2005. Human brain mechanisms of pain perception and regulation in health and disease. *Eur J Pain* 9(4): 463–484.

19. Qiao X, Sun G, Clare JJ, Werkman TR, Wadman WJ. 2014. Properties of human brain sodium channel α-subunits expressed in HEK293 cells and their modulation by carbamazepine, phenytoin and lamotrigine. *Br J Pharmacol* 171(4): 1054–1067.

20. Jo S, Bean BP. 2014. Sidedness of carbamazepine accessibility to voltage-gated sodium channels. *Mol Pharmacol* 85(2): 381–387.

21. Jokeit H, Okujava M, Woermann FG. 2001. Carbamazepine reduces memory induced activation of mesial temporal lobe structures: A pharmacological fMRI-study. *BMC Neurol* 1: 6.

22. Dib-Hajj SD, Rush AM, Cummins TR, et al. 2005. Gain-of-function mutation in Nav1.7 in familial erythromelalgia induces bursting of sensory neurons. *Brain* 128(pt 8): 1847–1854.

23. Lamm C, Decety J, Singer T. 2011. Meta-analytic evidence for common and distinct neural networks associated with directly experienced pain and empathy for pain. *Neuroimage* 54(3): 2492–2502.

24. Diederich NJ, Goetz CG. 2008. The placebo treatments in neurosciences: New insights from clinical and neuroimaging studies. *Neurology* 71(9): 677–684.

25. Hashmi JA, Baria AT, Baliki MN, Huang L, Schnitzer TJ, Apkarian AV. 2012. Brain networks predicting placebo analgesia in a clinical trial for chronic back pain. *Pain* 153(12): 2393–2402.

26. Tracey I. 2010. Getting the pain you expect: Mechanisms of placebo, nocebo and reappraisal effects in humans. *Nat Med* 16(11): 1277–1283.

27. Wager TD, Rilling JK, Smith EE, et al. 2004. Placebo-induced changes in FMRI in the anticipation and experience of pain. *Science* 303(5661): 1162–1167.

28. Zubieta JK, Stohler CS. 2009. Neurobiological mechanisms of placebo responses. *Ann N Y Acad Sci* 1156: 198–210.

29. Seymour B, O'Doherty JP, Koltzenburg M, et al. 2005. Opponent appetitive-aversive neural processes underlie predictive learning of pain relief. *Nat Neurosci* 8(9): 1234–1240.

30. Mesulam MM. 1998. From sensation to cognition. *Brain* 121(pt 6): 1013–1052.

31. Corbetta M, Shulman GL. 2002. Control of goal-directed and stimulus-driven attention in the brain. *Nat Rev Neurosci* 3(3): 201–215.

32. Segerdahl AR, Xie J, Paterson K, Ramirez JD, Tracey I, Bennett DL. 2012. Imaging the neural correlates of neuropathic pain and pleasurable relief associated with inherited erythromelalgia in a single subject with quantitative arterial spin labelling. *Pain* 153(5): 1122–1127.

33. Waxman SG, Merkies IS, Gerrits MM, et al. 2014. Sodium channel genes in pain-related disorders: Phenotype-genotype associations and recommendations for clinical use. *Lancet Neurol* 13(11): 1152–1160.

Learn from yesterday, live for today, hope for tomorrow. The important thing is not to stop.

—Albert Einstein

When $Na_V1.7$ was identified as a major player in pain and mutations of its *SCN9A* gene were shown to produce dramatic pain profiles in humans, a pain gene had been found. But science's arrow never stops flying. Sometimes it advances rapidly, and sometimes slowly. It is now whizzing ahead in laboratory experiments that are teaching us how ion channels work and how their dysfunction can cause disease. And, at the same time, it is slowly inching forward on another track, in studies on novel clinical approaches—small molecule blockers, gene therapy strategies, inhibitors based on modified toxins or antibodies—that will hopefully become new medications that put $Na_V1.7$ to sleep.

In one of these studies we are working with a biotech company called Convergence Pharmaceuticals (now part of Biogen) to evaluate their $Na_V1.7$ blocker, designed to inhibit sodium channels when they are *abnormally active*. Our studies have shown that the Convergence blocker inhibits the firing of trigeminal ganglion neurons, the cells that give rise to abnormal impulse activity responsible for trigeminal neuralgia, an often-devastating pain disorder in which patients suffer from attacks of lancinating pain focused on the face, sometimes described as feeling like blows from an axe. Phase II clinical studies on this new blocker are beginning to provide hints that it may reduce the number and intensity of pain attacks in trigeminal neuralgia (Zakrzewska et al. 2017). Much more needs to be done, but these results encourage me to think that, indeed, the genes of men on fire are pointing in the direction of new treatments for pain in "the rest of us."

Of course, we do not yet know what will happen next in clinical studies. Trials on larger numbers of patients, at other doses and for longer periods of time, are needed. Other disease indications need to be explored. And, as with all new medications, there is always the possibility that, in long-term studies, unexpected side effects may occur. As I speak with patients and their families, I share my sense of hope. And, I tell them that we will not reach our goal tomorrow. We need more numbers. In the end, the numbers will tell the story.

But, what if $Na_V1.7$ blockers fail to make it all the way to the clinic? My view is still optimistic because, even if pharmacological blockade or knockdown of $Na_V1.7$ prove not to be useful as a therapeutic strategy that can be used in the clinic, the search for a pain gene may nonetheless point toward new therapies. Validation of $Na_V1.7$ as a human pain gene has provided a template for establishing, in humans, that two other sodium channels meeting the criteria for being "peripheral" are also potential pain targets. $Na_V1.8$, discovered by John Wood at University College London and initially called SNS (Sensory Neuron Specific), is preferentially produced in DRG neurons (Akopian, Sivilotti, and Wood 1996), where it supports high-frequency firing (Renganathan, Cummins, and Waxman 2001). And, within human DRG neurons, $Na_V1.8$ plays an even more powerful role than it does in rodents (Han, Huang, and Waxman 2016). Several years after we published the first mutations validating $Na_V1.7$ as a pain gene, we followed a similar route and demonstrated that gain-of-function mutations of $Na_V1.8$ can produce painful peripheral neuropathies in humans, thus establishing its role as a human pain channel (Faber et al. 2012; Han et al. 2014; Huang et al. 2013). $Na_V1.8$ blockers are under development (Jarvis et al. 2007).

Sodium channel $Na_V1.9$, originally termed NaN (Na channel, Nociceptive) was first identified in my laboratory in 1998 by Dib-Hajj et al. (1998). It exerts a strong effect on the excitability of DRG neurons (Baker et al. 2003; Cummins et al. 1999; Herzog, Cummins, and Waxman 2001). Gain-of-function mutations of $Na_V1.9$ have now been found in patients with several familial disorders causing severe pain (Zhang et al. 2013), including painful neuropathy (Han et al. 2015; Huang et al. 2014). So $Na_V1.9$ is also a therapeutic target.

Even prior to knowing how the therapy part of the story will end, the search for a pain gene has been exhilarating. Driven by stories like those of two soldiers with similar nerve injuries, one resulting in excruciating pain and the other in mild tingling, the search for a pain gene encircled the globe. Beginning in 1965, the hunt for the gene led from Alabama to the Netherlands, then to Beijing, and then back to America. Propelled by detective work and by the development of new methods for investigating the genome, the search sifted through more than 20,000 genes, ultimately finding a master gene for pain. That gene encoded a sodium channel, a member of a family of molecules, essential for the workings of the nervous system, originally discovered in the squid. Over- or underactivity of sodium channel $Na_V1.7$, due to mutations of that gene, produce remarkable clinical syndromes of "men on fire" or, conversely, of people who cannot feel pain. Here, we have a wonderful example of the importance of elegantly crafted molecules for the workings of our bodies. And an exquisite example of our genetic heritage.

Our mining of the human genome, and our explorations of pain, continue at an almost-dizzying pace. Today as on most days, my laboratory—30 scientists strong—is a beehive of activity. Cell and molecular biologists, electrophysiologists, biophysicists, pharmacologists, geneticists, and clinicians, all buzzing with energy:

• In a laboratory without windows, a cell biologist surrounded by lasers and powerful microscopes is watching, in real time, as point-like flashes on a computer screen show her single sodium channels as they are plugged into the membranes of growing nerve cells, including pain-signaling neurons; hopefully we will soon understand, in greater detail, how different types of nerve cells build their membranes, each containing a precisely calibrated mixture of ion channels that enables them to communicate in their proper dialect.

• In a laboratory down the hall, we are trying to understand why, on very rare occasions, people with the man on fire syndrome lose the capability to maintain their body temperature. A photograph of a child with inherited erythromelalgia, recently hospitalized with hypothermia, hangs on the wall. Neither we nor other scientists around the world have understood this rare phenomenon. But now a light bulb has popped on in our minds, and we are beginning to learn how the sympathetic nerve fibers that control heat generation in fat cells fail to function properly as a result of $Na_V1.7$ mutations. Maybe we can figure out how to more effectively treat the hypothermia when it occurs.

• In a third module, we are studying the mutation from a teenager whose clinical picture is particularly enigmatic: episodes of severe pain separated by periods in which she does not feel pain and continues, for example, to walk on a leg with a newly, and severely, fractured limb; week by week, we are unraveling the complexities of the unusual mutant sodium channel that produces this complex picture.

• Nearby, in another windowless laboratory crammed with delicate equipment, two pharmacologists are assessing the effects of multiple drugs on various $Na_V1.7$ mutant channels. They talk quietly with each other, but not with the robotic patch clamper they are supervising. The robot speeds, by ten-fold, the number of drugs they can study each week.

- And in still another laboratory a channel biophysicist, a molecular biologist, and a geneticist are working together to unwrap the secrets of a family in which two people, both carrying the same mutation, suffer from inherited erythromelalgia. One suffers from severe pain, while the second has much milder pain. Lurking somewhere in the DNA of these two people, there may be "modifier genes" that cause pain in one to be more intense, and in the other less intense. There are more than 20,000 genes to interrogate, but this family may hold clues to understanding how pain is modulated. Perhaps we can find a gene that confers resilience to pain—it is hard to bridle the enthusiasm of my team as we sift through the possibilities.

On some nights it is hard to fall asleep, and on all mornings I wake up wondering, "What will we learn today?"

We are, in a sense, a product of the cells that make us up. And those cells reflect the instructions in our genes. As I look forward, I predict that the search for the pain gene will lead to new medications, devoid of central side effects or addictive potential, that will be used to treat pain both in people with the man on fire syndrome and in others. It will take years to find out whether this prediction is correct. But even at this point, I feel fortunate to be on a very special quest. The search for a pain gene has helped us to understand a part of what makes us sentient and alive. It has helped us to understand an experience that we all share. It has helped us to dissect God's megaphone, the megaphone of pain.

References

Akopian AN, Sivilotti L, Wood JN. 1996. A tetrodotoxin-resistant voltage-gated sodium channel expressed by sensory neurons. *Nature* 379(6562): 257–262.

Baker MD, Chandra SY, Ding Y, Waxman SG, Wood JN. 2003. GTP-induced tetrodotoxin-resistant Na+ current regulates excitability in mouse and rat small diameter sensory neurones. *J Physiol* 548(Pt 2): 373–382.

Cummins TR, Dib-Hajj SD, Black JA, Akopian AN, Wood JN, Waxman SG. 1999. A novel persistent tetrodotoxin-resistant sodium current in SNS-null and wild-type small primary sensory neurons. *J Neurosci* 19(24): RC43.

Dib-Hajj SD, Tyrrell L, Black JA, Waxman SG. 1998. NaN, a novel voltage-gated Na channel, is expressed preferentially in peripheral sensory neurons and down-regulated after axotomy. *Proc Natl Acad Sci USA* 95(15): 8963–8968.

Faber CG, Lauria G, Merkies IS, Cheng X, Han C, Ahn HS, Persson AK, et al. 2012. Gain-of-function Na$_V$1.8 mutations in painful neuropathy. *Proc Natl Acad Sci USA* 109(47): 19444–19449.

Han C, Huang J, Waxman SG. 2016. Sodium channel Na$_V$1.8: Emerging links to human disease. *Neurology* 86(5): 473–483.

Han C, Vasylyev D, Macala LJ, Gerrits MM, Hoeijmakers JG, Bekelaar KJ, Dib-Hajj SD, Faber CG, Merkies IS, Waxman SG. 2014. The G1662S Na$_V$1.8 mutation in small fibre neuropathy: Impaired inactivation underlying DRG neuron hyper-excitability. *J Neurol Neurosurg Psychiatry* 85(5): 499–505.

Han C, Yang Y, de Greef BT, Hoeijmakers JG, Gerrits MM, Verhamme C, Qu J, et al. 2015. The Domain II S4-S5 linker in Na$_V$1.9: A missense mutation enhances activation, impairs fast inactivation, and produces human painful neuropathy. *Neuromolecular Med* 17(2): 158–169.

Herzog RI, Cummins TR, Waxman SG. 2001. Persistent TTX-resistant Na+ current affects resting potential and response to depolarization in simulated spinal sensory neurons. *J Neurophysiol* 86(3): 1351–1364.

Huang J, Han C, Estacion M, Vasylyev D, Hoeijmakers JG, Gerrits MM, Tyrrell L, et al., and the Propane Study Group. 2014. Gain-of-function mutations in sodium channel Na(v)1.9 in painful neuropathy. *Brain* 137(Pt 6): 1627–1642.

Huang J, Yang Y, Zhao P, Gerrits MM, Hoeijmakers JG, Bekelaar K, Merkies IS, Faber CG, Dib-Hajj SD, Waxman SG. 2013. Small-fiber neuropathy $Na_V1.8$ mutation shifts activation to hyperpolarized potentials and increases excitability of dorsal root ganglion neurons. *J Neurosci* 33(35): 14087–14097.

Jarvis MF, Honore P, Shieh CC, Chapman M, Joshi S, Zhang XF, Kort M, et al. 2007. A-803467, a potent and selective $Na_V1.8$ sodium channel blocker, attenuates neuropathic and inflammatory pain in the rat. *Proc Natl Acad Sci USA* 104(20): 8520–8525.

Renganathan M, Cummins TR, Waxman SG. 2001. Contribution of Na(v)1.8 sodium channels to action potential electrogenesis in DRG neurons. *J Neurophysiol* 86(2): 629–640.

Zakrzewska JM, Palmer J, Morisset V, Giblin GMP, Obermann M, Ettlin DA, Cruccu G, et al. 2017. Safety and efficacy of a $Na_V1.7$-selective sodium channel blocker, in trigeminal neuralgia: A double-blind, placebo-controlled, randomised withdrawal phase 2 trial. *Lancet Neurol* 16(4): 291–300.

Zhang XY, Wen J, Yang W, Wang C, Gao L, Zheng LH, Wang T, et al. 2013. Gain-of-function mutations in SCN11A cause familial episodic pain. *Am J Hum Genet* 93(5): 957–966.

GLOSSARY

action potential   The all-or-none nerve impulse produced by neurons. During the action potential there is a rapid depolarization of the cell membrane, measuring about 100 millivolts (1/10 of a volt). Each action potential is brief, lasting about one millisecond (1/1,000 of a second).

activation   The opening of a sodium channel, so that it can admit a small flow of sodium ions. Activation of sodium channels is triggered by depolarization. Activation of the $Na_V1.7$ sodium channel is enhanced in inherited erythromelalgia by a hyperpolarizing shift in the voltage dependence of channel activation.

amino acids   The building blocks of proteins. There are twenty amino acids in humans. Amino acids line up in precise order, like links in the chain, to form a protein molecule.

axon   A nerve fiber.

channelopathy-associated insensitivity to pain   A rare genetic disorder in which affected individuals do not produce functional $Na_V1.7$ channels, as a result of mutations in the gene encoding the channel. Affected individuals do not feel pain and are notable for painless fractures, painless burns, painless childbirth, painless tooth extractions, etc.

current clamp   A method, often implemented using patch-clamp electrodes, for continuously monitoring the voltage within a nerve cell, so as to follow the electrical activity of the cell over time.

deactivation   The process by which a sodium channel closes after the stimulating depolarization is removed.

dorsal root ganglion (DRG) neuron   A sensory neuron, with its cell body contained within a ganglion or cluster of cells located next to the spinal cord, that sends an axon to peripheral parts of the body including muscle, bone, and skin. DRG neurons provide sensory input about the skin, muscle, bone, etc. to the spinal cord, where this information is relayed to the brain.

dynamic clamp recording   A variation of the patch-clamp recording method, in which specific currents (usually, currents attributable to a specific channel) are subtracted using computer methodology, while other currents (again, attributable to a specific channel or channel variant of interest) are added back by the computer to simulate, within real neurons, the effect of precisely calibrated amounts of the added currents.

erythermalgia   Another name for erythromelalgia.

erythromelalgia   A disorder characterized by burning pain, usually in the feet and hands, triggered by mild warmth and relieved by cooling. The pain is accompanied by reddening of the affected limbs.

excitability   Physiological term, referring to the capability of a cell to generate action potentials.

firing   The production of action potentials by a neuron. Firing can be evoked by various stimuli or can be spontaneous.

functional magnetic resonance imaging (fMRI)   A form of functional brain imaging that noninvasively assesses energy consumption on a regional basis, thereby indicating the degree of activity in various parts of the brain.

gain-of-function mutation   A mutation that enhances the function of the encoded protein. Gain-of-function mutations that cause inherited erythromelalgia enhance the function of the $Na_V1.7$ channel by making it easier to activate the channel and by slowing deactivation.

gene   A region of DNA, comprised of nucleotides. Genes are the basic units of heredity. Each gene contains the instructions for a particular protein molecule.

genome   The complete set of DNA within an organism, including all of its genes. There are more than 20,000 genes in the human genome.

hyperexcitability   A state of a neuron in which it generates more electrical activity than it does in its normal state. Threshold is reduced, and the frequency of firing may be increased, in hyperexcitable neurons, and spontaneous firing may occur.

hypoexcitability   A state of a neuron in which it generates less electrical activity than it should. Threshold is increased and the frequency of firing is reduced in hypoexcitable neurons.

idiopathic small fiber neuropathy (iSFN)   Small fiber neuropathy in which there is no apparent nongenetic cause. Also called cryptogenic small fiber neuropathy.

inactivation   A process by which, shortly after opening (within milliseconds), sodium channels enter a nonoperable (inactivated) state. Most types of sodium channels are inactivated by depolarization of the nerve cell membrane, but $Na_V1.8$ is relatively resistant to this form of an activation and remains available even when cells are depolarized.

induced pluripotent stem cell (iPSC)   A type of stem cell derived from a specific person and containing that person's DNA. iPSCs have the capability, if prompted with the right mix of chemicals, to redifferentiate into any desired type of cell.

inflammatory pain   Pain signaling the presence of tissue damage.

inherited erythromelalgia (IEM)   The inherited form of erythromelalgia. It has been estimated that about 5% of cases of erythromelalgia are inherited. IEM is caused by gain-of-function mutations that make it easier to activate sodium channel $Na_V1.7$.

intraepidermal nerve fiber   The tip of an axon innervating the epidermis.

intraepidermal nerve fiber density (IENFD)   The density, or number per square millimeter, of intraepidermal nerve fibers within a particular portion of the skin. IENFD is reduced in small fiber neuropathy.

linkage analysis   A method of genetic analysis that takes advantage of the presence of single nucleotide polymorphisms that provide markers of particular regions along specific genes.

loss-of-function mutation   A mutation that reduces or abolishes the function of the encoded protein. Loss-of-function mutations of $Na_V1.7$ cause channelopathy-associated insensitivity to pain.

"man on fire" syndrome   Erythromelalgia.

mutation   A change in the structure of a gene that results in a variant that can be transmitted to subsequent generations. Many mutations are caused by alteration of a single base within DNA, resulting in the substitution of an incorrect amino acid at a particular site within the mutant protein.

$Na_V1.7$ A "peripheral" sodium channel, preferentially produced in peripheral neurons such as dorsal root ganglion neurons, that boosts small stimuli and facilitates neurotransmitter release at the first synapse in the spinal cord, thereby setting the gain on these neurons. The $Na_V1.7$ sodium channel is encoded by gene *SCN9A*.

$Na_V1.8$ A peripheral sodium channel, relatively resistant to inactivation by depolarization, that produces the electrical current needed for high-frequency firing in dorsal root ganglion neurons. $Na_V1.8$ channels are encoded by gene *SCN10A*.

$Na_V1.9$ A peripheral sodium channel that depolarizes resting potential in pain-signaling dorsal root ganglion neurons and amplifies small depolarizing inputs to them. $Na_V1.9$ channels are encoded by gene *SCN11A*.

neuroma   A knot-like tangle of nerve fibers formed by abortively regenerating axons after traumatic nerve injury. Neuromas are sites of abnormal, ectopic nerve impulse generation, and can be very painful.

neuron   A nerve cell.

neuropathic pain   Pain due to disease or dysfunction of the nervous system, particularly the somatosensory system.

nociceptors   A subclass of dorsal root ganglion neurons that convey, within the healthy nervous system, pain messages from the periphery to the spinal cord.

nucleotides   The smaller molecules that make up DNA. There are four nucleotides, labeled A, T, G, and C. A string of three nucleotides is needed to code for an amino acid.

nucleus accumbens   A part of the brain involved in its response to reward and punishment.

paroxysmal extreme pain disorder (PEPD)   A rare genetic disease characterized by perirectal pain in infancy, triggered by stimulation in or around the rectum. In adulthood, the pain migrates to the area around the jaw and eye. PEPD is caused by mutations that impair inactivation of $Na_V1.7$.

patch clamp   A method for recording from nerve cells with the small electrode that establishes a high-resistance bond with the cell membrane.

peripheral neuron   A nerve cell whose cell body is not located within the brain or spinal cord. Dorsal root ganglion neurons and sympathetic ganglion neurons, with cell bodies located within clusters outside of the spinal cord, are peripheral neurons.

peripheral neuropathy   A class of disorders characterized by damage to, or dysfunction of, peripheral nerves.

SCN9A   The gene encoding sodium channel $Na_V1.7$.

SCN10A   The gene encoding sodium channel $Na_V1.8$

SCN11A   The gene encoding sodium channel $Na_V1.9$.

single nucleotide polymorphism (SNP)   A variation in DNA sequence that occurs when a single nucleotide (A, T, C, or G) at a particular site is changed. Depending on the substitution, the corresponding amino acid may be changed. SNPs do not necessarily cause disease. They can, however, provide markers that are useful in linkage analysis.

small fiber neuropathy (SFN)   A form of peripheral neuropathy that specifically affects small-diameter nerve fibers.

sodium channel   A large protein molecule, located within the membrane of nerve cells and muscle cells, that opens to permit a small flow of sodium ions into the cell when activated. Sodium channels are necessary for the production of nerve impulses.

spontaneous firing   The generation of action potentials by a neuron in the absence of any stimulus.

threshold   A measure of the point at which a neuron fires. Threshold can be measured in terms of membrane potential ("voltage threshold") or in terms of the amount of electrical current needed to evoke an action potential ("current threshold," also called "rheobase").

trigeminal ganglion neuron   A sensory neuron, with its cell body located in the trigeminal ganglion, that innervates the face.

trigeminal neuralgia   A disorder in which affected people experience paroxysmal attacks of severe knife-like pain involving the face.

voltage clamp   A method, often implemented by patch clamp, for recording small electrical currents within nerve cells. Voltage-clamp recording allows the activities of various types of ion channels to be assessed.

INDEX